ANTIGENS, LYMPHOID CELLS, AND THE IMMUNE RESPONSE

IMMUNOLOGY

An International Series of Monographs and Treatises

EDITED BY

F. J. DIXON, JR.
Division of Experimental Pathology
Scripps Clinic and Research Foundation
La Jolla, California

HENRY G. KUNKEL
The Rockefeller University
New York New York

G. J. V. Nossal and G. L. Ada, Antigens, Lymphoid Cells, and the Immune Response. 1971

ANTIGENS, LYMPHOID CELLS, AND THE IMMUNE RESPONSE

G. J. V. NOSSAL

THE WALTER AND ELIZA HALL INSTITUTE OF MEDICAL RESEARCH
MELBOURNE, VICTORIA, AUSTRALIA

and

G. L. ADA

DEPARTMENT OF MICROBIOLOGY
AUSTRALIAN NATIONAL UNIVERSITY
CANBERRA, AUSTRALIA

1971

ACADEMIC PRESS New York and London

ACADEMIC PRESS, INC.
111 Fifth Avenue, New York, New York 10003

United Kingdom Edition published by
ACADEMIC PRESS, INC. (LONDON) LTD.
Berkeley Square House, London W1X 6BA

LIBRARY OF CONGRESS CATALOG CARD NUMBER: 71-137602

PRINTED IN THE UNITED STATES OF AMERICA

290837

To F. M. Burnet, to whom we both owe so much.

CONTENTS

8. Interaction of Antigens with Cells of the Reticuloendothelial System

9. The Interaction of Antigen with Lymphoid Cells

Contents

FOREWORD

This book inaugurates the international series of monographs and treatises on "Immunology" which deals with major topics of current interest in the ever-expanding field of immunology. It marks a new venture by the Editors of the *Advances in Immunology* which aims to provide an adjunct series covering in greater depth the most timely and most important subjects in this discipline. Many of the outstanding immunologists who will be involved have already contributed chapters to the *Advances*. Immunology has become such a hybrid science, impinging on such variegated areas, that a distinct need has developed among its students for detailed coverage of central topics.

It is amply fitting that the series begins with a volume from one of the world's foremost immunology laboratories. The subject, too, is most appropriate since it represents such a central and fundamental theme of immunology. A high standard has been set and, if similar realization stems from subsequent volumes, the success of the series is virtually guaranteed.

F. J. Dixon, Jr.
H. G. Kunkel

PREFACE

The aim of this book is to present an up-to-date picture of what is known about the manner in which antigens stimulate an immune response. Such a monograph seems necessary because a large amount of precise and valuable information has accumulated in a short time and has not before been fully collated. We hope that the volume will be of value to a diverse group of readers. It is primarily directed to research workers, post-doctoral fellows, and graduate students in the field of cellular immunology. However, the field of immunology has such wide ramifications into spheres such as clinical medicine and surgery, biochemistry, and microbiology that few professional biologists or doctors can afford to ignore it entirely. We hope that our analysis of the interactions between antigen molecules and lymphocytes will suggest to students analogies to other biological information and control systems. We hope, also, that it will demonstrate to the biochemists and immunochemists who have so revolutionized the antibody problem over the last decade that their biological counterparts have also not been idle, and that the two schools can learn from one another.

Our volume deals with the nature and properties of antigens and with the functional anatomy and cell physiology of the mammalian lymphoid system which responds to antigens. The focal point of our attention is the confrontation between antigen molecule and responsive lymphocyte, and the crucial decision which must then be made between immunity or immunologic tolerance. While there is a conscious bias toward studies conducted in our own laboratories, we hope that we have summarized and integrated all the key information gathered on these topics since 1963. The scope and treatment of the subject matter and the kinds of technical information which are presented are fully summarized in Chapter 1. A speculative synthesis of the field in the final chapter should, we hope, be of fairly general interest.

It became clear to us in writing the volume that one of the key ways in which this book differs from most others in immunology is that it and the work it summarizes represent real collaboration between biologist and biochemist. We feel that this combined focusing of different background skills has not only enriched our professional lives, but represents the key to progress in our understanding of the life process for the foreseeable future.

G. J. V. Nossal
G. L. Ada

ACKNOWLEDGMENTS

Our sincere thanks are due to the following people for their help and support in this publication: our secretaries, Mrs. J. Box and Mrs. B. Money, for their painstaking and careful preparation of the manuscript; Dr. Margaret Pierce, Mrs. Judith Mitchell, and Mr. John Pye for their valuable help at various stages in the preparation of the manuscript; Mr. Andrew Abbot for his help with the electron micrographs; and all our colleagues at The Walter and Eliza Hall Institute for their cooperation and interest, many of them at a detailed level.

The original work for this publication was supported by the following grants and contracts: The National Health and Medical Research Council, Canberra, Australia; The Australian Research Grants Committee; the National Institute of Allergy and Infectious Diseases, AI-0-3958; and the United States Atomic Energy Commission, AT (30-D-3695).

Permission to reproduce some of the illustrations and tables was kindly given by the following: Dr. E. Diener, Dr. Patricia E. Lind, Dr. G. Möller, Dr. F. W. Putnam, Dr. G. R. Shellam, and Dr. R. B. Taylor, and by the editors of *Biochemistry, The Australian Journal of Experimental Biology and Medical Science, The Journal of Experimental Medicine, Immunology, Proceedings of the National Academy of Sciences,* and *Science.*

This is publication number 1386 from the Walter and Eliza Hall Institute.

INTRODUCTION: CENTRAL QUESTIONS IN CELLULAR IMMUNOLOGY

The decade of the 1960's brought a remarkable change to immunology. From the discovery of the multichain nature of the immunoglobulins, progressively more detailed knowledge of their structure soon followed, and the realization that Bence-Jones proteins were homogeneous immunoglobulin light chains stimulated extensive investigations into the amino acid sequence of first light and later heavy immunoglobulin chains. In 1969, the first sequence analysis of a complete immunoglobulin molecule became available, so that it is reasonable to conclude that the problem of antibody structure is nearing a definitive solution. In fact, it is becoming evident that many investigators who have contributed to our knowledge of antibody structure are turning their attention to cellular immunological problems. The way in which antigen affects lymphocytes and activates antibody production is still far from being fully understood, but methods of increasing sophistication have recently become available to help accelerate progress. While the main chemical truths about antibody structure are generally known to and accepted by cellular immunologists, it appears that the key discoveries about lymphocytes and antibody-producing cells made during the 1960's have been less fully digested by immunochemists. Thus we felt that, both from the point of view of advanced students in immunology, and of workers in immunochemistry wishing to delve deeper into cellular problems, the time was ripe for a book which summarized current knowledge about antigens, lymphoid cells, and the immune response. In particular, we will concentrate on the induction of antibody formation. We felt 1970 to be an appropriate publication time because studies on the fate of antigen reached a new stage of precision and value when radioautographic techniques were applied to them. This approach has now been in wide use for about 7 years, and while it is clear that it will continue to yield fruitful information, we believe that the broad principles determining the localization of injected antigen molecules have now been fairly fully uncovered and should be summarized.

The dominant research theme in the authors' laboratories over the past several years has been to seek an answer to the question: how does antigen work? In any broad overview of the problem of antibody formation it is usual to divide the immune response into three major compartments: (1) afferent; (2) central; (3) efferent. The first compartment is concerned with the mechanisms by which the "antigenic message" is brought to the lymphoid system which eventually responds by antibody production. The second deals with the origin, nature, and function of lymphoid cells and with the key question of the genetic basis of the information necessary for the synthesis of antibodies. The third covers the cellular events which follow an effective encounter between antigen and reactive lymphocyte, including the intervening steps of cell multiplication, differentiation, and migration. In this context, the main emphasis in this book will be on the afferent component. However, as our story unfolds, it will become increasingly clear that the above separation of the problem into three compartments is highly arbitrary and that the inductive function of antigen can only be understood if due regard is given to certain aspects of the central and efferent limbs as well.

When we commenced our series of investigations on the role of antigens in immunity in 1963, the tracing of radioactively marked antigen molecules through the body of an injected animal already had a long history. Yet, the yield of information truly relevant to inductive mechanisms had been slender. Nevertheless, it seemed to us that a detailed knowledge of where antigen was, and (perhaps more importantly) where it *was not*, during critical stages of immunological events, constituted information worth possessing. If nothing else, such information was a *sine qua non* for an eventual complete appreciation of inductive mechanisms. However, as we thought about the matter in 1963, two flaws in the majority of the then available literature on distribution of radioactive antigens became apparent to us. First, far too little attention appeared to have been given to questions of the nature, dose, and specific activity of the labeled antigens. Frequently large quantities of lightly labeled material had been injected with obvious loss of sensitivity; and the antigens chosen were materials of low inherent immunogenicity and possessing a tendency to permeate widely through extracellular fluids, resulting in high "noise levels." Second, relatively little use had been made of the very powerful tool of radioautography, let alone quantitative or high-resolution variants of the technique. We thus decided to design an extensive set of investigations using chiefly a pure protein antigen, flagellin, and its various polymerized and fragmented versions, rendered radioactive to as high a substitution level as practicable with the external label [125]I. The advantages and disadvantages of this type of labeling will be discussed in Chapter 4.

We will make no attempt at an exhaustive review of the extensive early literature on antigen tracing, as this has already been dealt with by Campbell and Garvey (1963) and we will not cover problems of delayed hypersensitivity or allograft rejection. However, immunological memory and immunological tolerance will naturally be considered. The many uncertainties which continue to surround cellular immune phenomena complicate considerably the task of authors wishing to deal logically with the subject. It is clear that the two broad categories of cells involved in interacting with antigens are phagocytic and lymphocytic cells, but the detailed relationships *between* the two categories remain problematical. For this reason we have deemed it best to discuss these two cell categories separately before attempting any speculative synthesis. Thus Chapters 4, 7, and 8 will be chiefly concerned with the reticuloendothelial cells which capture antigens, and 5, 6, 9, and 10 with lymphocytes and the effects which antigens may have on them. These seven chapters are preceded by two fairly general ones which discuss the nature of antigens and antibodies from the viewpoint of their function in the afferent limb of the antibody response. There has been a great expansion of interest in antibody production *in vitro* over recent years; while certain *in vitro* studies will be considered in Chapters 2 through 10, and particularly in Chapter 8, we hope to summarize most of the new knowledge on this subject in Chapter 11.

In Chapters 2 through 11 we will concentrate mainly on experimental findings and their immediate implications. In Chapter 12, we present a speculative synthesis of currently available information on mechanisms of induction of antibody formation, and will point out what we consider to be key questions requiring experimentation. Each chapter has its own summary, and these should constitute a useful guide for the reader interested in only certain facets of the book.

We trust that for some investigators this book may also serve a practical function and act as an aid in the planning of future experiments. Therefore we have included several appendixes which describe in detail some of our chief research techniques. It is not always possible to include the various little "tricks" of a particular method in a normal research paper, and we hope that some readers will find useful practical hints in this section of the book.

As already mentioned, we are currently in the midst of a phase of research in cellular immunology where *in vitro* studies of antibody formation have gained preeminence. We share the general view that the precise tools of tissue culture will contribute much to our understanding of immunocyte behavior but will attempt to point out throughout this book that *in vitro* and *in vivo* observations on lymphoid cells complement each other, and that both are necessary for a satisfactory understanding. Thus, it would be unwise to neglect a detailed consideration of lymphatic tissue architecture, such as is presented in Chapter 5.

A final reason for the presentation of this book comes from the enormous practical implications of cellular immunology. The urgent demands of clinical medicine often cannot await a complete scientific knowledge of a particular phenomenon. It is true that we do not know all about how antigen affects lymphoid cells, yet in the clinic this interaction is constantly being manipulated. It is clearly an interaction subject to manifold and subtle controls. There will be no attempt in this book to discuss clinical aspects of immunosuppression. However, we believe that an eventual satisfactory manipulation of the mammalian immune response will depend on the application of fundamental principles of immunogenicity and "tolerogenicity" that are our primary concern here. Therefore we hope that those interested in clinical control of immune processes will find in this volume material of value to them. At present, most immunosuppression is aimed at either the central or the efferent components of the immune response. There is one outstanding exception, as the brilliant success of passive anti-D antibody in the prevention of Rh-sensitization (Finn *et al.*, 1961; Freda *et al.*, 1964) must be considered as affecting the afferent limb. We predict that manipulation of the afferent limb of immune responses will play an increasing role in clinical practice. For this reason alone, it is proper to attempt to collate what we know about antigen and its *in vivo* effects.

CHAPTER 2

ANTIGENS AND THE AFFERENT LIMB OF THE IMMUNE RESPONSE

Antigens or immunogens are commonly defined as substances which, upon introduction into a suitable host, give rise to the formation of antibodies. This is a limited definition as it neglects those aspects of immunology in which an immune response appears to be mediated directly by cells. For the purposes of this monograph, however, we are interested primarily in the role antigen plays in antibody formation. We are especially interested in the fate of antigen both *in vivo* and *in vitro* so that those antigens which have been most used and adequately studied in this respect will be the main subject of the presentation. As emphasized in Chapter 1, this was until recently a neglected aspect of immunology.

Though most workers use the terms antigen and immunogen synonomously, it is becoming increasingly common to equate the term antigenic properties with the serological properties, i.e., the *in vitro* reaction between an antigen and antibody. In contrast, the term immunogenicity is now used more frequently to describe the ability of a substance to cause specific antibody formation in a suitable host or in tissue culture. Many biological macromolecules can act as immunogens but the two

major classes are proteins and polysaccharides. It is not the purpose
of this monograph to review knowledge about the many different types
of proteins or polysaccharides used in such studies. Rather we wish
to draw attention to those properties of a substance which are of importance in the expression of its antigenicity and immunogenicity. It
is necessary to stress this dual interest. There are many reports about
the properties of proteins, polysaccharides, and fragments thereof with
respect to their *in vitro* reaction with antisera prepared against the original antigen or against the fragments. It is only recently that interest
has been shown in the *in vivo* behavior of the antigen or fragment
and for purposes which will become clearer later in this chapter, proteins
or synthetic polypeptides have been the common choice for these studies.
Polysaccharides have rarely been used in this type of study and they
will be discussed only occasionally in this monograph.

It has been customary to consider immunogens as consisting of two
parts. The first concerned those portions of the molecule against which
the antibody formed specifically expressed its activity. Such areas were
called antigenic determinants. An antigenic determinant, when isolated,
should quantitatively react with antibody formed against that portion
of the intact molecule though it may do so at low efficiency. A chemical
compound added to the immunogen might also become a determinant.
The term hapten was introduced to describe such a compound and
referred to a substance of low molecular weight which would react
with specific antibodies but was unable to induce their formation unless
coupled to a "carrier" molecule. This distinction was made early and
is well described by Landsteiner (1946). In recent years, the concept
of the dual activity of an immunogen has been highlighted by two
developments: (1) by the work of polymer chemists who synthesized
polypeptides of tailored shape, size, and other characteristics. The study
of these substances led to the realization that the specificity of an immune response—either cell-mediated or antibody production—could be
directed against both the "haptenic" portion and the "carrier" backbone
of certain polymers (e.g., Benacerraf *et al.*, 1967; Schlossman, 1967).
(2) The more recent indication that the recognition by the host of
the haptenic and carrier portions of a molecule (both of which might
be represented in a simple protein) involved two different cells. This
is discussed more fully in Chapter 6. It is pertinent, however, to remark
here that, especially in the case of a naturally occurring protein, it may
be difficult to decide which portion of the molecule is the hapten and
which portion is the carrier. This may depend upon the nature of the
titrating agent. The possibility arises that the portion of the molecule

which is recognized as a hapten in one type of experiment may serve as a carrier in different circumstances. A term used by Sela, *immuno-dominant determinant*, may be useful in such circumstances.

Sela (1966) has suggested a division of immunogenic substances into three broad categories. (1) Synthetic immunogens, consisting of poly-peptide chains of varying degrees of complexity and the product of laboratory syntheses. (2) Artificial immunogens in which groups of different size and complexity are coupled to a carrier which might be a natural protein or polysaccharide. (3) Natural immunogens which are products of cells or microorganisms, unmodified by any synthetic procedure, though possibly modified by the isolation procedure. Of these three classes our attention will be directly mainly to synthetic and natural antigens, the study of one complementing that of the other.

I. Types of Immunogens

A. ARTIFICIAL AND SYNTHETIC POLYPEPTIDES

The use of haptens coupled to a protein or carbohydrate carrier al-lowed Landsteiner and colleagues to describe in some detail the speci-ficity of the antigen-antibody reaction. More recently, the influence of attached groups such as amino acids on the enhancement or depression of the immunogenicity of the protein has been studied in detail. Such studies have also indicated the size range of antigenic determinants.

Based on the work of several groups, Sela (1966) listed those amino acids which, when attached to proteins, were found to have such effects. For example, the addition of a few residues of tyrosine to a poorly antigenic material such as gelatin, substantially increased the immuno-genicity of the gelatin. The antibody formed to the modified protein had a specificity which was increasingly directed to the added tyrosine residues as more were attached. This reaction offers a method of obtain-ing a protein which could be labeled with radioactive iodide to a very high specific activity—a possibility which has not yet been tried but which could be useful in particular circumstances.

The reverse situation has also been exploited. Small molecules of natural origin, such as nucleosides (Ungar-Waron *et al.*, 1967), glyco-lipids (Arnon *et al.*, 1967), and an antigenically active peptide derived from lysozyme (Arnon and Sela, 1969) have been attached to synthetic polypeptides. Antibodies formed against these conjugates may react specifically with the "natural" hapten.

A study of artificial antigens has provided estimates of the size of combining sites for antibodies. For both polytyrosyl gelatin (Givol and Sela, 1964) and polyalanyl bovine serum albumin (Sage *et al.*, 1964), a peptide containing five amino acid residues has been suggested as a maximum size. Much effort has been put into the study of synthetic antigens. The literature is so extensive that no attempt is made to cover it, even in a superficial way. Maurer (1964), Sela (1966), and Schlossman (1967) have written articles to which readers are referred. A very large number of synthetic polypeptides has been described. A variety of factors such as amino acid composition, size, shape, rigidity, charge, and accessibility and positioning of particular groups have been shown to play a role either in their immunogenicity and in the properties of antibodies formed to them or in their tolerance-inducing properties. We discuss here a few cases which are of direct relevance to our story.

Of the many polypeptides synthesized, few have been used in studies involving antigen distribution and localization. One of particular interest in the multichain polypeptide (T,G)-A-L (Sela *et al.*, 1962). This polymer consists of a poly-L-lysine backbone with side chains composed of polymers of DL-alanine, at the end of which are attached L-glutamic acid and L-tyrosine residues. (T,G)-A-L 509 (mol. wt. about 230,000) contained about 200 tyrosine residues per mole. When injected in saline into mice, the polymer was not immunogenic but if injected emulsified in Freund's complete adjuvant antibody production occurred. The immunogenicity of the preparation was related to the content of tyrosine and to a lesser extent, glutamic acid.

Synthetic polypeptides, composed of D-amino acids, may also be immunogenic, though less so than a polypeptide composed of the corresponding L-amino acids. Gill *et al.* (1964) found that a polypeptide composed of D-tyrosine, D-glutamic acid, and D-lysine was immunogenic when injected with adjuvant into rabbits. Janeway and Sela (1967) found that the random linear copolymer, D-Tyr, D-Glu, D-Ala, elicited a primary response when injected with adjuvant into mice. Injection in saline caused a substantial degree of tolerance.

Although it had been suspected for a long time that the ability of an animal to form antibody to an immunogen was determined by its genetic constitution, this has been most clearly shown using synthetic antigens. Three groups in particular—Pinchuck and Maurer (1968), McDevitt and Sela (1965), and Benacerraf and colleagues (see Benacerraf *et al.*, 1967)—have used synthetic antigens and demonstrated that the recognition of a particular antigen may be controlled by a single, dominant gene. In extending their work, McDevitt and Sela and colleagues (see review by McDevitt and Benacerraf, 1970) have found that the gene controlling recognition of an antigen was, in some cases, linked to an allele of the H_2 locus which is concerned with the main pattern of histocompatibility antigens of the mouse. This rather unexpected relationship has been used by Jerne (1969) as a basis for a hypothesis concerning the origin of antibody diversity.

The role of size in determining the immunogenicity or otherwise of a substance has been elegantly examined using polypeptides. Schlossman and colleagues (Schlossman et al., 1965, 1966) prepared a series of dinitrophenyloligolysyl peptides which differed from each other regarding the size of the lysine carrier and the position of the hapten. The smallest substance which was regularly immunogenic was α-DNP-octa-L-lysine. It is of interest that α-DNP-octa-L-lysine was the smallest molecule in this series which could form stable hydrogen bonds in its folded configuration (Benacerraf et al., 1967).

B. Fibrous Proteins

In many of their properties, fibrous proteins appear to occupy an intermediate position between synthetic polypeptides and naturally occurring globular proteins. They occur naturally but have repeated amino acid sequences which result in repeating antigenic areas. Proteins of this type have been used infrequently in in vivo studies and will not be discussed.

C. Naturally Occurring Immunogens

Proteins which have been used extensively in in vivo studies may be divided into two groups, those which in nature probably occur mainly as the monomer, such as serum proteins and many enzymes; and those which in nature occur as a polymer consisting of an array of several or many protein units, arranged in such a fashion that a portion of the molecule is always adjacent to neighboring molecules, and portion is "exposed" to the external medium. Monomeric units may usually be obtained from the polymer by simple disaggregation procedures. A representative of this class is the flagellar proteins from various organisms, and particular attention will be paid to those from the Salmonella organisms. Tobacco mosaic virus (TMV) also belongs to this group and has been well studied.

D. Serum Proteins

Perhaps the most common of all antigens used in *in vivo* studies
are the proteins present to high levels in mammalian sera and are
therefore readily isolated in a pure state. A variety of serum albumins
and globulins is obtainable commercially and this ready availability has
been a great attraction for many workers. The structure of globulin
molecules will be discussed in the following chapter. Bovine and human
serum albumins have been studied in considerable detail by Lapresle
and co-workers (Lapresle and Webb, 1965, and earlier references) and
Porter and co-workers (see review, Porter and Press, 1962). These
studies are of interest because the investigators were concerned with
the antigenic activity of both large fragments and oligo peptides.
Fragments with molecular weights between 11,000 and 20,000 were obtained from both albumins. In inhibition tests, these had activities which,
on a molar basis, were as high as those of the original protein and
their activity was found to depend upon their conformation. Smaller
size fragments (mol. wt. 6600–7000) could be obtained from both proteins but these had considerably reduced serological activity. A limitation
to the further study of these proteins was the lack of knowledge of
their detailed structure.

E. Myoglobin

A logical sequence to these studies was to examine a protein whose
amino acid sequence and conformation was known. Kendrew *et al.*
(1961) and Edmundson (1965) had described these features for the
protein myoglobin and its derivatives from sperm whale and several
groups (Crumpton and Wilkinson, 1965; Crumpton, 1967; Atassi and
Saplin, 1968; Atassi and Caruso, 1968; Atassi, 1968a,b) have studied
the antigenic properties of fragments in some detail. Crumpton and
colleagues isolated antigenically active fragments from enzymic digests
(carried out at 2°C) of apomyoglobin. The reader is referred to the
review of Crumpton (1966) for details but the main points of interest
which were found are as follows. Myoglobin possesses a minimum of
four antigenic sites. The serologically active peptides come from helical
and nonhelical portions of the molecule. One of these is at the C-terminal
end of the molecule and this has, in particular, been investigated in
some detail. In general, when inhibition tests were used to define the
activity of a peptide, larger peptides were found to be more active as
inhibitors than were the smaller peptides. The evidence was consistent

with the interpretation that though an antigenic site might be small, the presence of adjacent amino acids could maintain these amino acids which formed the antigenic site in a conformation which was similar to that present in the intact parent molecule. The size of an antigenic site was probably between 3 and 5 amino acids. It was suggested that an isolated antigenic fragment must retain the conformation present in the parent protein in order to compete stoichometrically with the parent protein in an inhibition test. Loss of the appropriate conformation

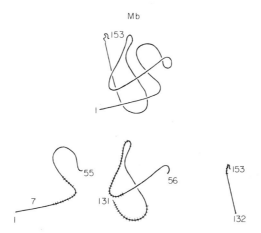

FIG. 2.1. A schematic line drawing of the mode of folding of the sperm whale myoglobin polypeptide chain. The position of cleavage at methionines −55 and −131 are indicated and the peptides obtained are dissected apart for clarity. The position of tryptophan −7 is also indicated on segment 1–55. The approximate locations of the reactive tryptic peptides are shown by the marking on the main line. (After Atassi and Saplin, 1968.)

would be reflected by a decrease in the serological activity of the isolated fragment.

Attassi and colleagues have found rather similar results. After tryptic digestion, four peptides were obtained which could inhibit the reaction between the intact antigen and its antibody. Three of these four peptides came from external "corners" of the molecule. When myoglobin was cleaved at both methionine residues by treatment with cyanogen bromide, three peptides were obtained (Fig. 2.1). Residues 1–55 and 56–131 gave immune precipitates with antisera to the intact protein but residue 132–153 showed only inhibitory activity. Almost all the serological activity of the intact antigen was recovered in the three peptides. The tryptophan at residue 7 was not found to be an essential part of an antigenic site as modification of this residue did not affect serological activity. If both tryptophan residues (7 and 14) were substituted, antigenic reactivity was drastically decreased and the spherical shape of the molecule was changed. Titration of the tyrosine 103 did not affect the serological activity of the peptide 56–131, but titration of tyrosines 145 and 151 abolished the inhibitory activity of peptide 132–153.

Although these studies have brought us closer to a definition of an antigenic site in a protein molecule and to an appreciation of the comformational requirements, little attempt has been made to take direct advantage of this information to further our knowledge of the immunogenic behavior of the molecule. This is in part because the parent proteins themselves are poor immunogens and in some species, antibody to them is produced in detectable amounts only if the protein is injected with, for example, Freund's complete adjuvant. For many purposes, it is more advantageous to use proteins which cause antibody formation without the simultaneous injection of added adjuvants. For reasons that are not yet clear, it is frequently the case that bacterial and viral proteins are highly immunogenic in vertebrates. Two such proteins which have been studied in some detail are the unit protein from tobacco mosaic virus particles and the protein, flagellin, present in flagella from *Salmonella* organisms.

F. TOBACCO MOSAIC VIRUS PROTEIN

Tobacco mosaic virus (TMV) and its unit protein have been intensively studied by two groups—Anderer and co-workers in Tubingen and Benjamini and colleagues in San Francisco. Anderer (1963) prepared up to twenty peptides from the *vulgare* strain of this virus. Some of these were effective in inhibiting a TMV-anti-TMV antibody precipitating system. Peptides 18–23 and 123–134 were most efficient but peptides 62–68 and 142–158 had some activity. It is supposed that peptides 18–23 contributed to the exposed surface of the virus particle. Anderer and Schlumberger (1965) synthesized a peptide similar in sequence to the natural one 153–158. Antiserum to this peptide precipitated the virus showing that the peptide must be exposed in the virus particle. The same authors later showed (Anderer and Schlumberger, 1966) that antisera to artificial antigens with the C-terminal amino acid or dipeptide as haptenic groups would still cross-react with the virus containing the homologous C-terminal amino acid.

In their studies, Benjamini and colleagues measured the ability of TMV peptides to react with antiserum to the unit viral protein. It was found (Benjamini *et al.*, 1964) that the tryptic peptide, residues 93–112, was able completely to inhibit the fixation of complement by the complex composed of TMV *protein* and anti-TMV *protein* antibody. Further investigation showed (Young *et al.*, 1966) that certain portions of this peptide were not required for immunological activity to be demonstrated. The peptide was still active after removal of three residues from the N-terminus or of two residues from the C-terminus. The di-, tri-, tetra, penta, hexa-, hepta-, octa-, and nonapeptides (Young *et al.*, 1967) of the C-terminal decapeptide of residues 93–112 peptide (Stewart *et al.*, 1966) were synthesized. All were acetylated with acetic-C^{14} anhydride and the labeled acetyl peptides were tested for specific binding with anti-TMV protein sera. The C-terminal pentapeptide and all larger peptides were found to possess immunological activity while the shorter peptides lacked significant activity. It was subsequently shown that the N-terminal portion of the pentapeptide conferred hydrophobicity on the C-terminal portion. N-octanoyl-Ala-Thr-Arg was synthesized and was found to bind strongly to the anti-TMV protein whereas Ala-Thr-Arg had little activity (Benjamini *et al.*, 1969).

The different findings of the two groups have been discussed by Rappaport (1965) and Crumpton (1967) and will not be considered here, except to point out the obvious differences in the assay systems used by the two groups.

The results of these and other investigations showed that an antigenic determinant might contain only 3–5 amino acids (see Kabat, 1966) and even one or two amino acids might, in special circumstances, show some activity as illustrated by the results of both groups.

G. FLAGELLA PROTEINS OF *Salmonella* ORGANISMS

As flagellar proteins have been much used in the authors' laboratories and as many of the findings are presented and discussed later in the monograph, the properties of these proteins will be described in some detail.

Salmonella organisms carry two major antigenic systems—the O or somatic antigen which is lipopolysaccharide present on the surface of the bacterial body; and the H or flagellar antigens carried by the protein, flagellin, the unit protein present in the flagella. Strains of *Salmonella* are classified in the Kaufman-White scale according to the specificity of antibody raised in animals following injection in saline of whole organisms. The flagella particle itself consists of linear arrays of the protein flagellin together with varying amounts, usually between 1–5% (w/w), of substances composed of carbohydrate and lipid. Flagellin is readily prepared from flagella by disaggregation (Appendix I) leaving an insoluble residue containing the carbohydrate and lipid. The flagellin may be polymerized to form a polymer (polymerized flagellin) which, in the electron microscope, appears to have a similar structure to the flagella particle. Flagellin from several strains of *Salmonella* has a molecular weight of about 40,000. McDonough (1965) has carried out amino acid analyses of flagellin from different strains and some general findings are worth comment. Cysteine and tryptophan are absent in all and histidine in some strains. Methionine, proline, phenylalanine, and tyrosine are present in low amounts. There are many arginine and lysine residues and some strains have the substituted lysine residue, ϵ-*N*-methyllysine. Flagella are relatively resistant to trypsin (Kobayashi *et al.*, 1959) as is also polymerized flagellin (J. Pye, personal communication). Flagellin from *Salmonella adelaide* (SW 1338) has a tryptic-resistant core (Ada *et al.*, 1967). Flagellin from this organism contains no histidine, 3 methionine residues, and 11 of the 25 lysine residues are methylated. Treatment with cyanogen bromide (CNBr) yields 4 major fragments together with partial breakdown products (Parish and Ada, 1969a). From amino acid analyses and the positions of the different components in the gel after polyacrylamide gel electrophoresis, the fragments were estimated to have molecular weights as follows: fragment A, 18,000; fragment B, 12,000; fragment C, 5500; and fragment D, 4500. Fragment A contained 1 arginine and 10 of the 11 methylated lysine residues. Antisera were raised in rabbits against the polymer, flagellin, the complete CNBr digest, and three of the isolated fragments. Using four different serological tests, it was found that fragment A contained in apparently unaltered form all the antigenic determinants which were normally expressed in the flagellin molecule or the polymer particle (Parish *et al.*, 1969). Reaction with iodide at small extents of substitution showed that in flagellin, the tyrosine residue in fragment D was more readily substituted than those in fragment A. By contrast, in polymerized flagellin, the tyrosine residues of fragment A were more readily substituted (Parish and Ada, 1969a). Taken together the serological and iodination data were consistent with the interpretation that in polymerized flagellin, the fragment A portion of the flagellin molecule was exposed to the external environment. It suggested that amino acid sequences in fragment D and possibly also in fragments B and C were not so exposed. In *S. adelaide* flagellin, the ratio of ϵ-*N*-methyllysine/lysine was 11:25 whereas this ratio in fragment A was 10:11, suggesting that methylation of the lysine residues occurred *after* the polymerization process.

Figure 2.2 shows in simplified diagramatic form the way in which it is considered fragment A is disposed in the flagellin molecule and in particles of polymerized flagellin or flagella.

Polymerized flagellin, flagellin, and fragment A (from *S. adelaide*) differ in their immunogenic- and tolerance-inducing properties. Poly-

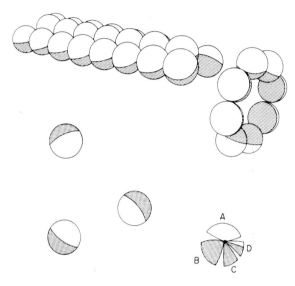

FIG. 2.2. A simple diagram showing a possible arrangement of flagellin molecules in a particle of polymerized flagellin (adapted from a model proposed by Lowy and Hanson, 1965). Each ball represents a single molecule of the monomer, flagellin. In the top part of the diagram is seen three adjacent linear arrays of flagellin molecules, as they might occur in the polymer (each particle of polymer consisting of eight such linear arrays) and an end-on view of a polymer particle. The clear portion of each molecule represents that segment of flagellin exposed to the "external medium," the hatched area that segment either opposed to adjacent flagellin molecules or exposed to the "internal medium." The lower part of the diagram shows three separate molecules of flagellin and one molecule of flagellin split by cyanogen bromide treatment in four fragments, A, B, C, and D. It is considered that the exterior portion of the molecule in the polymer consists mainly of fragment A, which contains the demonstrable antigenic activity of the flagellin molecule.

merized flagellin is highly immunogenic in rats, a single injection (in saline) causing initially an IgM and then an IgG response. Flagellin is also immunogenic though only an IgG response occurs (Nossal *et al.*, 1964a). Both are effective in causing a secondary response (Nossal *et al.*, 1965a). In contrast, fragment A is poorly immunogenic in adult rats when injected in saline (though good antibody titers result if adjuvants are used). If given as a series of injections in saline into adult or young rats, fragment A is effective at inducing specific tolerance which may be complete when tested by a subsequent injection of flagellin and almost complete if the animals are challenged with polymerized flagellin (Parish and Ada, 1969b). Those findings and a possible interpretation in terms of antigen–cell interaction are discussed later (Chapters 10 and 12).

H. HEMOCYANIN

Hemocyanin is frequently used as an immunogen because there are sensitive methods available for the detection of anti-hemocyanin antibodies and injection of small amounts of the protein into experimental animals results in antibody formation. Furthermore, the possibility of previous casual contact of laboratory animals with this protein is negligible. This protein occurs in two phyla of invertebrates, Mollusca and Arthropoda and is present in solution in a variety of polymeric forms. Svedberg and Pedersen (1940) have described their physical properties in some detail but little is known of the chemical basis of their antigenic and immunogenic activity.

I. COMPLEX NATURAL ANTIGENS

As well as the synthetic and natural antigens just described, there are a group of preparations which can be classified as complex natural antigens. These include whole bacteria, viruses, and red cells. For certain purposes in immunology, they offer a compromise between conflicting reasons for choosing a suitable immunogen. For detailed studies on the fate of the immunogen, their very complexity argues against their use. They are in widespread use primarily because they are good immunogens and because there are sensitive methods available for the estimation of antibodies to them. All virus particles are complex in structure and contain one or more proteins. One in common use for the reasons outlined above is the T2 coliphage. This is a DNA-containing virus and contains many different proteins. The most sensitive method of antibody estimation is neutralization of the infectivity of the phage particles and the antibody responsible for this neutralization has a specificity directed toward a protein in the tail of the viral particles.

Perhaps the most common preparation in use in immunological laboratories is the intact red blood cell, again for similar reasons. The invention of the plaque technique for estimation of antibody-forming cells (Jerne and Nordin, 1963; Ingraham and Bussard, 1964) has provided a method of exquisite sensitivity for the measurement of the antibody response. Despite this, there has been a considerable lag in the isolation and characterization of the components in the red cell membrane which confer upon it the antigenic and, in part, the immunogenic properties.

1. Properties of Proteins which Influence Their Immunogenicity

The study of synthetic polypeptides has led to some understanding of the role which amino acid composition, disposition of groups, the conformation of the molecule, charge, and other factors may play in the determination of immunogenicity (Sela, 1966). We are more ignorant concerning the properties which determine the immunogenicity of natural substances such as proteins. Some factors of importance are (1) the substance must be regarded as foreign by the host animal. This means in all probability that there are cells present with receptors which recognize the foreign determinant. Furthermore, it is also likely that the cell receptors concerned must have a high affinity for the antigenic determinant if the cell is to be stimulated by the antigen (Siskind and Benacerraf, 1969). Univalent antigens are not immunogenic (e.g., Rajewsky et al., 1969). It is presently considered that the induction of optimal antibody formation may in some cases require the cooperation of at least two cell types, possibly derived from the bone marrow and thymus, and both of which express specificity in their reaction with the immunogen (see Chapter 6). This implies that two rare cells must meet. If the immunogenic molecule is bound to the surface of one cell (by a "haptenic" group), the chance of this cell now meeting another particular cell, as required by this hypothesis, may be proportional to the number of *different* determinants on the "carrier" portion of the immunogen. Possession of many different determinants may therefore be a factor in favor of an antigen being a good immunogen. (3) Size is often considered to be an important factor. A strict relationship between immunogenicity and size has not been shown, possibly because above a certain value size per se is not of critical importance. The presence on particles such as bacterial flagella, viruses, and probably cell membranes of repeating patterns of determinants may be of greater importance. For example, bacterial flagellin, aggregated in a random fashion by a cross-linking reagent, is much less immunogenic than the

same preparation polymerized in linear arrays to form repeating units
(C. R. Parish, personal communication). The presence of repeating antigenic determinants may well be important in determining the extent
to which an antigen can not only react with but also stimulate an antigen
sensitive cell.

II. Choice of Immunogen

There are factors other than immunogenicity which need to be considered in choosing an antigen suitable for both *in vivo* and *in vitro*
studies. One is the method to be used to detect the antigen after injection
into an animal or addition to a cell suspension. A second consideration
is the sensitivity of methods available for the detection of antibody to
the antigen.

A. Detection of Immunogen by Direct Visualization

Viruses, bacteria, or cells with a characteristic size, shape or other
properties have been detected within cells or tissues after injection into
animals. Such an approach may best be regarded as being qualitative
rather than quantitative but still may yield information of particular
importance. To quote a recent application, Litt (1967) has studied the
fate of injected foreign red cells upon their entrance into guinea pig
lymph nodes. Very shortly after injection, phagocytosis of some injected
cells by medullary macrophages could be observed. Such cells stayed
intact for some time whereas red cells penetrating to the diffuse cortex
of the node could be seen to be lysed very rapidly, an occurrence possibly due to complement-dependent lysis and considered by Litt to
reflect the rapid synthesis of anti-red blood cell antibody. Ferritin has
been used as an antigen in many investigations (e.g., Wellensiek and
Coons, 1964). Because of the density of the iron core of ferritin, the
particle may easily be identified in electron micrographs of tissue sections
and its position within a cell accurately determined. The resolution is
rather better than that obtained in radioautography. Disadvantages are
(1) that the identification of the particle depends upon the iron core
rather than the antigenic protein coat and, (2) that a cell may need
to contain many particles in order that several may be identified with
certainty in the necessarily thin section required for electron microscopy.

B. Detection due to Innate Properties

An obvious approach has been to utilize the antigenicity or immunogenicity of the injected material. Humphrey and White (1964) have given estimates of the relative sensitivities of various immunological procedures for the estimation of antigens and Campbell and Garvey (1963) have quoted several examples of the use of such techniques to estimate the presence of antigenic or immunogenic material in tissues some time after injection. Although once of fairly wide use, such procedures have been used more recently in conjunction with an antigen labeled with an attached marker. Such methods had their greatest use in showing the presence or absence of intact or active fragments of an antigen in tissues and hence the distribution of the substance throughout the body. Infectious agents can be followed in the body by infectivity measurements provided replication of the agent is avoided or masking of activity does not take place. Enzyme activity can be used, especially if methods of great sensitivity are available, (e.g., β-galactosidase; Rotman, 1961) but from the point of view of determining the role of antigen in the induction of antibody formation, the fate of the material in the body should be determined by its antigenic rather than its enzymic properties.

The immunofluorescent technique introduced by Coons et al. (1942) has made a major contribution to our knowledge of antigen distribution and is now one of the most widely used procedures in immunological laboratories. The technique is specific and in tissue sections or cell smears has great resolution. The most serious objection to the technique for the present purpose is the relatively low sensitivity. Though exact figures do not seem to be available concerning the number of molecules needed to give an easily detectable reaction, the technique has been shown to be at least 10,000 times less sensitive than is radioautography of tissues containing antigen labeled with carrier-free preparations of radioactive iodide (Miller and Nossal, 1964).

C. Detection due to Added Markers

Early workers determined the gross distribution patterns of proteins in animals by using proteins to which were attached a dye substance, such as Evans' Blue, and thereafter following the chromophore. Though such a procedure was obviously of great value, the dye has now been replaced by radioactive isotopes. Labeling protein with radioactive isotope has become now a very widely used technique because of the great specificity and the sensitivity of detection. As the knowledge gained by the use of this technique is a major reason for the writing of this monograph, a short discussion of some aspects of the technique is warranted here.

The first requirement for this approach is the availability of the protein in a pure form. Until this is achieved it may well be impossible to interpret the results as part or even all of the label may be on a contaminating protein in the preparation. One may extend this requirement a step further—that the marker should be irreversibly attached to that part of the protein which carries the antigenic determinants. Complete confidence in the use of a label to follow the fate and localization of an antigen in tissues can only be obtained if the label itself is part of an antigenic determinant (Humphrey et al., 1967).

The choice of the isotope to be used depends upon several factors. For ease of detection in tissues or extracts, a γ-emitter is desirable because of the great ease of scintillation counting to determine radioactivity. On the other hand, as location in individual cells will be determined by autoradiography, a weak β-emitter is desirable. Here a compromise must be made between the high resolution obtained with a very weak emitter such as tritium, and the low efficiency of grain formation of such a weak β-emitter. To minimize possible changes in the properties of the antigen and to obtain effective labeling, the isotope should be available as a preparation in which most atoms of the element are radioactive. A further consideration is the rate of disintegration of the isotope used. The extent of substitution necessary to achieve a particular specific activity is a function of the half-life of the isotope—the shorter the half-life of the isotope, the lower will be the required extent of substitution. In addition, it is desirable that the isotope be introduced into the molecule without changing the chemical or physical properties of the molecule. With naturally occurring antigens, this might be done biosynthetically but high specific activity labeling of proteins in this way has not yet been reported. Similarly, direct exchange procedures, e.g., tritiation, applied to proteins have not been successful.

The isotope which most nearly satisfies these conditions is ^{125}I which emits both γ- and β-rays. The β-rays have a higher energy than those of ^3H and hence some resolution is lost, but the grain yield in autoradiographs of conventional histological sections is eight times higher than that of ^3H (Ada et al., 1965). ^{35}S has been used extensively in earlier work (Campbell and Garvey, 1963) but its use is restricted to the labeling of haptenic groups. Labeling of proteins to high specific activity has been obtained only with isotopes of iodine. Many proteins can be labeled to have specific activities of 10–100 mCi/μg. The synthetic polymer (T,G)-A-L has been substituted with ^{125}I to very high specific activities (2.5 mCi/μg; Humphrey and Keller, 1970).

The method most used to achieve efficient labeling of proteins with low concentrations of iodide (the direct oxidation technique) may damage a protein (McConahey and Dixon, 1966) due to oxidation of methionine residues (Parish and Fetherstonhaugh, 1970). Alternatively, in some cases, iodination may be carried out enzymically (Marchalonis, 1969).

The amino acid residues labeled (mainly tyrosine) may not be part of an antigenic determinant in the protein so that fragmentation of the molecule might result in separation of the labeled fragment from antigenic fragments (Nossal et al., 1965a). Deiodination might occur in vivo, resulting in unlabeled, but otherwise intact antigen, though evidence showing that this occurs in lymphoid tissue has not yet been reported.

As an example of the potential of biosynthetic labeling procedures, Ehrenreich and Cohn (1968a) reported the biosynthesis of rabbit hemoglobin containing leucine-^{3}H. The specific activity ranged from 0.005–0.02 mCi/mg which is too low for most aspects of in vivo studies. In contrast, Humphrey et al. (1967) were able to prepare a batch of the polypeptide (T,G)-A-L which contained alanine-^{3}H and which had a specific activity of 3–3.5 μCi/μg. This was used in in vivo studies.

D. Detection of Antibody to the Injected Immunogen

It will be apparent that there is a twofold purpose in studying the fate of immunogen in tissues. The first is to define the manner in which the immunogen is handled by the body. The second is to relate the immune response which develops to the particular localization pattern of the immunogen. For both purposes, it is necessary to determine the levels of antibody formed to the injected material. It is most desirable to have a sensitive method for the detection of antibody as this may be of crucial importance in determining whether a state of immunity or partial tolerance exists in the animal.

It is beyond the scope of this chapter to describe the many methods available for the detection of antibodies or of antibody-forming cells. Some will be mentioned in later chapters.

E. A PERFECT IMMUNOGEN?

It might be thought that in a study of the role of immunogen in the immune response, it would be ideal if we could use a protein or synthetic polypeptide which was highly immunogenic in animals when injected without adjuvant. We would wish to have a sensitive method for the estimation of antibody formed against this immunogen and be able to label it to high specific activity with an isotope, preferentially ^{125}I, which should become attached to a tyrosine(s) residue(s) which in turn formed part of an antigenic determinant. This would require that we knew not only the amino acid sequence and conformation of the molecule but the nature and disposition of antigenic determinants within it. The availability of such an immunogen, though advantageous, would not automatically provide a solution to all our questions. It is inevitable that relevant information will continue to be provided piecemeal through the study of a number of systems, each of which may be eminently suitable for elucidating a particular facet of the immune response. The behavior of an immunogen in a new environment cannot always be confidently anticipated from their known behavior in a previously studied system. For example, mice of the CBA strain, if thymectomized at birth, in adult life respond normally to bacterial flagella but poorly to sheep red blood cells (SRBC) (Miller and Martin, 1970). In contrast, Lewis rats thymectomized at birth, in adult life respond normally to SRBC but poorly to flagella (Lind, 1970).

III. Summary

Some synthetic polypeptides and proteins used as natural antigens were discussed with particular reference to properties which influence their antigenic and immunogenic properties. Though the evidence from various studies suggests that an antigenic determinant might be as small a sequence as 3–5 amino acid residues, other portions of the molecule contributed to their activity. The use of synthetic polypeptides has enabled an analysis to be made of many factors which contribute to the immunogenicity of a molecule. On the other hand, we are still rather ignorant why some naturally occurring proteins are more immunogenic than others. Factors which are probably important are the "foreignness" of the antigenic determinants, the presence of many different determinants and, in particulate antigens, the occurrence of repeating patterns of antigenic determinants.

Their innate immunogenicity in animals or in tissue culture is one of several factors which influence our choice of a suitable immunogen for studying the *in vivo* behavior of antigens. A satisfactory method for tracing such material *in vivo* must be available and if as has become standard practice, the material is to be labeled with radioactive isotope, the isotope and method of labeling chosen. ^{125}I is a compromise choice for most purposes. Though many questions could be more satisfactorily answered if the "perfect" antigen were available, it seems likely that many different antigens will be continued to be used, each offering in particular circumstances some advantage over the others available.

ANTIBODIES AND THE AFFERENT LIMB OF THE IMMUNE RESPONSE

The main product of the interaction of an antigen and the appropriate cells in the body are antibodies. In this chapter we are interested not so much in the mode of synthesis of antibodies, but rather on the effect their presence may have on the development of the immune response. In this context a brief description is given of their structure and biological properties. For a more detailed statement on antibody structure, readers are referred to a recent review (Edelman and Gall, 1969).

I. The Structure of Immunoglobulins

Immunoglobulins may occur in five major classes which in human sera are called IgG, IgM, IgA, IgD, and IgE. These classes differ one from the other in properties such as size, charge, valence (antigen binding), carbohydrate content, size of constituent amino acid chains, and so on. For this monograph we are interested mainly in two classes, IgG and IgM, as antibodies in these two classes have received most attention as far as structural studies are concerned. So far as is known, most classes of immunoglobulins have the same unit structure consisting of heavy (mol. wt. 50,000–70,000) and light (mol. wt. 22,000) chains held together by disulfide bonds. In IgA, there is an additional component called the transport piece. The accepted structure for IgG (mol. wt. 150,000) is shown in diagrammatic form in Fig. 3.1.

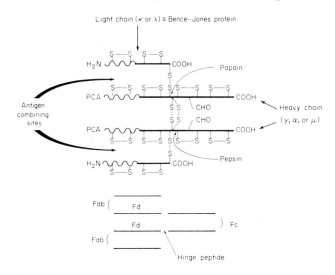

FIG. 3.1. Two diagrammatic representations of the structure of the IgG molecule. In the upper diagram (after Putnam, 1969), some features of the chemical structure of the molecule are presented. There are four interchain and twelve intrachain disulfide bonds. The variable portions (amino acid sequence) of the chains are confined to the N-terminal half of the light chains and to the PCA-terminal quarter of the heavy chains. The approximate positions of cleavage by pepsin and by papain of the heavy chains is shown. On the lower diagram is shown the nomenclature assigned to the different fragments obtained, in part, by papain digestion. The hinge peptide refers to a region of the heavy chains which is considered to allow flexibility in conformation of these fragments with respect to one another. It is believed that the combining sites of the molecule for antigen is a function of amino acid sequences in the variable regions of the light and heavy chains (upper diagram).

Two identical halves, each consisting of a light and a heavy chain are joined together by two disulfide bonds. The light and heavy chains in each half are also held together by a disulfide bond. The chains may be separated and then isolated if these bonds are first cleaved and then alkylated to prevent rejoining. If prepared under appropriate conditions (Fleishman et al., 1962; Marchalonis and Edelman, 1968) the dissociated chains may retain some of the biological activity of the original molecule. This applies particularly to the heavy chain, which in many cases appears to retain preferentially the antigen binding capacity of the molecule. This method of breakdown of the molecule does not involve splitting peptide bonds.

A second type of procedure is to act upon the IgG molecule with proteolytic enzymes. If papain, activated with a sulfydryl reagent is used, peptide bond cleavage occurs near the center of the heavy chain (Fig. 3.1), and three major subunits are recovered (Porter, 1959). Two of the subunits are identical and each contains an antigen-combining site. The two pieces are named Fab. The third piece is named Fc and if prepared from IgG of some species, notably rabbit, is readily crystallizable. If the Fab subunit is itself reduced, a light chain is recovered together with a residual portion of the heavy chain, and this portion is called the Fd fragment. The approximate position of cleavage of IgG by pepsin is shown in Fig. 3.1. If IgG is acted upon by pepsin at about pH 5, a fragment is isolated which corresponds closely to the Fab fragment resulting from papain digestion but has almost twice the molecular weight (100,000) (Nisonoff et al., 1959). It can be converted by reduction of one disulfide bond into two fragments, each of molecular weight 50,000, which are only slightly larger than Fab and are called Fab¹. The original peptic fragment is therefore (Fab¹)₂. A fragment corresponding to Fc is not recovered as this portion of the IgG molecule is split into smaller fragments by pepsin. Trypsin also will cleave mildly reduced and amino ethylated IgG into two active Fab units and a crystallizable Fc fragment (Givol, 1967).

A third method of cleavage of the IgG molecule is to use the reagent cyanogen bromide (CNBr) which selectively cleaves the peptide bond adjacent to a methionine residue. Because most proteins contain rather few methionine residues, this reagent has been most useful in splitting peptide chains into large fragments which are frequently of a suitable size for subsequent amino acid sequencing. This procedure has been of particular use in the sequencing of the heavy chains of IgG. Under certain conditions, IgG may be cleaved by reaction with CNBr and fragments recovered which have biological activity. Cahnmann et al. (1966) showed that at relatively low concentrations of CNBr, one peptide bond in IgG is split and this yields three fragments similar in their behavior to Fab or Fc. The similarity in size of the Fab fragments which result from the action of three different enzymes and of CNBr indicates that all these cleavages occur in the same region of the heavy chain. This region—the so-called *hinge region*—may be more accessible than others. The sequence of amino acids in this region is now known and the probable sites of action of these reagents known (Smyth and Utsumi, 1967; Givol and De Lorenzo, 1968).

One of the remarkable results of these various procedures has been the recovery of large fragments of the IgG molecule which still retain antigen-binding activity. Fab, Fab[1] and (Fab[1])$_2$, if prepared from antibody to a known antigen, all retain the ability to react with that antigen. Fab and Fab[1] are univalent and (Fab[1])$_2$ divalent. A question which has engaged much attention is the relative roles of the light chain and Fd fragment in the reaction with antigen. Though there are well-established exceptions, the usual finding has been that the Fd fragment or isolated heavy chain carried the main binding site for antigen and that the light chain plays a complementary or modifying role (Edelman, 1964). It is generally found that maximum antigen-binding activity requires both the light and heavy chains. As the antigenic determinants of several proteins have been shown to contain as few as 3–5 amino acids, it is supposed that the antigen binding sites of antibodies might also be small in size and involve only 1–2% of the total amino acids (about 1500); thus one site in the light and heavy chains together might contain less than 20 amino acids. The precise position in either chain of these sites is not known but it is believed that amino acid sequences in the N-terminal halves of the light and heavy chains are involved. The heterogenicity in the amino acid sequences of antibody molecules is confined to the N-terminal half of the light chain and the N-terminal quarter of the heavy chain.

The presence of the Fc piece in IgG confers several biological activities on the intact molecule. A few of these are the ability to bind complement, to react with cell surfaces, to pass across the placenta, and to mediate passive cutaneous anaphylaxis in guinea pigs (e.g., Isliker et al., 1965). Some of them will be discussed in more detail later. It has rarely been shown that an Fc fragment, isolated from an IgG preparation, retains biological activity.

Though the structure of the IgG molecule is conventionally drawn as in Fig. 3.1, the molecule is known to exist in the shape of the letter Y with the two light chains and the Fd portions forming the upper arms and the Fc portion the lower segment. Electron micrographs suggest that the binding site for antigen is at the upper tip of each arm (Valentine and Green, 1967). The IgG molecule is flexible at a position near the disulfide bonds linking the heavy chains, and Smyth and Utsumi (1967) have shown that this may be due to the presence in this area of the heavy chain of the amino acid sequence, Pro-Pro-Pro. It can thus be imagined that reaction of the IgG molecule with antigen is unlikely to hinder, by a steric mechanism, the Fc portion in its reaction with either complement or the cell surface. Reaction of antibody with antigen results in a conformational change of the globulin molecule. Presumably the size of the antigen reacting with the antibody affects the magnitude of this change.

Within any species, all classes of antibody have the same light chains. In humans, two serologically distinct light chains are found and these are nominated κ and λ chains. Mice and rabbits have also been shown to have two classes of light chains. Antibodies of the different classes have distinct serological specificities and this is a property of their heavy chains which are referred to as γ, μ, α, δ, and ϵ according to their origin IgG, IgM, IgA, IgD, and IgE, respectively.

There are conflicting reports on the structure and activity of subunits of IgM. It is acknowledged that reduction of IgM yields ten subunits— the area of conflict is in the activity of these subunits. Reduction of horse IgM antibody against Type 1 pneumococcus polysaccharide yielded 6.3 S subunits which combined with but did not precipitate the antigen (Hill and Cebra, 1965). Reduction and alkylation of rabbit IgM antihapten antibody yielded 6 S subunits which had the same total number of antigen-binding sites as the parent molecule (Onoue et al., 1965). Miller and Metzger (1966) found subunits of a human IgM paraprotein to be structurally similar to IgG, that is, to have two light and two heavy chains, making it likely that the IgM molecule contained ten antigen-binding sites. In contrast, evidence for ten heavy and fifteen light chains in human IgM paraprotein has been reported (Suzuki and Deutsch, 1966). Upon mild reduction, units of 8 S were found and these were considered to contain two heavy and three light chains. After mild reduction of a purified rabbit anti-Forssman IgM, Frank and Humphrey (1968) obtained subunits which appeared to consist of a single light and heavy chain. Only half of these subunits possessed specific binding sites for Forssman antigen and these sites were of low avidity in contrast to the high avidity of the parent molecule. It was suggested that the IgM molecule contained 10 units each of molecular weight 90,000 so that the heavy chain had a molecular weight of 70,000. It thus apeared that each anti-Forssman IgM molecule had five effective binding sites.

The reason for the ineffectiveness of the remaining five sites was not clear although it has been suggested (Ashman and Metzger, 1969) that the differences lay not within individual molecules but between different molecules. In very detailed studies, Ashman and Metzger (1969) studied a human Waldenstrom macroglobulin which was found to bind nitrophenyl derivatives. Their evidence was conclusive that this protein had a valence of 10. Like other IgM proteins studied, it was composed of five subunits linked by single disulfide bonds. Limited tryptic digestion yielded 5 moles of $F(ab^1)_2$ μ or 10 moles of Fab μ fragments which had valences of 2 and 1, respectively (see below).

It may well be important that IgM has a large number of high-affinity binding sites. (1) Firm binding would occur with those immunogens which have closely spaced, repeating antigenic determinants, such as occur in protein polymers and perhaps on cell surfaces (Chapter 2). (2) There is increasing evidence that at least some receptors for antigens on antigen reactive cells are IgM (see Chapter 10). This may aid the effective binding of antigen.

Papain digestion of a human IgM yielded two types of fragments (Onoue et al., 1968); Mihaesco and Seligmann, 1968). One of the fragments resembled the Fab fragment of IgG as it consisted of a light chain and part of a μ chain which was not present in the Fab-like fragment and therefore was considered to correspond to an Fc piece. Tryptic digestion yielded Fab-like fragments which had antigen-binding activity (Miller and Metzger, 1966). Peptic digestion yielded three fragments, all related structurally to the Fab-like fragment obtained by papain digestion of IgM (Kishimoto et al., 1968).

II. Some Biological Properties of Antibodies

A. Cytophilic Properties

The roles which antibodies play in the body are manifold, but in the context of this monograph we will be concerned with only some of these. Apart from the ability to react with antigen, a major property of immunoglobulins is to react with cells. Boyden and Sorkin (1961) first drew attention to the fact that if normal rabbit spleen cells were exposed to rabbit antibody raised against HSA, some of the anti-HSA antibodies could be adsorbed onto spleen cells. Such antibodies were called cytophilic and were detected by exposing the coated cells to radioactive antigen. The reaction was specific and occurred more extensively at 0° than at 37°C. Cytophilic antibody represented only a portion of the whole IgG preparation. Boyden (1964) went on to show that only some cells were coated by antibody and these were identified as macrophages. Lymphocytes, polymorphonuclear leukocytes or fibrosarcoma cells were not affected. Berken and Benacerraf (1966) found that the cytophilic activity for macrophages was a property possessed by most, if not all, the complement binding IgG_2 populations of guinea pig antibodies. Fractions of rabbit and mouse IgM were inactive. Benacerraf et al. (1963) had earlier shown that the antisera of guinea pigs immunized with hapten-protein conjugates contained two populations of precipitating antibodies which differed in their electrophoretic mobility on agar gel and starch block electrophoresis. White et al. (1963) made similar observations. Both groups reported that the IgG_1 antibodies were able to sensitize guinea pigs for passive cutaneous anaphylaxis (PCA) and for systemic anaphylaxis, but were unable either to fix complement in the presence of antigen or to sensitize antigen-coated erythrocytes for lysis by complement. Complement fixation was a property of the IgG_2 antibodies. The two immunoglobulins differed in their Fc fragments and this agreed with earlier observations that the Fc fragments of 7 S antibodies contained complement fixing and passive anaphylactic sensitizing activities (Ovary and Karush, 1961). Using a system devised by Boyden (1964) in which erythrocytes as antigen were allowed to react with macrophages, Berken and Benacerraf (1966) showed that rabbit and mouse antisera to sheep erythrocytes also contained cytophilic antibodies and that cross-sensitization could occur. Peptic digestion of guinea pig IgG_2 antibodies to sheep erythrocytes destroyed the ability of the antibodies to adsorb to macrophages and it was inferred that the ability to attach to macrophages resided in the Fc fragment of the molecules. Heavy chains, prepared by reduction and alkylation of the antibody molecules, were inactive but a possible reason for this was the fact that the original IgG_2 preparation had a low affinity for the macrophages. Nussenzweig and Benacerraf (1964) showed that the different mobilities of guinea pig IgG_1 and IgG_2 antibodies was most likely due to charge differences in the Fc portion of the molecules. This was later extended by Lamm et al. (1967) and by Lamm (1969). The two classes of immunoglobulins were found to contain similar Fab and $(Fab^1)_2$ fragments, identical light chains, and dissimilar Fc fragments. Some peptides, however, appeared to be common to both Fc pieces. It would be interesting to know whether in fact the isolated Fc or heavy subunits were adsorbed to the macrophages. Benacerraf (1968) went on to show that a more sensitive way of demonstrating the reaction was to mix the erythrocytes with antibody beforehand and then to react the complex with macrophages. The binding of the complexes to the macrophage was firmer than the binding of the antibody alone. Possibly, formation of the complex resulted in a change in conformation of the IgG molecule involving the Fc portion an this resulted in firmer binding. As expected, the erythrocyte in such a complex could be lysed by complement. Such a procedure however may have measured in addition the presence of opsonizing antibody. Benacerraf considered that the possibility of cytophilic antibody playing a role in the pathogenesis of delayed type hypersensitivity would be greater if such antibody reacted first with the antigen involved.

Nelson (1969) has recently reviewed in detail all but the most recent studies on cytophilic antibodies including the many contributions of his own group. These include the production and properties of cytophilic antibodies in different species and a study of factors which affect the attachment on these antibodies to macrophages. The detailed mechanism of interaction between immunoglobulin and the plasma membrane of macrophages is unknown.

The Fc fragment of immunoglobulins contains carbohydrate residues and intrachain disulfide groups. That the latter may play a role (such as a disulfide bond interchange) is suggested by Benacerraf's observations that the reaction of antibody with macrophages is weakened by the prior reduction and alkylation of the antibody molecule. On the other hand, this effect may simply be due to a change in conformation of the antibody molecule, in which case the disulfide bonds would play an indirect rather than a direct role. Possible groups in the macrophage membrane which might play a part in the reaction have been investigated by Howard and Benacerraf (1966), Davey and Asherson (1967), and Kossard and Nelson (1968a,b). Phospholipid is involved and the presence of sulfhydryl groups may be necessary. The results of experiments using oxidizing reagents suggested that carbohydrate and/or methionine residues in the cell membrane may play a role. It is unlikely that a large protein component is directly involved.

Using red cells sensitized with an IgG anti-Rh_0 antibody, Huber and colleagues (Huber and Fudenberg, 1968; Huber et al., 1969) have demonstrated that monocytes and hepatic and splenic macrophages from humans all possess receptors for IgG. This receptor is not present either on lymphocytes or on lymphocytes stimulated in vitro with phytomitogens. This receptor may well be similar to or even the same as the macrophage receptor for cytophilic globulins. The importance of this finding is that it documents a functional marker which clearly distinguishes between members of two cell lines which sometimes have embarrassingly similar morphological characteristics.

B. OPSONIZATION

It is often considered that a general property of antibodies is to promote phagocytosis of antigen by macrophages (opsonization) though there does not appear to be a complete documentation of this property. In fact, it is now clear that cytophilic antibodies in mice are macroglobulins (Parish, 1965; Nelson and Mildenhall, 1967; Nelson et al., 1967) whereas opsonizing antibodies are IgG (Tizard, 1969). Different workers have studied the ability of IgM and IgG preparations to opsonize a variety of preparations. Robbins et al. (1965) found that IgM antibodies were better at enhancing the in vivo clearance of S. typhimurium than were IgG antibodies. Rowley and Turner (1966) estimated the number of molecules of antibody required to promote phagocytosis of one bacterium of Salmonella adelaide by mouse peritoneal macrophages. A maximum figure of eight molecules of IgM per bacterium or 2200 molecules of IgG per bacterium were calculated and it was probable that the actual number of bound molecules per cell was lower. Solomon (1966) found that IgG and IgM antibodies of equal hemagglutinating activity had similar opsonizing activity as measured by the clearance of goat erythrocytes in chick embryos. In contrast, other investigators, working with other systems have found IgG antibodies to be more effective than IgM antibodies (Gerlings-Petersen and Pondman, 1965; Smith et al., 1967; Rabinovitch, 1967a,b). For example, Rabinovitch found that if glutaraldehyde-treated horse red blood cells were allowed to attach to macrophages, addition of anti-horse cell IgG antibodies allowed prompt uptake of the red cells by the macrophages whereas anti-horse cell IgM antibodies did not stimulate this uptake.
Fragments of IgG antibody have decreased opsonizing activity (Spiegelberg et al., 1963). Rowley et al. (1965) found that papain or peptic digests of rabbit IgG antibodies raised against Salmonella adelaide organisms were only capable of opsonizing the organisms when used at a concentration of 1000 times higher than the minimal effective dose of the original IgG molecule. These results again infer that the Fc portion of antibodies, in general, may play a role similar to that of the Fc piece in cytophilic antibodies. If so, does complement play a role in this interaction? Rowley et al. (1965) could find no evidence for a direct role of complement. It would be of interest to know whether the guinea pig IgG_1 antibody which neither fixes complement nor appears to possess cytophilic activity but is involved in the passive cutaneous anaphylactic (PCA) reaction, is capable of promoting phagocytosis of the antigen against which it is raised.

C. Follicular Localization of Antigen

The second example where reaction of antigen with antibody may have a profound effect on the fate of the antigen *in vivo* is the phenomenon of antigen localization in the follicles of lymphoid tissues. This reaction will be described in detail in Chapter 7, after a description of the anatomy and ultrastructure of lymphoid follicles. It can be mentioned here that the Fc portion of the molecule is also implicated in this reaction although in syngeneic systems, the reaction may involve an additional host factor.

D. Lymphocyte-Associated Antibodies

The presence of antibody on the surface of lymphocytes could also influence the fate of injected antigens. It is now well documented that lymphocytes have antibodies on their surface and the nature of this antibody will be discussed in detail in a later chapter. In the present context, the question arises whether this antibody has been adsorbed to the lymphocyte. Sorkin (1964) earlier suggested that cytophilic antibody could be adsorbed to lymphocytes but Boyden (1964) could find no evidence for this. Uhr (1965) reported that lymphocytes could be passively sensitized with an antigen–antibody complex if complement was present. Unanue (1968) showed that macrophages and lymphocytes do not have common antigens at their surface. Furthermore lymphocytes, even though they assume, on transformation into blasts, many of the properties of macrophages such as phagocytosis, glass adherance, and ability to adsorb cytophilic antibody (Coulson *et al.*, 1967) still do not react with antimacrophage serum. Merler and Janeway (1968) studied the properties of antibodies isolated from human small lymphocytes but could not decide whether or not they represented cytophilic antibody. There is, in short, little convincing evidence that antibody is adsorbed to the surface of lymphocytes.

There is more recent evidence for the presence of immunoglobulin on the surface of lymphocytes from unimmunized animals (Byrt and Ada, 1969; Ada *et al.*, 1970) and this is discussed in detail in Chapter 9.

III. The Influence of Antibodies on the Immune Response

Combination of antigen with antibody is one factor which could influence profoundly the fate of injected antigen. As we will later discuss the antibody response to a given antigen in terms of the fate of the injected antigen, it is desirable to record the extent to which antibody may influence the immune response.

Several studies have compared the ability of germfree and conventional animals to mount an antibody response to a variety of antigens, ranging from bacteria to soluble proteins. In each case, the germfree animals were able to respond to antigenic stimulus. For example, Bauer *et al.* (1966) showed that conventional mice gave a more rapid antibody response to two antigens, *Serratia marcescans* and horse ferritin than did germfree mice although 14 days after the injection, both groups had similar antibody titers. The difference was attributed to an enhancing effect of the microbial flora on macrophage function in the conventional mice but it is also possible that the effect was due to opsonins, not detected by the normal method of titration. Sterzl *et al.* (1965) showed that germfree piglets raised on a synthetic diet responded normally to antigen injection, the antigen used being heterologous erythrocytes. On the other hand, Rowley (1970) has studied the susceptibility of different hosts to infection by Type III *Streptococcus pneumonia* or *Salmonella typhimurium*. The resistance to infection by some strains was correlated with the presence of natural antibody in the serum (which aided opsonization) and to the subsequent accelerated immune response. However, it seems reasonably certain that the presence of opsonins is not mandatory for antigen to induce antibody formation.

It has been known for many years that mixing antigen with excess antibody prior to injection can suppress the antibody response as measured by the subsequent appearance of antibodies in the serum. In their studies on the effect of passive administration of specific antibody with antigen, Uhr and Baumann (1961a,b) pointed to the possibility that antibody formed during an immune response could act as a "feedback" mechanism. One study where such an effect has been documented under physiological conditions is that of Britton and Möller (1965) and Britton *et al.* (1968) who showed cyclic variations in serum antibody titers (19 S) and the number of plaque-forming cells in mice after an injection of *Escherichia coli* lipopolysaccharide. It was considered that high 19 S antibody levels resulting from the initial antigen injection stopped further 19 S antibody synthesis so that antibody titers fell. When a sufficiently low level of antibody was reached, persisting immunogenic lipopolysaccharide in the system initiated a further cycle of 19 S antibody production.

The addition of antibody to particular systems has allowed a closer examination of the role it plays. Of primary importance is the finding, supported by abundant evidence, that the effect of antibody in inhibiting the primary response to an antigen is specific, indicating that most likely the initial step in the suppressing effect is reaction of antibody with antigen. Uhr and Baumann (1961a) considered that antibody need not have reacted with antigenic sites on the antigen, though Dixon *et al.* (1967) found that when key hole limpet hemocyanin (KLH) was administered in adjuvants, a great excess of antibody (enough in fact to react with all antigenic sites) was necessary to suppress the antibody response.

Both the ability to prime for a secondary response and to trigger a secondary response could also be inhibited by specific antibody but to achieve effective inhibition was much more difficult. It is commonly noted that amounts of antibody which completely suppress a primary response to an antigen have no detectable effect on the triggering of a secondary response (e.g., Uhr and Baumann, 1961b; Rowley and Fitch, 1964; Ada *et al.*, 1968).

In determining the effectiveness of different classes of antibodies to suppress antibody induction, several difficulties arise. (1) Innate differences in the capacity of antibodies of different classes to perform a particular function such as hemagglutination, immobilization of bacteria, and so on; (2) The need to make comparisons on a stoichometric basis; (3) Differences in avidity which for different classes of antibody may vary during an antibody response (e.g., Webster, 1968a,b); (4) Unequal suppression of different antigenic determinants on the same molecule (Brody *et al.*, 1967); (5) Different biological half-lives of antibody classes. No single investigation has considered all these aspects so it is not surprising that different results have been reported. For example, Pearlman (1966) found IgG and IgM antibody of equivalent antigen-combining capacity to be equally effective in suppressing the formation of antibody to sheep red blood cells in rabbits and Rowley and Fitch (1964) found a similar situation in rats. With more purified preparations, however, Möller and Wigzell (1965) found only 7 S antibodies to be efficient at suppressing the immune response to sheep red blood cells. Henry and Jerne (1968) found a primary response in mice to sheep red blood cells to be enhanced by IgM and to be suppressed by IgG. They interpreted their results as a competition between IgM and IgG molecules for antigenic determinants as appropriate mixtures of IgG and IgM antibodies resulted in an antibody response of the normal size. Readers are referred to the excellent review of Uhr and Möller (1968) for further information. There is general agreement on the marked inhibition which passively transferred IgG can induce. There is still some uncertainty about the effects caused by transferred IgM.

There is little information on the detailed mechanism whereby anti-body suppressed the antibody response. Dixon *et al.* (1967) did not observe a direct adverse effect of passively administered antibody on potentially responsive cells. Rather, the close parallelism between the amount of passive antibody needed to suppress the subsequent antibody response and the size of the antigenic challenge suggested that the pas-sive antibody acted by neutralizing the effect of retained antigen. Brody *et al.* (1967) demonstrated that injection of antibody to one antigenic determinant on a molecule did *not* inhibit antibody production to a second, distinct antigenic determinant on the *same* molecule. Similar results were obtained by Cerottini *et al.* (1969) who studied the for-mation of antibody to the Fab and Fc portion of IgG which had been injected in Freund's incomplete adjuvant. Antibody to particular deter-minants, if injected 1 hour prior to or 7 days after injection of IgM into rabbits, specifically inhibited antibody production to the correspond-ing determinant. These results argue against the simple interpretation that antibody-antigen complexes formed in this way are simply destroyed and eliminated from the system. The findings favor rather the interpreta-tion that formation of a complex between the antigen and the injected antibody inhibits the possibility of reaction between the antigen and some cell receptor, presumably antibody. Such an interpretation might not require that the injected antibody to be effective, must be intact; that is, isolated antigen binding fragments of IgG, lacking the Fc piece, would still be effective as suppressing agents. Such has generally been found to be the case (Tao and Uhr, 1966a; Fitch and Rowley, 1968; Cerottini *et al.*, 1969).

In contrast, Rowley and Fitch (1964) had previously found results which favored a different interpretation. These authors showed that the exposure of normal spleen cells *in vivo* or *in vitro* to specific antibody against sheep red cells suppressed the response of the spleen cells to this antigen in X-irradiated recipients. That is, potential antibody form-ing cells (antigen reactive cells) were rendered unresponsive to the antigen in the presence of antibody. Recent *in vitro* studies using poly-merized flagellin as antigen (Feldman and Diener, 1970) have shown that exposure of cells to antibody alone has no effect on their subsequent immune reactivity, but that transient exposure to mixtures of antigen and antibody can lead to a loss of subsequent reactivity to normally immunogenic concentrations of antigen. They tentatively interpret this effect as being due to the building up of a lattice of antigen and antibody at the surface of the antigen-reactive cell, which could well alter the nature of the signal at the cell surface from immunogenic to tolerogenic. This matter will be taken up in detail in Chapter 11.

Broadly speaking the two available methods for specifically depressing an antibody response to an antigen is the induction of tolerance and antibody-mediated suppression. It is not unreasonable to think that a similar mechanism might operate in each case. From a practical point of view, passively administered human IgG anti-D (anti-RL$_0$) has been of great value in the suppression of Rh immunization (World Health Organ. Bull., 1967).

IV. Summary

In this chapter, we have considered the structure of antibodies and the role of antibodies in the afferent aspect of the antibody response. Both IgG and IgM are composed of polypeptide chains joined together by disulfide bonds. IgG has two antigen-combining sites for antigen situated near the N-terminal amino acid ends of the chains. Three fragments are obtained by papain digestion of IgG—two Fab pieces which are univalent and an Fc piece which has diverse biological properties, including the ability to react with cell membranes. IgM molecules have ten binding sites for antigen; in some cases, five only may be effective.

Some properties of cytophilic antibodies are described. These antibodies react with the plasma membrane of macrophages and this binding is rather more firm if an antigen–antibody complex is first formed. Complement probably does not play a role. It is inferred that the Fc portion of the antibody molecule is involved in the reaction with the cell membrane. On the cell membrane, phospholipid and possibly sulfhydryl groups may play a part in the reaction. In guinea pigs, this type of antibody is confined to the IgG class. So far, there is little firm evidence for antibodies which are cytophilic for lymphocytes.

Antibodies of either the IgG or IgM class may enhance phagocytosis, but the presence of natural antibodies or opsonins does not appear to be always necessary for antigens to induce antibody formation. In contrast, it has been generally found that passively administered antibody depresses a primary antibody response. It has a lesser and sometimes undectable effect on the secondary antibody response. Antibody formed during an immune response may act to inhibit further antibody production. The net result of the antibody is to "subtract" antigenic determinants from the system. Whether the mechanism of this effect is simply at the antigen level (afferent) or extends to the antigen reactive cell (central) is still under investigation. IgG appears to be more effective at inhibiting the antibody response than is IgM and there is some evidence that the latter may in fact enhance the antibody response.

CHAPTER 4

ORGAN DISTRIBUTION OF ANTIGENS

In this chapter we are concerned with the gross overall pattern of antigen distribution between organs after injection of antigens and with the rate of elimination of antigens and their breakdown products from the body. The basic question asked is—how does the body handle foreign material? The topic has been studied in increasing detail over a period of half a century. We will describe basic patterns of antigen distribution and consider variations in this pattern which occur in a variety of situations, e.g., in the presence of antibody, the influence of adjuvants, in neonatal and tolerant animals, and so on.

Perhaps more than any other topic in this monograph, gross organ distribution patterns of antigen after normal routes of injection were essentially established even before the use of isotopes as biological tracers. This early work has been reviewed by Campbell and Garvey (1963) and we will only occasionally and briefly mention some of the information established by early workers. The work of principally the last 6–7 years has been characterized by the almost exclusive use of radioactive isotopes as markers. Their introduction allowed great expansion to occur so that a wide variety of substances could be studied, irrespective of whether these substances possessed an easily demonstrable biological activity or physical property. With reservations to be discussed, the behavior of foreign substances in the body could be assessed more accurately, more easily, and more frequently over longer periods of time and often irrespective of the complexity of the milieu in which the substance was present. This most recent phase has been characterized by two considerations: (1) an attempt to study more closely antigen behavior patterns in specific organs, particularly lymphoid organs; and (2) the use of relatively small amounts of antigens, approximating more closely to "physiological levels." This was made possible by the availability both of "carrier-free" preparations of commonly used isotopes, particularly iodide, and more efficient methods for their incorporation into or attachment to biological substances.

I. Reliability of Radioactive Iodide as a Marker for Proteins

No entirely satisfactory method of labeling proteins with isotope is available (see Chapter 2). In early work (see Campbell and Garvey, 1963) haptens of various types were attached to proteins. These might contain ^{35}S or ^3H and the linkage of haptens to protein was considered to be insusceptible to enzymic degradation. Until very recently, however, radioactive haptens substituted with isotope to high specific activity were not generally available. Because of its general suitability and the great ease of labeling proteins with radioactive iodide, much recent work has used iodinated proteins or synthetic polypeptides as test antigens. As most of the results referred to in the monograph are based on the use of iodide-labeled antigens and as it seems probable that their use will increase, some discussion on the reliability of this label is warranted. Several questions need to be answered. (1) Does labeling affect the biological properties of this protein? (2) Could it be shown that the attached iodide was associated with an antigenic determinant of the protein? (3) Did deiodination of the protein occur *in vivo* and if so, was the liberated iodide reutilized?

Many workers have studied the effects of iodination on the properties of proteins (frequently serum proteins) as revealed either by the behavior of the iodinated protein in serological tests or by the survival of the protein in the blood after intravenous injection. Provided the extent of substitution of the protein was about 1 gm atom of iodide per 30,000 gm of protein or less, it was generally found that the properties of the protein were unchanged. Also, such trace-labeled proteins were found to behave similarly to unlabeled protein after intravenous

injection, at least for some days (Campbell and Garvey, 1963). Apart
from the extent of substitution of the protein with iodide, McConahey
and Dixon (1966) have also pointed out that the method of iodinating
the protein may affect its properties.

The distribution of iodide in iodide-labeled proteins has rarely been
studied. Flagellin (*S. adelaide*) contains six tyrosine residues, five of
which are in a portion of the molecule (fragment A) which contains
all demonstrable antigenic determinants. The sixth residue is in fragment
D (cf. Chapter 2). At extents of substitution between 0.1–1 atom
iodide/molecule of protein, tyrosine residues in both portions of the
molecule become substituted. When preparations of polymerized flagellin are iodinated, tyrosine residues in fragment A are preferentially
substituted (Parish and Ada, 1969a). The synthetic polypeptide, (T,G)-
A,L contains tyrosine residues (cf. Chapter 2) which form part of the
antigenic determinant of the molecule. Consequently, iodide residues
in a molecule such as (T,G)-A,L are a valid marker for studies on
the fate of such molecules *in vivo*.

Does attached iodide remain asociated with tyrosyl residues of proteins
in vivo? After injection of protein tagged with radioactive iodide to
an animal, a large proportion of the injected radioactivity is found in
the thyroid gland. Administration of excess carrier iodide to the animal
minimizes this accumulation of the radioactive iodide (Wormall, 1930).
Diiodotyrosine injected into rats may be deiodinated in the thyroid
(Tong *et al.*, 1954). Iodotyrosine itself is an unnatural amino acid and
is not utilized by cells (Ryser, 1963). It is known that radioactive iodide
associated with specific antigen may be recovered from popliteal lymph
nodes many weeks after the injection of ^{131}I-labeled flagella into the
hind footpads of rats (Ada and Williams, 1966). This finding does not
answer the question of whether some antigen which had been deiodinated might also be present. However, there does not appear to be any
evidence to support this possibility. When thyroxine labeled with [131]I
was incubated with liver slices in the absence of excess carrier iodide,
the label was subsequently recovered as triiodothyronine and this was
taken as evidence for the deiodination of thyroxine (Albright *et al.*,
1954). Carpenter *et al.* (1967) showed that the deiodinases of kidney
did not affect the iodinated D-polymer (D-Glu[55], D-Lys[39], D-Tyr[6]) which
was retained in the kidney. Humphrey and Keller (1970) labeled the
polypeptide (T,G)-A-L (cf. Chapter 2) to a very high specific activity
(2.5 mCi/μg) with ^{125}I and injected this into mice. The mice failed
to respond to this antigen although other animals responded well to
the same antigen labeled with [127]I. This result was interpreted as a

specific inactivation of sensitive cells by the radioactive antigen and suggests that at least much of the label remained associated with the polypeptides. There are also now several reports showing that the break-down product of iodide-labeled proteins ingested by cultured sarcoma cells (Gabathuler and Ryser, 1967) or by macrophages (Cohn, 1966; Ehrenreich and Cohn, 1968a) is iodotyrosine, not free iodide, and this is most simply explained as being the result of proteolysis rather than deiodination of the protein. Several groups have failed to show reutil-ization of radioactive iodide, particularly if carrier iodide was present (Laws, 1952; Cohen et al., 1956; Carpenter et al., 1967). Finally Humphrey et al. (1967) have described an experiment in which the synthetic antigen, (T,G)-A-L (cf. Chapter 2), was prepared so that alanine residues in the side chains were substituted with ^{3}H and terminal tyrosine residues were substituted with ^{125}I. At various times after injec-tion into mouse foot pads, radioactivity in the popliteal lymph nodes was determined and expressed as a ratio ^{125}I:^{3}H. There was an early loss of ^{125}I relative to ^{3}H but in time, the ratio returned to the original value. The experiment does not clearly distinguish between the alterna-tives of deiodination and peptide bond cleavage to remove iodotyrosine to explain loss of radioactive iodide. It may have been possible to make such a distinction if, in addition, the alternative form of the synthetic polypeptide—in which the alanine side chains were linked to the poly-lysine backbone by tyrosyl residues (Sela, 1966)—had been used.

In conclusion, there remains some uncertainty in the interpretation of experiments in which proteins labeled with ^{125}I are injected and radioactivity in various tissues determined. However, until it has been shown that deiodination of labeled, injected protein and/or reutilization of the label (iodide or iodotyrosine) occurs to any appreciable extent, it is reasonable to assume that the protein to which radioactive iodide is bound in tissues is antigen derived. Unless the pattern of labeling of a protein with iodide is known in some detail, one cannot presume the absence of unlabeled, antigenic fragments of the protein in injected animals. Whether such fragments might be immunologically important is discussed in Chapter 8.

II. Routes for the Carriage of Substances throughout the Body

There are several commonly used routes for the injection of foreign substances into the body—intravenous, intraperitoneal, subcutaneous, and intramuscular. Unless adjuvants are used, most of the foreign substance is not retained at the site of injection but becomes distributed throughout the body, irrespective of the route of injection and, in most cases, the nature of the injected material. This spread occurs via two circulatory systems—the vascular and the lymphatic.

The general features of blood circulation are well known. The major tissues which have been examined for antigen distribution are the liver, spleen, bone marrow, kidney, and lymph nodes. Fenner (1968) has described the essential features of the liver, spleen, and bone marrow which allow foreign substances access to certain cells in each tissue. In these tissues, veins and arteries are connected by sinusoids and the injected substance, brought to a tissue by the blood, is carried through the sinusoid where it comes into contact with phagocytic cells which may, more or less efficiently, ingest it. In the spleen, however, there is a zone of cells known as the "marginal zone" which is important in antigen handling and is discussed more fully in Chapters 6 and 7.

Lymphatic vessels drain much of the exposed surface of the body and substances introduced subcutaneously, e.g., into the hind footpads of laboratory animals, are carried by the lymph toward the venous system. En route, the lymph "percolates" through one or more lymph nodes via sinusoids which are again lined by phagocytic cells. These cells may ingest the material. An additional factor is the rate of diffusion of a substance through the basement membranes of a vessel, the diffusion rate being proportional to the radius of the substance. Particles or very large molecules may primarily escape from capillaries into extravascular spaces through intercellular gaps found in the vessels of some organs (Bennett et al., 1959).

It is obvious that two major factors in the distribution throughout the body of a foreign substance injected by any route is the ability of the macrophages to trap and to retain or to digest the substance. Relevant known factors influencing the trapping efficiency of this process are the molecular size of the injected material, the charge of the substance, and the presence or absence of opsonins or specific antibodies.

III. Distribution of Injected Substances throughout the Body

A. In Unprimed Animals

Broadly speaking we will be considering two types of foreign substances. The first type comprises those that are able to persist in the extracellular fluid compartment of the body. Examples of these are foreign serum proteins, such as albumins and γ-globulins, and some of the synthetic polypeptides. The second type comprises those antigens which are rapidly phagocytosed so that after intravenous injection, they have a short half-life in the circulation. Examples of these are the flagellar antigens, polypeptides composed of D-amino acids, and many of the high molecular weight or particulate antigens.

After injection of a substance of the former type, there are three phases of antigen clearance and these are best observed after intravenous injection—an initial equilibration phase, a period of slow elimination due to catabolism of the free antigen, and a period of more rapid loss when specific antibody is formed as a result of the antigen injection. This third phase is due to phagocytosis of the immune complexes by reticuloendothelial cells. Glenny and Hopkins (1923) first described such a pattern and the technique—immune elimination—has come into wide use as a sensitive method for the detection of antibody formation after injection of this type of antigen.

Nakamura et al. (1968) have listed the half-life in the plasma of rabbits of a series of plasma proteins (and their derivatives), having molecular weights of 50,000 to 950,000 and which had been labeled with ^{131}I or ^{125}I and injected intravenously. The average plasma half-life varied from 1.4 days for humans β_{1C}-globulin to 6 days for rabbit 7 S γG-globulin. These authors were concerned primarily in investigating the factors responsible for the distribution of plasma proteins between intra- and extravascular compartments. As expected, the amount of plasma protein in the extravascular space after equilibration correlated exponentially with the effective hydrodynamic diffusion radius of the plasma protein. The extravascular space itself appeared to be heterogeneous, some compartments accepting only small proteins. The authors placed considerable emphasis on this study as they considered that immunological phenomena may well depend upon the concentration of the substance in the extravascular space.

In contrast to these results, other substances (the second type mentioned above), after injection into conventional animals, may have very short half-lives in the circulation. For example, flagellin (1 μg) injected intravenously into adult rats disappears rapidly from the blood. Only 1–2% of the radioactivity injected was present in the blood 12 hr after injection, and 0.01–0.02% at 48 hr. The corresponding values for radioactivity in the spleen were 0.07 and 0.02%, respectively (Shellam, 1969b). The antigenically active peptide from flagellin (fragment A, mol. wt.

18,000) also had a short half-life in the circulation of adult rats (Ada and Parish, 1968). Poly-γ-D-glutamic acid, either free or complexed with methylated bovine serum albumin, also had a short half-life in the blood, less than 10% of the injected amount being present 12 hr after injection (Roelants et al., 1969).

Footpad injection of animals has been widely used because the popliteal node which drains this injection site has proved to be particularly suitable for studies of antigen localization. The rate of diffusion of the substance may be a major factor in the drainage of substances from the footpad (Herd and Ada, 1969a). Bernstein and Ovary (1968) have suggested that the molecular size of an antigen is one of the factors concerned in the absorption of antigens from the gastrointestinal tract.

Table 4.I contains results from five different investigations on the distribution of a variety of labeled proteins which were injected into the footpads of rats or rabbits. The main points emerging were: (1) The popliteal nodes contained as much or more radioactivity than did any other lymph node examined, despite the small size of this node, and frequently as much or more radioactivity than did the spleen. The liver might contain about the same amount of label as did the draining lymph node or very much more, depending on the nature of the antigen. After injection by this route, the proportion of antigen present in the major lymphoid organs rarely exceeded a few percent of the total injected. This is in agreement with results obtained by earlier workers (see Campbell and Garvey, 1963). The total lymphoid tissue of both rabbits and rats is known to be less than 1% of the total body weight (Hellman, 1914; Sjovall, 1936; Andreasen, 1943). (2) There was little direct correlation between the predicted immunogenicity of an antigen preparation and the degree to which it was trapped by the draining lymph nodes. (3) In some cases, it was likely that size of the antigen played a part— flagella particles were trapped more efficiently than were flagellin molecules. In other experiments, it was shown that heat-coagulated human serum albumin, injected into the hind footpads of rats was trapped to a much greater extent than was native human serum albumin (Lang and Ada, 1967b). Although a relationship between size of a substance and its uptake by lymphoid organs has not been rigorously established, it is a general finding (e.g., Dresser, 1961a; Frei et al., 1965) that aggregated or denatured substances are phagocytosed more readily than are the native substances. (4) Antigens may be retained in lymphoid tissues for varying lengths of time. For example, labeled flagella may be detected in rat lymph nodes for some months after injection whereas a foreign serum protein, labeled to a similar extent, and even if aggre-

TABLE 4.I

The Proportion of Radioactivity Present at the Injection Site and in Different Tissues After Hind Footpad Injection of Various Proteins Labeled with ^{125}I or ^{131}I into Rats or Rabbits

Antigen	Amount (μg)	Animal	Time after injection	Feet	Popliteal nodes	Iliac (aortic) nodes	Mesenteric nodes	Spleen	Liver	Blood	Lung	Reference
Flagella	1	Rat[a]	4 hr	50	0.5			1	2.5	14	0.4	Ada et al. (1964b)
Hemocyanin (Maia squinado)	20	Rabbit	24 hr	15	0.08					3		Humphrey and Frank (1967)
			4 days	0.5	0.01					0.08		
			14 days	0.3						0.01		
Flagella	10	Rat[a]	48 hrs		0.27	0.12	0.02	0.32	0.35			Ada et al. (1964b)
Flagellin	5				0.04	0.02	<0.01	0.03	0.41			
Horse ferritin	1				0.04	0.006		0.02				
Rat hemoglobin	1				0.25	0.09		0.05	0.63			
Flagella	1–2	Rat	24 hr	5	0.3							Ada and Williams (1966)
			10 days	0.6	0.1							
			40 days		0.05							
Flagellin	1–2	Rat	24 hr	0.53	0.05							Ada and Lang (1966)
			10 days	0.02	0.05							
			27 days	0.016	0.0035							
Hemocyanin (Maia squinado)	5		48 hr	0.21	0.12							
			17 days	0.026	0.012							
Human serum albumin	5–10		48 hr	0.29	0.01							
			8 days	0.055	0.0017							
Human serum albumin	10		3 days	0.37	0.02	0.003			0.315	0.07		Lang and Ada (1967a)
			8 days	0.037	0.005	0.007			0.04			

a These animals were not fed carrier iodide in their drinking water.

gated before injection, is detected in the draining lymph node after footpad injection for a period of only a few days after injection.

Footpad injection of antigen is frequently found to result in a good antibody response to the antigen so this route of injection is often used. It must be stressed, however, that it is difficult to determine the exact kinetics of antigen retention in a lymph node which drains such an injection site as the radioactivity present in the node is a composite of different factors. Among these are the continuous and asynchronous arrival of antigen into the node, specific retention mechanisms, local antigen degradation, and escape of antigen and antigen degradation products via the efferent lymph or circulation.

While the immunologist usually studies the fate of antigen after injection by subcutaneous or intravenous routes, it is likely that the natural route of entry of antigen is commonly by the gastrointestinal or respiratory tracts. It could be thought that antigen entering the body via a natural route might be handled in a different pattern. It is reassuring to find that this appears not to be the case. Cooper and colleagues (Cooper and Thonard, 1967; Cooper et al., 1967) studied the distribution of labeled antigen in rats after direct instillation into the lumen of isolated segments of the intestinal tract. Animals injected in this way produced serum antibodies in amounts similar to those elicited by parental injection. Using ^{125}I-labeled flagella (S. adelaide), about 20% of the injected radioactivity rapidly left the loop. The remainder was lost very slowly so that 70% was still present 8 days after instillation. The level of radioactivity in the spleen or mesenteric lymph node, was at any time examined, less than 1% of the total instilled. When ^{51}Cr-labeled endotoxin was instilled, both the rate of disappearance of label from the instillation site and the subsequent low level in lymphoid organs was of the same general pattern observed when antigen was injected in the footpad of rats. In an extension of the work, Cooper and Turner (1967) injected antigen directly into Peyer's patches of rats. With ^{125}I-labeled flagella, there was a rapid loss of radioactivity from the injection site, about 3% remaining at 48 hr. ^{51}Cr, which had been used to label sheep red blood cells or stroma, was retained to a much greater extent. In either case, other lymphoid organs were found to retain relatively little of the injected antigen. However, the kinetics of antibody formation following injections of antigen into Peyer's patches was different from that described after parental injection of antigen and these authors considered this modified response might be a true reflection of the response of a particular lymphoid tissue to antigenic stimulation.

IV. Influence of Natural Antibody on Antigen Distribution

The presence in the body of "natural" or specific antibody or the prior addition of specific antibody to an antigen preparation, may have a pronounced effect on the subsequent distribution of the antigen through the body (and within tissues, as will be discussed in a later chapter). There are at least two reasons for this. The first is that antigen—antibody complexes may be very much larger than the antigen itself and thus be more efficiently taken up by phagocytic cells within tissues. A second reason is the particular ability of immunoglobulins to react with phagocytic cells probably by means of the Fc portion of the molecule. This reactivity may be enhanced in the case of antigen–antibody complexes (Chapter 3). It is worth noting that this property may be unique to this type of molecule and for this reason, immunoglobulins per se are best not considered as *typical* antigens if it is wished to study antigen distribution and localization.

The role that opsonins play in the clearance of large particles, including living bacteria, from the circulation has been under intensive study for more than half a decade, and is beyond the scope of this monograph to discuss this aspect. Rowley (1962) and Boyden (1965) have reviewed this aspect and their groups have made notable contributions in this field (cf. Chapter 3).

The distribution of injected flagellar antigens between the organs of conventionally raised rats is influenced by opsonins. Some idea of the extent of influence of opsonins in the pattern of distribution has been gauged using three different approaches, in each of which an absence or diminution of opsonins is presumed to occur; (1) The use of germfree rats. (2) X-irradiation of rats. (3) Chronic thoracic duct lymph drainage of rats. Details of the histological localization pattern of flagellar antigens will be given later (Chapter 7); here the effect on organ distribution is briefly reported. (1) Germfree and conventional rats (75–115 gm) were injected in the hind footpads with ^{125}I flagella (0.8 μg). At times later than 24 hr after the injection, the levels of radioactivity in the popliteal nodes and in the spleen, but not in the serum, were slightly lower in the germfree rats than in the conventional rats (Miller *et al.*, 1968, and unpublished). It is probable that larger differences would have been observed if flagellin, rather than flagella, had been injected. (2) Jaroslow and Nossal (1966) investigated the distribution of labeled flagellar antigens in X-irradiated rats. Rats were given 450 r of whole body irradiation and 24 hr later either ^{125}I-flagella (100 μg) was injected into the hind footpads (exp. A) or ^{125}I polymerized flagellin (10 μg) was injected intravenously (exp. B). In both experiments, the spleens of irradiated rats were found to contain less radioactivity than was present in the spleen of control rats and this was most marked 8 days after the injection (exp. B). The results were interpreted as reflecting a decrease in the level of opsonins due to destruction of lymphocytes, but direct damage to reticulo endothelial cells could not be excluded. (3) Chronic drainage of the rat via the thoracic duct also reduced opsonin levels. Williams (1966a) showed that follicular local- ization of labeled flagellin was depressed by 75% following thoracic duct drainage of rats. The evidence was consistent with the notion that the opsonin for flagellar antigens may be an IgM (Williams, 1966b) and this fits in with the demonstration (Reade *et al.*, 1965) that an opsonic antibody directed against another species of *Salmonella* bacteria was an IgM. When Wistar and Shellam (1969) examined directly the serum levels of various immunoglobulin classes of the rat following chronic thoracic duct drainage, they found a profound decrease in the levels of both IgM and IgG.

V. Influence of Specific Antibody on Antigen Distribution

Specific antibody, either added to an antigen or present in the host animal, usually changes the normal distribution pattern of an injected antigen. This effect has been so well documented in the earlier literature that only a few recent observations will be quoted. It was mentioned earlier in this chapter that immunoglobulins are atypical in their innate localization patterns. This is seen even on a gross organ distribution pattern. Herd and Ada (1969a) studied the trapping and retention of rabbit IgG and IgG subunits in rat popliteal lymph nodes after foot- pad injection. There was a good correlation between the molecular weight of the different preparations and their rate of drainage from the footpad but not with their trapping or retention in the node. How- ever, a comparison of various pairs of subunits, e.g., Fab vs. Fc, or L chain vs. H chain, suggested that the presence of the Fc piece in an IgG fragment or subunit was important for the trapping and retention of that fragment.

The *in vivo* interaction of specific antibody with an antigen results in the formation of antigen–antibody complexes. If the antigen used is one which normally persists in the circulation, antigen–antibody complexes formed near equivalence or in antibody excess are very rapidly eliminated from the circulation whereas complexes formed in antigen excess persist in the circulation for longer periods of time, though not as long as either antigen or antibody persist if injected alone (Weigle, 1958). Complexes between the antigen (BSA) and fragment of the specific antibody which lacked the Fc piece were less rapidly eliminated than the BSA–IgG complexes, thus implicating the Fc portion of the IgG molecule in the immune elimination of the antigen–antibody complex. Complexes between the antigen and specific fragment of IgG which lacked the Fc fragment were eliminated from the circulation at the same rate as the antigen alone. In the *absence* of antigen, these same fragments were rapidly eliminated, suggesting that their value as prophylactic agents would be limited (Spiegelberg and Weigle, 1965).

Lymph nodes draining injection sites also trap higher proportions of an antigen if specific antibody is present. In one series of experiments, groups of adult rats were either injected with anti-flagella antiserum or had received a previous injection of flagella or flagellin. Rats in both groups and also in a control group were then injected into the hind footpads with ^{125}I-labeled flagella or flagellin and the amount of radioactivity in the popliteal lymph nodes determined. The presence of antibody, either injected or resulting from the prior injection of antigen, increased the proportion of injected radioactivity trapped in the node by two- to threefold in the case of flagella and up to sixfold when flagellin was used (Nossal et al., 1965b). Still larger differences were observed if an antigen such as HSA or BSA was used which, if injected by itself, was known to be trapped very poorly. After footpad injection, the differences in retention in popliteal and iliac nodes and in the liver were as high as 30 to 40-fold, according to the ratio of antigen and antibody in the injected complex (Ada and Lang, 1966; Lang and Ada, 1967a). If the rat anti-HSA IgG was treated with papain and the $(Fab)_2$ fragment mixed with HSA and injected, this complex was trapped more efficiently than HSA alone but to a much lesser extent than was the HSA-IgG complex (Herd and Ada, 1969a).

Circulating antigen–antibody complexes may be toxic to tissues. Relatively large aggregates of antigen and antibody may be deposited within the alveolar capillaries of the lung, so obstructing blood flow and causing anaphylaxis. Different tissues are involved in different species. Similarly, the union of antigen and antibody, when one is present in the circulation and the other is deposited in the skin, may cause a tissue reaction (Arthus reaction). Serum sickness, either of an acute or chronic type, occurs when a large amount of a "circulating" antigen is given as a single or as multiple injections. In order to cause serum sickness, an antigen must be (1) sufficiently immunogenic to induce an antibody response and (2) capable of persisting in the circulation until antibody is formed so that relatively large amounts of antigen-antibody complexes are formed. Antigens which do not persist in the circulation do not cause serum sickness although they may be good immunogens. Glomerulo-nephritis occurs due to the deposition of the complexes in the kidney glomerulus (Unanue and Dixon, 1967). As the tissues involved in these reactions are not immunological targets but merely receptacles for the deposition of the complex, these conditions will not be discussed further.

VI. Influence of Adjuvants on Antigen Distribution

Injection of an antigen with an adjuvant usually enhances the antibody responses. To what extent does the presence of the adjuvant affect the distribution of the antigen? Bacterial endotoxin, injected either separately or with antigens, could not be shown to have any influence on antigen distribution. Sweet et al. (1965) injected ^{125}I-bovine γ-globulin (BGG) into mice with or without endotoxin. No difference was noted in the half-life of the antigen in the blood or in the amount of radioactivity in the liver, spleen, lungs, or kidneys between the two groups of mice. Pierce (1967) found that injection of endotoxin into rats did not influence the rate of elimination of injected ^{125}I-labeled BGG in the circulation. Ada et al. (1968) injected native HSA, heat-denatured HSA, or a complex of HSA and rat anti-HSA IgG into the hind footpads of rats with or without endotoxin. Injection of the endotoxin did not affect the levels of radioactivity in the draining lymph nodes in any case.

As would be expected, premixing antigen with an oil-based adjuvant such as Freund's complete adjuvant does influence the antigen distribution pattern. Three investigations have been recently carried out. The antigens were (T,G)-A-L, a synthetic polypeptide, molecular weight about 230,000 (McDevitt et al., 1966; see Chapter 2) flagellin from S. adelaide, molecular weight, 40,000 (Lind, 1968; see Chapter 2) and bovine encephalitogenic polypeptide (BEP), molecular weight 3500 (Lamoureux et al., 1968). Each was labeled with ^{125}I, emulsified in Freund's complete adjuvant and injected into the hind footpads of mice, rats, or guinea pigs, respectively. The rate of drainage from the footpads and the amount of radioactivity in the draining lymph nodes, spleen, and the serum were estimated and compared with values from animals injected with the preparation in saline. In Fig. 4.1 is plotted the results from two of these investigations. Values for the ratio, radioactivity in tissues after injection in adjuvant/radioactivity in tissues after injection in saline are compared with time. The major findings were: Injection in adjuvant very profoundly decreased the rate of drainage of antigen from the injection site. This was a relatively short-lived effect with the

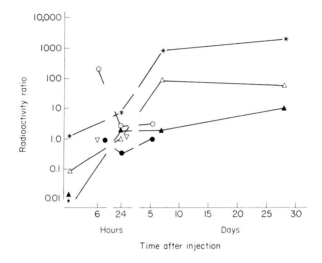

Fig. 4.1. A comparison of the retention of two preparations, [125]-I-flagellin and [125]-I-BEP (brain encephalitogenic polypeptide), in different tissues after injection into rat hind footpads either in saline or in Freund's complete adjuvant. Radioactivity ratio = radioactivity in tissue after injection in adjuvant/radioactivity in tissue after injection in saline. Antigen: Flagellin, ✻ hind footpad; △ popliteal nodes; ▲ spleen. Brain encephalitogenic polypeptide (BEP); ⊙ hind footpad; ▽ popliteal nodes; ● spleen.

low molecular weight BEP, but was very pronounced when flagellin was used. Because of the slow drainage of antigen from the footpads, it might have been expected that the draining nodes and spleen would contain little antigen because of the slow rate of entry of antigen to these tissues. However, the amount of antigen in these tissues was higher than in controls (especially in the case of flagellin), indicating that the antigen injected in the adjuvant was better retained in these tissues. The reason for this enhanced retention is immediately apparent from radioautographs of the tissues concerned—the antigen is still associated to a large extent with oil droplets (Chapter 7). Less data is available from the experiments with (T,G)-A-L but the overall picture appears similar to that reported for flagellin.

VII. Antigen Distribution in Tolerant Animals

Interorgan distribution of antigens in tolerant animals is the same as that in untreated animals. Azar (1967) injected human IgG (^{131}I-HGG, 200 μg) intraperitoneally into adult mice, some of which were control animals whereas others had been previously injected with and made tolerant to this antigen. The radioactivity was estimated in several tissues, including spleen and lymph nodes at 4, 8, 24, and 48 hr, after injection. Except for a difference in antigen content of the thymus at 4 hr between the two groups (when the tolerant animals had higher values), both groups of mice had similar levels of antigen in the organs examined at various time intervals after injection. Humphrey and Frank (1967) injected ^{125}I-labeled hemocyanin (M. squinado, 20 μg) or ^{125}I-labeled HSA (1 mg) into the footpads of rabbits, groups of which had been made and shown to be tolerant to either of these antigens. No consistent difference in the antigen content of popliteal nodes in the control and tolerant animals for each antigen was found. Ada et al. (1965) injected ^{125}I-flagellin (S. adelaide) into the footpads of rats which either were normal or had been rendered tolerant to this antigen. The radioactivity in popliteal and iliac lymph nodes and in the spleen were determined but no significant difference in isotope content of their organs from the two groups were noted. It seems safe to conclude that the pattern of distribution of injected antigens between the organs of tolerant and normal animals is similar as judged by the radioactivity content of organs.

VIII. Antigen Distribution in Fetal and Young Animals

Antigens which have a long half-life in the circulation of adult animals appear to behave rather similarly in young animals. Humphrey (1961) and Deichmiller and Dixon (1960) studied the catabolism of I-labeled albumins and γ-globulins after injection into baby rabbits. The half-lives of rabbit or of human serum albumins in the blood was found to be similar (about 6 days) in rabbits of any age; however, both rabbit and human γ-globulins were catabolized more rapidly in older than in younger animals. This was not an invariable finding as the half-life of human γ-globulin was shown to be similar in baby and adult guinea pigs (Humphrey and Turk, 1961). Robbins *et al.* (1963) measured the rate of degradation, organ deposition, and blood clearance of azo albumins and of internally labeled (^{35}S) rabbit serum albumin in newborn, 6-, and 30-day-old rabbits. Newborn rabbits catabolized the azo proteins less efficiently than did 6- and 30-day-old rabbits. However, rabbits in the three groups showed little difference in their ability to metabolize the rabbit albumin and the proportion of injected radioactivity in the spleen and liver was 0.01 and 1.6–4.7%, respectively, 24 hr after the injection.

Reade and Jenkin (1965) showed that the rate of uptake of particulate material, such as bacteria and carbon black, by the reticuloendothelial system of fetal rats varied both with the age of the fetus and the type of particle. The reticuloendothelial system showed with time an increasing ability or capacity to phagocytose the particles but even in fetal rats, active phagocytosis occurred (Reade and Casley-Smith, 1965). Janeway and Humphrey (1969) have studied the retention of a D-amino acid polypeptide (p[D-Tyr, D-Glu, D-Ala], 247) in newborn and adult mice. The polypeptide was taken up rapidly and retained by macrophages in the liver, spleen, and lymph nodes of newborn mice with an efficiency of the same order as that of adults. Despite these results a clear distinction in the ability of cells of adult and newborn rats to retain and catabolize injected substances has been observed, particularly using flagellar antigens (Mitchell and Nossal, 1966). Following a single intraperitoneal injection of either flagellin, polymerized flagellin, flagella, or bovine serum albumin (each labeled with ^{125}I) into neonatal rats, nearly 1 week elapsed in each case before 90% of the radioactivity was excreted. In contrast, rats given multiple injections of flagellin since birth and injected at 8 weeks (when tolerant) with radioactive flagellin excreted 90% of the radioactivity in 8 hr. As judged by isotope levels, the rate of catabolism of each antigen in neonatal rats was fairly similar during the first 2 weeks after birth. During the first week after an injection (at birth), no organ examined had a higher specific activity (counts/sec/mg tissue) than did the blood. After this time, there was evidence of retention of the labeled antigens, particularly in kidney but also in liver, spleen, lung, and lymph nodes, but not in thymus. Only a small proportion of the injected label was found in lymphoid tissues at any time. Radioautographic examination confirmed the absence of significant phagocytosis of labeled antigens in spleen or lymph nodes during the first week after birth. Furthermore, addition of specific anti-body to labeled flagellin before injection did not result in readily demon-strable phagocytosis of the antigen within 24 hr. However, other studies (Ada, unpublished) have shown that complexes formed between bovine serum albumin–anti-BSA IgG may be taken up by cells in the spleen of 1-day old rats though rather less well than occurs in the spleens of adult rats.

The examples available are too few to allow a simple conclusion to be drawn. Newborn animals can phagocytose foreign substances but their phagocytic cells seem to display a sense of discrimination even more remarkable than those of adult animals. This aspect deserves further study.

IX. Antigens and the Thymus

The thymus is a primary lymphoid organ which plays a central role in the functioning of the animal's immune system but which itself is not a center for antibody production. In an early investigation, Marshall and White (1961) showed that if antigens were injected directly into guinea pig thymus, antibody was subsequently formed; accordingly, they suggested that a "barrier" existed between the blood stream and the thymic parenchyma which restricted the passage of antigens, injected by other routes, to the thymus. Several investigators have since shown (see Clark, 1964a,b) that a variety of antigens, injected by conventional routes into animals could penetrate to the thymus, although many of these had to be injected in rather large amounts (1–10 mg) in order that their presence in the thymus could be demonstrated. Blau and Veall (1967) studied the distribution of antigens, paying particular atten-tion to the thymus. Both ^{125}I homologous serum albumin and human IgG were injected (0.1–7 mg) intracardially into guinea pigs. At 2–7 days after injection, the concentration of injected protein in the thymus was similar to that in the spleen. Blau (1967) went on to show that Hassall's corpuscles in the guinea pig thymus actively phagocytosed the injected antigen. Nossal and Mitchell (1966) however, showed that the extensive phagocytosis of antigens, injected by usual routes, in other organs of the body would create a "barrierlike" effect. In their work, human serum albumin or flagellar antigens were injected intravenously into adult or newborn rats in doses of 10–100 μg. In newborn rats, all antigens readily reached the thymus; in adult rats, a significant propor-

tion of the albumin but very low amounts of the flagellar antigens penetrated to the thymus. Similarly, Janeway and Humphrey (1969) found
that the D-amino acid polymer, D-TGA 247 (see p. 53) which was
efficiently phagocytosed in other tissues did not penetrate to the thymus.

Nossal and Mitchell (1966) proposed that persisting tolerance to an
antigen might depend upon that antigen reaching all lymphoid organs
including the thymus. Others (e.g., Staples et al., 1966; Argyris, 1968)
have also suggested that the thymus, representing a source of immature
lymphoid cells, may be involved in the process of induction of tolerance.
More recently, Mitchison (1969) has produced evidence that thymic
cells can indeed be rendered tolerant in vivo.

Although there are many gaps in our knowledge, there is substantial
evidence that it may be unnecessary for antigen to reach the thymus
for either antibody production or tolerance to occur. Tolerance to
flagellin in neonatal rats (Shellam and Nossal, 1968) and in adult rats
(Ada and Parish, 1968) has been achieved using extremely low doses
of either flagellin or the fragment A of flagellin, respectively. Particularly
in the latter work when less than 10^8 molecules of antigen were injected
into the rats, it is most likely that antigen could not reach the thymus
in significant amounts. Second, the D-amino acid polypeptide (D-TGA
247) which induced tolerance in adult rats hardly penetrated into the
thymus (Janeway and Humphrey, 1969). Third, a variety of antigens
has been shown to react in vitro with lymphocytes from spleen (Naor
and Sulitzeanu, 1967; Byrt and Ada, 1969; Humphrey and Keller, 1970),
and from thoracic duct lymph, peritoneal exudate, and from bone marrow, but to a lesser extent with lymphocytes from thymus (Byrt and
Ada, 1969; Humphrey and Keller, 1970). These findings will be discussed
in more detail in later chapters.

X. The Distribution of Enantiomorphic Polymers

Some naturally occurring substances contain D-amino acids but a much
greater variety of D-amino acid polypeptides can be made by synthetic
procedures. A study of both types has shown particular distribution
patterns uncharacteristic of their L-isomers. Gill and colleagues have
made detailed studies (Gill et al., 1965; Papermaster et al., 1965; Carpenter et al., 1967). Some results of Gill et al. (1965) are presented
as an illustration. These authors compared the metabolic fate of poly
L-Glu^{58}, L-Lys^{36}, L-Tyr^6, and poly D-Glu^{55}, D-Lys^{39}, D-Tyr^6 (mol. wt. about

93,000). Each was labeled to an extent of about 1 atom isotope/mole with ^{131}I and 10-mg amounts injected without adjuvants into the ear veins of separate rabbits. Equilibration in the vascular system took place in 30–40 seconds. By 3–4 days, in each case, any radioactivity still in the serum was present either as free iodide or as iodopeptides (not distinguished). When urinary excretion of radioactivity stopped (7–10 days and 15–20 days in the case of the L- and D-polymers, respectively) the animals were killed and radioactivity in the organs measured. Liver, spleen, and kidney contained almost all of the retained radioactivity (lymph nodes and thymus none). The retention of radioactivity, in terms of the amount injected, was in the following proportions for liver, spleen, and kidney, respectively: L-polymer 1.0, nil, 0.1; D-polymer, 6, 0.4, 30. The amount of the L-isomer degraded was independent of dose (up to 60 mg) whereas the metabolism and excretion of the D-polymer was dose-dependent. These results showed that animal tissues contained D-proteases which were restricted in amounts and probably not inducible. Janeway and Humphrey (1967) studied the distribution in mice of 247, p(D-Tyr, D-Glu, D-Ala) and 253, p(L-Tyr, L-Glu, L-Ala) both labeled with [125]I. The D-polymer was broken down 22 times more slowly than the L-polymer and some of the D-polymer appeared to be excreted intact into the urine. After footpad injection, 200–1000 times as much D-polymer as L-polymer was retained in draining lymph nodes and spleen. As was also found by Gill et al. (1965) and Carpenter et al. (1967), the kidney and liver retained much of the D-polymer. In the kidney, the D-polymers were present inside the proximal convoluted tubules. The continued excretion of D-TGA 247 over some days implied that small amounts were continually circulating in the blood, although most in the blood was taken up by macrophages. In both situations described, the antigens were injected without adjuvant. The different behavior of the L- and D-isomers is of special interest with regard to the different immunological responses initiated by them (see Chapter 10).

Roelants et al. (1969) have reported results which are very different from the above. Poly-γ-D-glutamic acid as derived from *Bacillus anthracis*, has an average molecular weight of 33,000, and is poorly immunogenic. If complexed with methylated bovine serum albumin, and injected as an insoluble complex into rabbits, antibodies are formed which react against the D-polymer. Roelants et al. wished to see if the free polymer and the complex were handled differently by the body. The polymer was tritiated and injected either as the insoluble complex (M_{36}-³H-MBSA) or adsorbed onto alum (M_{36}-³H-alum). Within 20 days after the injection of M_{36}-³H-alum, 80% of the radioactivity had been excreted.

The corresponding figure for M_{36}-^{3}H-MBSA was only 20%. A comparison of retention patterns in the tissues at this time was also revealing. Of the amount of M_{36}-^{3}H-alum injected, 0.13% was in the spleen and 1% in the kidney, with M_{36}-^{3}H-M-BSA, about 16% was in the spleen and up to 70% in the kidney. In the spleen, both types of preparation were present mainly in large mononuclear cells presumably macrophages.

XI. Metabolism of Synthetic Polymers in Responder and Nonresponder Hosts

The use of synthetic polymers has also clarified our understanding of the influence of the host's genetic constitution on the antibody response. The effect was particularly clear-cut in the experiments of Levine and Benacerraf (1964) and Benacerraf *et al.* (1967) who studied the ability of responder and nonresponder guinea pigs to degrade DNP-poly-L-lysine conjugates. After footpad injection of labeled conjugates into guinea pigs in both groups, comparable amounts of the conjugates were present in the draining lymph node macrophages of both groups. Furthermore, both responder and nonresponder guinea pigs were equally able to degrade the conjugate, as shown by additional experiments with spleen extracts and the presence of low molecular weight products of the antigen in the urine. Thus, the inability of nonresponder guinea pigs to make antibody to the conjugate did not appear to be at the level of conjugate degradation.

XII. Discussion and Summary

Most work in the last 5 years or so on the distribution of antigens in the body has used radioactive isotopes as the marker of choice for tracing antigens and with few exceptions, radioactive iodide has been used. It is well to be aware that there are still unknown factors in assessing the validity of studies using iodinated antigens. On the one hand, it seems unlikely that iodinated antigens are deiodinated or that free iodide is reutilized in lymphoid tissues; on the other hand, little is known about the distribution of attached iodide in labeled antigens and in many studies, it has not been excluded that a labeled tyrosine is part of an "immunologically silent" portion of the molecule. At present, however, there is no reason to question seriously the observed organ distribution patterns of different antigens, especially as many similarities are seen when the behavior of antigens labeled in various ways is compared.

This being so, the first conclusion is that with most proteins and synthetic polypeptides, injection by almost any route results in a fairly rapid dissemination through the body. In adult animals, most of the injected substance is rapidly broken down and the products excreted. It is as though the main aim of the body was to get rid of the injected material. This frequently is so successfully done that after 48 hr, the proportion of injected substances in lymphoid tissues is much less than 1% of that injected. There are two main factors which will influence this. One is the extent to which the substance will be ingested by phagocytic cells. If not ingested, the substance may well persist in the body fluid for some time. Once ingested, can the material be digested? Longest retention of substances occurs when the substance is resistant to digestion and this behavior is generally shown by substances such as pneumococcal polysaccharides or polypeptides composed of D-amino acids. A striking example was the persistance in the spleen and kidney of an insoluble complex of poly-γ-D-glutamic acid and methylated bovine serum albumin.

One of the most important questions we can ask is—what proportion of the injected substance becomes involved in the induction of an immunological response? It is sometimes considered that the only portion of the injected substance so involved is that portion present in lymphoid tissues. This is an oversimplification. The amount of antigen present in lymphoid tissues has been shown to be sufficient for this purpose as organ cultures of lymph nodes or spleen from immunized animals support antibody production. In addition, from quite different considerations, McConahey et al. (1968) have suggested that less than 1% of the dose of hemocyanin (2 mg) which was used to immunize rabbits, was actually involved in inducing the formation of antibody. The demonstration by Baker et al. (1966) that a single injection of 10^{-15} gm of endotoxin into rabbits induced antibody formation highlights the point that in most experiments, much of the antigen injected into animals does not play an inductive role in antibody formation.

The complexity of the circulatory and drainage systems in the body is such that, after injection by the standard routes, adequate kinetic studies of antigen uptake and release from tissues are almost impossible to carry out. Qualitatively, we know that particulate antigens are taken up and/or retained in lymphoid tissues more efficiently than are soluble antigens but we do not possess quantitative information on this point. The technique of Morris and colleagues (e.g., Hall and Morris, 1962, 1965) of inserting fistulas into the afferent and efferent lymph ducts of sheep popliteal nodes will allow a more quantitative approach to many questions concerning the handling of antigens in particular lymphoid tissues.

In view of the inadequacy of our knowledge in this regard, are the observed organ distribution patterns shown by antigens meaningful? The answer is probably, yes, as the pattern may change dramatically in certain cases and this is accompanied by a corresponding change in the immune response. Tolerant and normal adult animals show similar antigen distribution patterns. Neonatal animals (which are the easier to make tolerant) are less efficient at phagocytosing some antigens than are adult animals. The presence of antibody, which inhibits a primary antibody response, may greatly increase the uptake and retention of antigen in tissues. Injection of endotoxin with antigen (which enhances the immune response) has no demonstrable effect on the antigen distribution pattern. Emulsification of antigen in Freund's complete adjuvant greatly decreased the drainage rate of the antigen from the injection site and allowed persistence of antigen in the tissues for a long period. Obviously differences in the observed immune responses which result from these different treatments is not explicable simply in terms of the antigen distribution patterns although these must contribute to an eventual understanding.

Later chapters will describe localization patterns of antigens within tissues. For reasons described above, only lymphoid organs have been closely examined. In some cases, the patterns seen are so well defined that they encourage speculation concerning the role which antigen in particular cells may play in inducing particular immune responses.

CHAPTER 5

THE FUNCTIONAL ANATOMY OF THE LYMPHOID SYSTEM

In this chapter and the next, we will consider lymphoid cells and lymphoid organs. First, we will consider the structure of the various lymphoid organs, not solely from the viewpoint of morphological description, but rather to give us insight into the functional capacity of each organ, and of the specialized microanatomical environmental niches in each organ. Also, an anatomical approach will be a necessary prerequisite for our study, in Chapter 7, of antigen localization patterns. In Chapter 6 the emphasis will shift to single lymphoid cells as functional entities. However, considerable overlap in subject matter between the two chapters is inevitable.

A schematic overview of the various functional compartments of the lymphoid system is given in Fig. 5.1. With a degree of conscious oversimplification of the problem, we can consider it in three levels. First, certain organs and notably the bone marrow contain a pool of undifferentiated stem cells which act as the reservoir from which all lymphocytes are ultimately derived. Second, the primary lymphoid organs (notably the thymus) exist as sites of further functional maturation and intense division of lymphoid cells, and not as sites of antibody production. Finally, the widely deployed peripheral lymphoid system

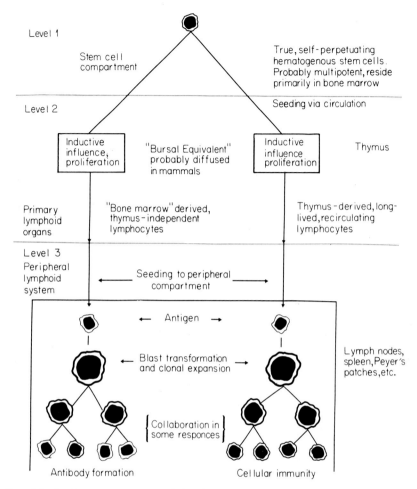

Level 1

Stem cell
compartment

True, self-perpetuating
hematogenous stem cells.
Probably multipotent, reside
primarily in bone marrow

Level 2

Seeding via circulation

Inductive
influence,
proliferation

"Bursal Equivalent"
probably diffused
in mammals

Inductive
influence
proliferation

Thymus

Primary
lymphoid
organs

"Bone marrow" derived,
thymus-independent
lymphocytes

Thymus-derived, long-
lived, recirculating
lymphocytes

Level 3
Peripheral
lymphoid
system

Seeding to peripheral
compartment

← Antigen →

← Blast transformation →
and clonal expansion

Lymph nodes,
spleen, Peyer's
patches, etc.

[Collaboration in
some responses]

Antibody formation

Cellular immunity

FIG. 5.1. A schematic overview of the three main functional compartments of the lymphoid system.

is where lymphoid cells respond to antigenic signals by executive immune responses such as antibody formation and delayed hypersensitivity-type cellular reactions.

I. The Genesis of Lymphocytes

A. FETAL ORIGIN

Classical hematologists and morphologists believed that lymphocytes came from fixed reticular cells in lymphatic tissues. Despite the extremely thin evidence which supported this view, it went relatively unchallenged, until the intensive research on the biological effects of ionizing radiation which followed World War II drew attention to the extraordinary recuperative powers of the lymphatic tissues of sublethally irradiated animals (Bloom, 1948). Various studies, particularly ones involving shielding of one lymphoid organ (Jacobson, 1952) soon revealed that progenitors of lymphoid cells could circulate. A detailed picture has emerged only recently, and we owe it largely to the studies of Ford, Loutit, Micklem, and collaborators at Harwell (Micklem *et al.*, 1966; Loutit, 1960) and of Moore and Owen (Moore, 1967; Moore and Owen, 1967a,b). It reveals a constant renewal of the dividing cell population of all lymphoid organs by cells immigrating via the circulation. The pool of stem cells in the adult animal resides largely in the bone marrow and its origins can be traced back to the early embryo.

For a time it seemed that many lymphocytes were the progeny of embryonic thymic epithelial cells (Auerbach, 1961). However, while Moore's experiments confirmed that the thymus is the first organ to become lymphoid in the embryo, he showed that the thymic anlage, while still entirely of epithelial nature, was colonized by large hemocytoblastlike cells which migrated into it, commencing at a time of embryogenesis that was sharply defined for each species. Parabiosis and cell transfer studies, employing chromosomal markers, showed that these immigrant cells, and not the epithelial cells, were the ancestors of the thymic lymphocytes. The blast progenitors are believed to be derived from hemangioblast cells residing originally in the blood islets of the yolk sac. Cells of similar morphology to those which colonize the thymus are also found to enter the anlagen of organs such as the avian bursa of Fabricius, the spleen, and the fetal liver. It is quite possible that each of these stem cells possesses the potential to differentiate down various pathways, e.g., toward erythropoiesis, myelopoiesis, or lymphopoiesis, and that the direction taken by each particular cell depends on the local environment in which it lodges, and on the inducers which it encounters there.

Auerbach (1970) has accepted the general picture presented by Moore, and has stressed that there exist many situations in embryogenesis where cells assume specialized functions after an appropriate "induction" of a mesenchymal cell population by cells of epithelial origin. Tubule formation by nephrogenic mesenchyme after induction by cells of the ureteric bud is a classic example. Thus, the mesenchymally derived hematogenous stem cells may receive some inductive instruction from fetal thymic epithelial cells leading to the construction of a thymic

cortex. There is reason to believe that the epithelial cells can continue
to exercise their inductive role throughout life.

B. Bone Marrow as Chief Source of Lymphoid Stem Cells in Adult Life

Seeding of stem cells into lymphoid organs does not cease at birth,
but in fact is a continuous feature of adult lymphocyte physiology. In
adults, the stem cell pool resides chiefly in the bone marrow, though
cells of similar function exist in the spleen. The gradual export from
these sources of lymphocyte progenitors can be charted by means of
chromosomal marker and parabiotic techniques (Ford, 1966; Micklem
et al., 1966). The morphological form which the progenitors assume
in the adult is not known, though it seems likely that they are lymphocytes. Furthermore, the mature lymphoid organs thus colonized already
contain large numbers of dividing lymphocytes, so the dependence of
indefinitely continuing lymphopoiesis on further cell inflow can only
be demonstrated in experiments which run for weeks or months.
Nevertheless, the gradual replenishment of both primary and secondary
lymphoid organs by bone marrow-derived cells is vital to the functional
integrity of these organs.

For practical purposes we can regard the adult bone marrow, with
its stem cell pool, as the first compartment of the lymphoid system.
These stem cells are not antigen-reactive (or immunocompetent) in the
conventional sense. Before achieving the capacity to respond to antigens,
they must differentiate further, presumably under the influence of inducers in primary lymphoid organs such as the thymus. This process
requires cell division and maturation, and takes a minimum of 2 to
3 weeks (Miller and Mitchell, 1967).

We must now turn to the second category or hierarchy of lymphoid
organs, namely the thymus, the avian bursa of Fabricius, and its possible
mammalian analogs.

II. Primary Lymphoid Organs

A. General Features and Functions

There are only two organs which can with certainty be designated
as primary lymphoid organs. These are the thymus and the avian bursa

of Fabricius. The two chief features which distinguish these organs from lymph nodes are (1) the absence in them, of executive immunological events such as antibody formation and (2) the fact that in them the intensity of lymphopoiesis, i.e., of mitosis among primitive lymphoid cells, is independent of antigenic stimulation. A third noteworthy feature, but one which is also present in organs such as the tonsils (the nature of which is still the subject of debate), is a prominent compartment of epithelial cells.

The most commonly held view of the function of these primary lymphoid organs is that they are sites of differentiation of antigen-reactive or immunocompetent cells (Miller, 1967; Warner and Szenberg, 1964). They receive stem cells from the bone marrow, which multiply extensively and differentiate to small lymphocytes, many of which are then seeded into the circulation and join the pool of lymphocyte present in the peripheral compartment. There is good evidence that small lymphocytes do leave the thymus (Nossal, 1964; Weissman, 1967), but it is also clear that large numbers of thymus cells die locally without subserving any obvious immunological function (Metcalf and Wiadrowski, 1966). The purpose of this local birth and death process is still a matter for conjecture. It has been found that mitotic figures in the thymus tend to cluster around some specialized cells, possibly of epithelial origin, which may be secretors of one or more humoral factors that act as a stimulus (Metcalf and Ishidate, 1962; Mandel, 1969).

B. The Thymus

Considerable new insight into the function of primary lymphoid organs has been gained through experiments involving extirpation of the organ at an early time of life. Miller (1961) found that removal of the thymus from mice on the day of birth caused a failure of correct and full development of immunological potential. This could be restored both by thymic grafts, and by grafts enclosed in a cell-impermeable Millipore diffusion chamber (Osoba and Miller, 1963; Miller et al., 1966). More recently, restoration of the immunodeficiency resulting from thymectomy has been claimed following repeated injections of thymic extracts (Trainin and Linker-Israeli, 1967), lending some support to the hope that an eventual purification of the active factor(s) will ensue. While these experiments involve an action of "thymic hormone" at a distance, it is more plausible to assume that in an intact animal, the inductive effect is mediated within the thymus itself, and causes a previously uncommitted stem cell to become an antigen-reactive lymphocyte.

In the decade following Miller's original discovery, an enormous amount of work on the immunological functions of the thymus has been performed. As this has been extensively reviewed by colleagues from our own laboratory (Metcalf, 1966; Miller and Osoba, 1967) and elsewhere (Good and Gabrielsen, 1964; Wolstenholme and Porter, 1966), it will not be considered at length here. However, we must discuss a frequently heard, major objection to the above interpretation of the nature and function of primary lymphoid organs. It concerns the failure of dramatic effects following thymectomy in many circumstances. If the thymus is so vital, for example, why does thymectomy in the human appear to be so harmless? This objection must be dealt with in two sections, pertaining to neonatal and adult thymectomy.

Neonatal thymectomy in some species and strains of animal appears not to affect the immune response of the test animal to the antigen(s) used by the investigator. For example, removal of the thymus in the sheep, even during embryonic life, appears not to hinder subsequent immune responses (Silverstein, 1970; Cole and Morris, 1970). Possible answers to this objection are, in principle, fourfold. First, the immune response under study may not be under thymic control, but may depend on nonthymus-derived cells. This is unlikely to be a satisfactory explanation in all cases, or, at least if it is, the role of the thymus in some species must be a very minor one. Second, the operation may have come too late. Certain long-lived antigen-reactive cells may have seeded out of the organ before surgical intervention and stand in readiness to respond. This may well hold in certain experiments. Third, accessory thymic tissue may be present and may assume increased function after thymectomy. This view appears to be gaining increasing experimental support. Finally, it is possible that under the stress of thymectomy, other cells in other organs gradually take over the function of the thymic medullary cells. It is known that if neonatally thymectomized mice are held germfree, and are thus protected from the infections which might otherwise kill them, a gradual, incomplete recovery of immune responsiveness ensues (Miller et al., 1967). This result in no way negates the importance of the normal thymus. It simply reveals that, if necessary, the animal can make use of unknown accessory mechanisms that, presumably, lie dormant within it. It is possible but not certain that the third and fourth mechanisms are in fact identical.

Adult thymectomy superficially appears to have little effect. However, this is in all probability due to the long-lived nature of antigen-reactive cells and to the importance of immunological memory in many allegedly primary immune responses. Two separate studies (Metcalf, 1965; Miller,

1965) have shown that while adult thymectomy in the mouse has little immediate effect on the immune response, a deficiency does become manifest after several months, and increases in severity thereafter. This is consistent with the idea that antigen-reactive cells once seeded out from the thymus no longer require its hormonal influence to respond to antigens. In man, it appears that small lymphocytes can live for many years. This suggests that the immunological effects of thymectomy in the adult human may not manifest themselves for a long period. We are not aware of any study of the immune responsiveness of a group of thymectomized humans conducted, say, 10 or 20 years after the operation. Such an investigation would be of profound interest.

Another facet which may militate against obvious deleterious effects of adult thymectomy relates to the degree of cross-reactivity among antigens. A normal adult animal has a large amount on antigen-driven lymphocyte production going on in its peripheral compartment. Much, and perhaps most, of this activity depends not on virgin cells recently seeded out from the thymus, but on "memory" lymphocytes, born in the peripheral lymphocyte compartment itself. After adult thymectomy, the seeding of new, virgin antigen-reactive lymphocytes may cease; but the proliferation of lymphoid cells already present in the peripheral compartment will continue in response to those antigens entering from the environment. In fact, the total amount of new lymphocyte formation in the peripheral lymphoid organs may show little change. If a new antigen is injected, it may well exhibit some cross-reactivity with one or more antigens that the animal has already met. In this case it would act as a stimulus to the relevant memory cells. If the cross-reacting antigen were a commonly present one, e.g., a constituent of a commensal intestinal bacterium, there would be a reactive population present even years after adult thymectomy.

C. The Avian Bursa of Fabricius and Possible Mammalian Analogs

One of the more puzzling aspects of the lesion which follows neonatal thymectomy is its patchiness. The animals which survive to adult life after this operation fail almost entirely to respond to some antigens, but respond normally, or nearly so, to others. In general, cellular immune responses such as allograft rejection are affected more profoundly than humoral antibody responses, though antibody formation to certain antigens is subnormal. Research on the immune responses of chickens has helped to shed light on this problem. The administration of androgenic hormones in embryonic life to this species can cause failure of development of the bursa of Fabricius, of the thymus, or of both organs. Studies from the Hall Institute (Szenberg and Warner, 1963; Warner et al., 1962) showed that "hormonally bursectomized" chickens failed to form humoral antibodies but maintained their power to reject skin allografts. By contrast, "hormonally thymectomized" birds with intact bursal function failed to reject grafts but formed antibody in normal fashion. This demonstrated a dissociation in immunological responsiveness, with the thymus being necessary for correct development of cell-mediated immunity and the bursa of humoral immunity. Warner and Szenberg proposed that the lymphoid system in birds was in fact composed of two broad cellular families. The one, under thymic control, was responsible for delayed hypersensitivity, skin homograft rejection, and related cellular phenomena. The other, under bursal control, was concerned in antibody production.

This general thesis has, in recent years, gained considerable support through an extensive series of studies from Good's laboratory (Perey et al., 1967, 1968; Perey and Good, 1968; Sutherland et al., 1964). This group has combined surgical ablation of lymphoid organs with sublethal whole body X-irradiation, avoiding some of the complexities of interpretation which might arise from hormonal destruction of bursa or thymus. They have argued strongly that the dissociation into two lymphoid cell families is present also in mammals, the germinal center plasma cell family being responsible for antibody production and dependent on some bursal equivalent, and the recirculating small lymphocyte pool being largely thymus-dependent and involved in cellular immunity. This thesis is supported by the existence of a variety of clinical immunological deficiency disorders, which Good terms "experiments of nature," and which mimic the deficiencies of birds deprived, respectively, of bursa, thymus, or both organs.

What is the mammalian bursal equivalent? The situation is certainly complex. While the thymus is necessary for the development of cell-mediated immunity, its ablation also occasions failed development of certain humoral immune responses. There does not appear to be a single organ possessing functions analogous to that of the bursa. There is some evidence that, in rabbits, early removal of the appendix and all Peyer's patches results in effects similar to those of bursectomy in the chicken (Perey et al., 1968). This has led to the view that the gut-associated lymphoid tissue exerts bursa-like functions in the control of the humoral immune response. However, this view has not gained universal acceptance, particularly as gut-associated lymphoid collections display two vital differences from true primary lymphoid organs. They *are* sites of antibody production and cell division in them *is* dependent on antigenic stimulation. The Peyer's patches of germfree animals, for example, are quite small and contain few dividing cells; after antigenic stimulation, however, they show intense mitotic activity and become factories producing both antibody-forming and memory cells (Cooper and Turner, 1967, 1968). It is possible that the inductive function of the bursa has been generalized and diffused in mammals. For example, it is possible that certain specialized cells in germinal centers cause lymphoid differentiation in bone marrow-derived cells (Bos, 1967). After irradiation, the germinal centers can be rapidly reconstructed from bone marrow but not from thymic cells. In the chapters which follow, we shall refer frequently to "bone marrow-derived" versus "thymus-derived" lymphocytes. In most cases, we will consider that the bone marrow-derived cells are really the equivalent of cells which, in birds, would be regarded as under bursa control.

III. Peripheral Lymphoid Organs

A. General Features and Functions

We are now in a position to look at the functional anatomy of the organs in which antibodies are formed and the cells mediating delayed hypersensitivity and homograft reactions are born. This comprises lymph nodes, spleen, Peyer's patches, pharyngeal and palatine tonsils, appendix, and milky spots of the omentum. Whether or not some of these tissues also exert a bursa-like inductive function, all are sites predominantly of antigen-driven division and cellular differentiation, with well-developed antigen-trapping and lymph filtration mechanisms. A characteristic common to these organs is that they are of small size in germfree animals, and that they swell during regional infections or immunization. The latter, normal response has frequently been incorrectly termed by some name which implies a pathological state, e.g., "sinus catarrh." Indeed, gross hypertrophy may be an indication of a disease, but some degree of cyclical swelling and regression is normal, reflecting the ebb and flow of minor infections in "conventional" animals or humans. As laboratory mammals live under conditions that are far less hygienic than ideal, it could be argued that the organs of specific pathogen-free (SPF) animals more closely approach the norm for people in developed communities. In both normal and SPF animals, some organs are, by virtue of their location, inherently more likely to be sites of antigenic barrage than others. Thus, mesenteric lymph nodes always possess the hallmarks of immunization, namely large, active germinal centers and abundant plasma cells; peripheral lymph nodes such as the popliteal are more frequently quite small and lacking these hallmarks.

In the descriptions which follow, we will discuss the "conventional" adult outbred Wistar rat. Though species and strain differences in detailed organization of lymphatic tissue can readily be noted, the most important features of functional anatomy are common to all the placental mammals. A more extensive treatment of many of these points can be found in the book of Yoffey and Courtice (1970).

B. Lymph Nodes

1. General Features

For a detailed description of the histology (Yoffey and Courtice, 1956) and ultrastructure (Clark, 1962; Han, 1961, Moe, 1964) of lymph nodes, the reader is referred elsewhere. Our purpose here is to outline those features of lymph node architecture which are of special importance to an understanding of antigen-trapping mechanisms (Nossal et al., 1968a,b) and lymphocyte physiology (Gowans and McGregor, 1965). Figure 5.2 is a schematic view of a section through a lymph node which has been subjected to antigenic stimulation. Differences between its appearance and that of unstimulated nodes will be described in the text.

Lymph nodes have a cortex, divided into lymphoid follicles and diffuse cortex; and a medulla, divided into medullary sinuses and cords. The first key point to note is that though each of these regions presents quite typical features, there is a remarkable absence of sharp anatomical boundaries in lymphatic tissue and cells appear to possess the capacity to move freely from one compartment to the other. Also, it is often impossible to state precisely where the border between two adjacent areas, e.g., diffuse cortex and medullary cord, can be found.

The basic pattern of lymph flow can be readily established by injecting subcutaneously a molecule which is radioactively labeled but not palatable to phagocytic cells; the animal's own serum albumin is a good example (Ada et al., 1964b,c). The lymph reaches the node via an afferent lymphatic, which, just proximal to the node, breaks up into a number of delicate branches. They terminate in the circular sinus, which is, in fact, a lined shell of fluid that surrounds the whole node. As this sinus is in free communication with the efferent lymph vessel, a proportion of the arriving lymph escapes the filtering action of the node. However, the bulk of the flow has to pass through the medullary sinuses. Lymph can reach the sinuses via well-defined channels called trabecular sinuses, which are, however, not extensively developed in the rat. In this species, typical medullary sinuses often extend quite superficially into the cortical region and communicate directly with the circular sinus. Finally, as the inner lining of the circular sinus is quite porous (Clark, 1962), a substantial proportion of the lymph percolates

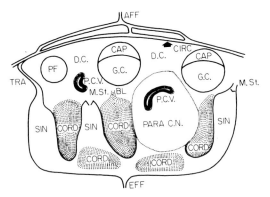

FIG. 5.2. Schematic view of a section through an antigenically stimulated lymph node. AFF, afferent lymphatic vessel; CIRC, circular sinus; TRA, trabecular sinus; PF, primary lymphoid follicle; D.C., diffuse cortex of lymph node; G.C., germinal center; CAP, antigen-trapping area of "cap" of germinal center, rich in dendritic follicle cells; P.C.V., postcapillary venule; M.St, "muddy stream" area where lymphocytes leave cortex and enter medullary sinus through valvelike area; BL, areas where blast cells can be seen, possibly moving from germinal center into medullary cord; PARA C.N., paracortical nodule which hypertrophies during cellular immune responses; CORD, medullary cord of lymph node rich in antibody-forming cells; SIN, medullary sinus, rich in macrophages and prime site of antigen capture; EFF, efferent lymphatic.

through the substance of the cortex, filtering between tightly packed lymphocytes before reaching the medulla. The lymph leaves the node via an efferent lymphatic. We must now consider each of the main structural elements in somewhat more detail.

2. The Circular Sinus

This is a delicate structure which can easily be damaged during dissection of the node prior to fixation. Its outer wall consists of a layer of flattened endothelial cells and a minimum of surrounding adventitial tissue. Its inner wall is formed, in fact, by the outermost cell layer of the lymph node substance. There are many monocytic and macrophage cells, and on occasion these show a contorted appearance, as if they were in active transit between sinus and node at the moment of killing. Some of the lining layer consists of rather nondescript ovoid cells with a large nucleus and little cytoplasm. At other places the outermost cell of the node, and thus the sinus lining cell, is a typical small or medium lymphocyte. In view of the known capacity of such cells to move, it is difficult to understand what actually holds the surface of the node in place. Clearly it appears to be a site of extensive cellular traffic. In the lumen of the sinus, one can see occasional monocytic and lymphocytic cells, and also small cell fragments which Söderström has termed lymphoglandular bodies (Söderström, 1967; 1968). At certain defined stages of active immunization, namely between 4 and 24 hr after antigen injection, considerable numbers of polymorphonuclear leukocytes can also be seen.

3. The Lymphoid Follicles (Fig. 5.3)

Some 20–50 μ subjacent to the inner sinus lining, lymphoid follicles can be found. These are spherical aggregations of lymphocytes and reticular cells which will be discussed in greater detail in Chapter 7. In germfree animals, these structures are poorly developed and it is difficult to distinguish exactly the follicles from the surrounding diffuse cortex. However, their presence can be demonstrated by a functional test that we will consider in Chapter 7 which has allowed the concept of "primary" lymphoid follicles to emerge clearly. In conventional animals, most follicles have been the site of at least limited immunological stimulation. It is convenient, but not altogether logical, to divide the follicles into two categories: *primary follicles*, in which no germinal center is obvious on a methyl green-pyronin-stained section; and *secondary follicles*, in which a pyroninophilic germinal center is surrounded by a cuff of small lymphocytes. In fact, there exists a continuous gradation of structures from the vestigial primary follicles of germfree rat popliteal lymph nodes to the very large germinal centers of the Peyer's patches or mesenteric lymph nodes of conventional rats. The features which speak for a minimally stimulated follicle are paucity of pyroninophilic or dividing cells, paucity of "tingible-body" macrophages, small size, and lack of clear demarcation from surrounding tissue. Such primary lymphoid follicles constitute the great majority of the follicles seen in the popliteal lymph nodes of young adult rats housed under good conditions. Intentional stimulation with a single injection of a powerful antigen then allows one to follow the progressive change to a secondary follicle (Nossal et al., 1964b).

A germinal center can only be understood if one grasps its nature as a reactive structure which develops in a primary follicle after antigenic stimulation. This fact has been frequently obscured in the past because of the presence, in the lymphatic tissue under study, of germinal centers prior to the antigen injection. These naturally occurring germinal centers are not to be thought of as autonomous lymphocyte factories similar to the thymus. Their presence reflects a state of "background" immunological stimulation of the test animal. The different lymph nodes of the body show this "physiological" germinal center formation to differing

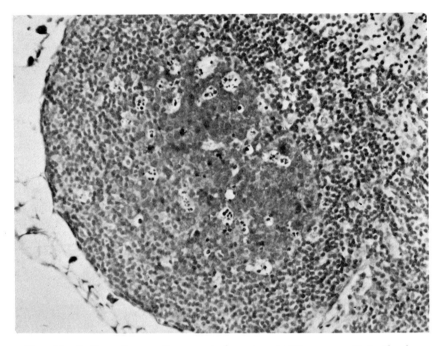

Fig. 5.3. Section of an active germinal center; ×400 approx. Note the large, tightly packed lymphocytes in the center, and the "moth eaten" appearance characteristic of tingible body macrophages in the surrounding small lymphocytes.

extents. The least activity will be encountered in distal limb nodes such as the popliteal or epitrochlear; the most, in the mesenteric nodes. Other nodes which invariably show large germinal centers include the caudal mesenteric pelvic node found just distal to the bifurcation of the aorta and the mediastinal nodes draining the bronchial tree. Inguinal and axillary nodes are somewhat variable but normally show relatively few germinal centers: iliac nodes and lumbar nodes are usually more active than the popliteal but less than mesenteric and mediastinal. In any case,

the investigator wishing to study germinal center physiology after antigenic stimulation must first carefully familiarize himself with the median
level of development which preexists in the lymph node he wishes to
study.

For the first 24–36 hr after intentional immunization, histological sections of lymph nodes show little change in the primary follicles. By
2 days, small numbers of large, pyroninophilic cells with prominent
nucleoli can be seen in the follicle, particularly in its deeper portions.
There is some evidence (Austin, 1968) that these are derived by transformation of immigrant lymphocytes. By 3 to 4 days, sections reveal
small aggregations of these pyroninophilic cells which have come to
lie adjacent to each other; the strong possibility exists that at least a
proportion of these are the descendants of the immigrant cells seen
at 2 days. At this time, the two-dimensional section shows profiles of
ca. 5 to 15 cells, implying three-dimensional nests of up to ca. 60 cells.
By day 4 to 5, with strong antigenic stimulation, this nest has the appearance of a typical young germinal center. There are rapidly dividing
lymphoid cells, and a very characteristic cell has made its appearance
in the "tingible body" macrophage or TBM. This is a phagocytic cell
with a diverse variety of inclusions, many of which appear to contain
constituents of degenerating lymphocytes. Nuclear debris in various
stages of digestion is a prominent feature. The inevitable presence of
cells of this type in an active germinal center suggests that the rapid
multiplication of lymphocytes in the region is always accompanied by
considerable cell death. At this stage, the number of large and medium
sized lymphoid cells in the germinal center is several hundred. If repeated antigenic stimuli are given, this number can grow to some
thousands within 1 to 2 weeks. In the absence of further injections,
however, the center has an innate tendency to regress. It attains a maximal size at a time which depends on the nature and dose of the original
immunization, varying from ca. 1 to 4 weeks, and then slowly diminishes
in size. The lymphoid cell proliferation diminishes at a somewhat faster
rate than the disappearance of TBM. Thus, during the regression phase,
centers can be seen with relatively few dividing cells but many TBM.
At late stages after immunization, "burnt out" secondary follicles can
be seen, which resemble primary follicles, but contain at their center
TBM and excess reticular cells.

As germinal centers grow, they presumably compress surrounding
structures. Structural elements of the lymph node stroma around the
center are stretched, and this gives the impression of a very sharp border
to the edge of the center, as seen in a histological section. Nevertheless,

electron microscopic examination fails to reveal a "capsule" around the center, and no anatomical barrier to cellular traffic is apparent at the edge. Growth of the center is also accompanied by reactive changes in the reticular cell population, which we shall consider in greater detail in Chapter 7. In a fully developed germinal center, the reticular cells are found in highest concentration on the side of the center which faces the circular sinus. In a good methyl green–pyronin-stained section, this reticular cell-rich area of the center can be seen as a salmon-pink "cap" over the more reddish, lymphocyte-rich remainder. Superficial again to this cap, is a cuff or collar of small lymphocytes, once thought to be the progeny of the center, but now known to consist mainly of long-lived cells.

On Fig. 5.2, an area of cortex has been labeled "BL." This is to illustrate a possibility suggested by certain rather rare tissue section profiles. In these, the distance between germinal center and medullary plasma cell cord is short (50 μ or less), and a string of pyroninophilic blast cells can be seen between center and cord. This appearance strongly suggests that it is possible for immature lymphoid cells to travel between these two anatomically distinct regions. However, one cannot draw firm kinetic conclusions from a survey of static sections, particularly in the absence of cellular labels, and it must be admitted that the fate of the many progeny cells resulting from the intense lymphopoiesis in germinal centers is still speculative. We shall return to this question below.

4. Diffuse Cortical Tissue of Lymph Node and Paracortical Nodules

The tissue which separates the follicles from each other and also from the medulla is known as the diffuse cortical tissue of lymph nodes, or simply as the diffuse cortex. After certain types of antigenic stimulation, and particularly after procedures which evoke a state of cellular immunity (delayed hypersensitivity), this area hypertrophies considerably (Scothorne and McGregor, 1955; Oort and Turk, 1965). Enlarged areas of cortex sometimes have a nodular appearance, and have been termed paracortical nodules (PCN). These PCN may penetrate deeply into the substance of the node. Indeed, they may be so extensive as to assume a greater total volume than the medulla. The diffuse cortex consists largely of tightly packed small lymphocytes, though after antigenic stimulation blasts and other large lymphoid cells are seen in substantial numbers. In this location, the dividing cells show no tendency to cluster into nests or centers. One of the outstanding features of this area is a special type of venule which has been called the "postcapillary venule"

(PCV; Fig. 5.4). It is characterized by a high, cuboidal endothelium, a narrow lumen which contains a disproportionately high concentration of lymphocytes, and a convoluted, characteristic shape (Marchesi and Gowans, 1964). Small lymphocytes can frequently be seen actually within the endothelial cells themselves. The diffuse cortex is otherwise noticeably avascular. The paucity of arterioles and capillaries, the dense packing of lymphocytes, and the obvious relative resistance to rapid lymph permeation all lead to a low oxygen and high carbon dioxide tension in this region.

The diffuse cortex is strikingly poor in phagocytic cells in comparison with other areas of the node. Macrophages and polymorphonuclear lymphocytes are encountered only occasionally.

There are no distinct limits to the diffuse cortex. It merges almost imperceptibly with the medullary cords. Also, a communication exists between the cortex and the medullary sinuses (see Fig. 5.2, M.St.). This has been studied in detail by Söderström who has given the picturesque name of "muddy stream" to certain regions of such communication. The appearances are of a gradually diminishing packing of lymphoid cells which finally spill into the sinus. At times, shreds of delicate fibrous tissue lend a valvelike appearance to the junction. The suggestion is that lymphoid cells stream slowly out of the diffuse cortex and into the sinus, the passage being slowed still further by a valve.

5. Medullary Cords (Fig. 5.5)

These are structures which penetrate from the diffuse cortex into the medulla of the node, interdigitating between the sinuses. In the absence of antigenic stimulation, they are not prominent, consisting only of scattered plasma cells usually close to a blood vessel. Two days or so after primary immunization, pyroninophilic cells appear, possibly through migration from the adjacent cortex, though again this is impossible to prove. Proliferation of plasma cell precursors continues, reaching a peak 5 to 7 days after antigen injection, when the cords are crowded with immature and mature plasma cells. Lymphocytes are also present, frequently exhibiting more cytoplasm than the usual small lymphocyte. The cords also contain some macrophages, but these are present in much smaller numbers than in the medullary sinuses.

As with the other structural elements of the node, the cords do not exhibit sharp borders and movement of cells from cord to sinus and vice versa is highly probable. Indeed, it has been shown that antibody-forming cells appear in efferent lymph in considerable numbers (Cunningham et al., 1966). These are usually not plasma cells but various types

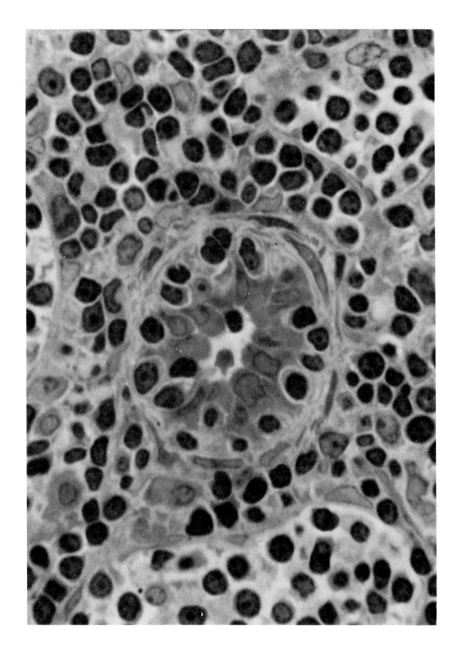

FIG. 5.4(a). Light microscopic section of a postcapillary venule (×1000) for comparison with Fig. 5.4(b) (See facing page.)

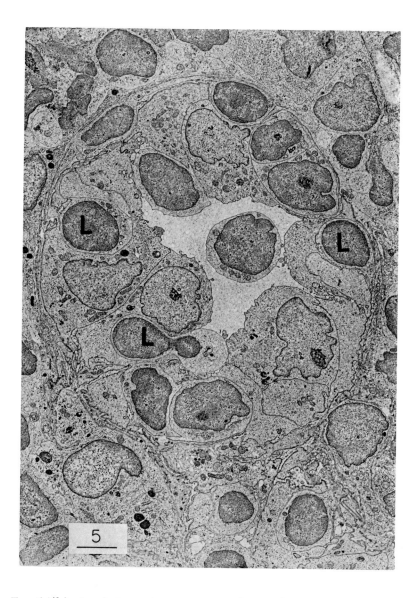

FIG. 5.4(b). An electron microscopic view of a similar venule. Note the many small lymphocytes actually inside the cytoplasm of the high, cuboidal endothelial cells. L, small lymphocytes.

of lymphocytes, suggesting that the typical mature plasma cell tends to remain in the node where it was formed. Antibody-forming lymphocytes of various sorts, however, appear to be capable of leaving the cords, entering the sinuses, reaching the efferent lymph, and finally settling in another lymph node.

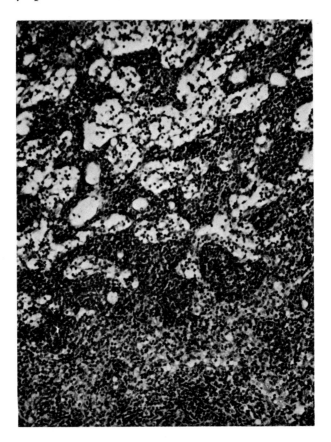

FIG. 5.5. A low power view of the lymph node medulla to show interdigitating areas of medullary cords and medullary sinuses. ×100.

6. Medullary Sinuses (Fig. 5.5)

Medullary sinuses are the major filters of lymph nodes. They consist of lymph-filled spaces lined by elongated macrophages, and containing numerous cells. In the unimmunized animal, many macrophages and a few lymphocytes lie within the sinus. Sometimes contiguous sheets of macrophages can be seen straddling the sinus. Mast cells also are present, as are very occasional polymorphonuclear leukocytes.

Intentional immunization causes a series of changes in lymphoid sinuses. There is, between 4 and 24 hr after antigen, a transient crowding of the sinuses with neutrophil (and some eosinophil) polymorphonuclear leukocytes, the intensity being dependent on the intensity of the antigenic stimulus. There is a gradual increase in mast cell content (Miller, 1964b), and it is our impression that the number of macrophages also rises, although this is not well documented. Macrophages which have ingested antigens undergo a series of typical ultrastructural changes which will be described in Chapter 7.

Lymphoid cells are found in substantial numbers in the sinuses after immunization, and naturally will, from time to time, be seen in close proximity to a macrophage. However, we have not been able to convince ourselves of any definite formation of "rosettes" of lymphocytes around macrophages in the medulla, in either the sinuses or the cords (Nossal et al., 1968a).

The sinus lining layer of macrophages appears to be both porous and mobile, reflecting again the absence of tight compartmentation in the lymphoid system.

C. The Spleen (Fig. 5.6)

1. General Features

Good descriptions of the structure of the spleen have recently been published (Weiss, 1964; Snook, 1964) and again we wish only to review the key points. The spleen differs from lymph nodes in the following chief features: (1) it has certain nonlymphoid functions, including erythropoiesis, myelopoiesis, and disposal of aged red cells, which occur in the sinuses of the red pulp, and will not concern us further; (2) it receives and deals with foreign materials via the blood rather than the lymphatic circulation, and thus has no portal of entry corresponding to the afferent lymphatics and circular sinus; and (3) though macrophages are present in the red pulp sinuses, there is really no structure in the spleen which corresponds to the lymph node medullary sinuses, with their capacity to filter and retain antigenic material. Instead, as we shall see, a different type of structure with antigen-trapping power is present, termed the *marginal zone*. There are also three types of structures which are the splenic analogs of structures we have already described in lymph nodes namely: (1) the lymphoid follicles (primary and secondary) of the splenic white pulp; (2) the diffuse lymphoid tissue of the white pulp, which has been termed the periarteriolar lymphocyte sheath, but has many features in common with the diffuse cortex of lymph nodes; and (3) the cords of the splenic red pulp, which are the chief sites of antibody production in the spleen and correspond to lymph node medullary cords.

Some features of splenic architecture are shown in Fig. 5.6, which is a modification of the concept of Snook (1964). The spleen consists

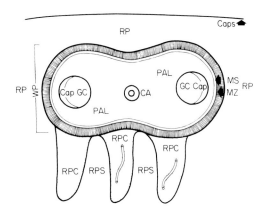

FIG. 5.6. A schematic view of the organization of the spleen as seen through a section from an immunized animal. CAP, capsule; RP, red pulp; WP, white pulp; MZ, marginal zone; MS, marginal sinus; PAL, periarteriolar lymphocyte sheath; CA, central arteriole; GC, germinal center; CAP, caplike area of germinal center rich in dendritic follicle cells; RPC, red pulp cords rich in antibody-forming cells; RPS, red pulp sinuses engaged in erythrocyte destruction and some erythropoiesis and myelopoiesis.

of islands of lymphatic tissue or *white pulp* in a "sea" of red pulp which is made up of alternating sinuses and cords. As with lymph nodes, the cords are not prominent in antigenically unstimulated animals. White pulp is separated from red pulp by a *marginal zone*, which surrounds the *marginal sinus*.

2. Arterial Supply

The white pulp is believed to develop around the adventitia of blood vessels in an expansion of the periarteriolar sheath of fibrous tissue and reticulum. Indeed, in each white pulp island the *central arteriole* is a prominently visible structure. It is characterized by a narrow lumen and thick wall, with high, somewhat cuboidal endothelial cells. Branches of such arterioles go in varying directions. Some spill directly into the red pulp sinuses; others nourish the red pulp cords. An important termination is into a vascular channel which totally surrounds the white pulp and separates it from the marginal zone, termed the marginal sinus. Germinal centers often contain capillary branches of the central arteriole, but the diffuse lymphoid tissue of the white pulp, like its counterpart in lymph nodes, is relatively avascular.

The marginal sinus bears some similarities to the circular sinus surrounding lymph nodes. Admittedly it is a blood vascular rather than a lymphatic channel, but it also is a portal from which antigens (in this case blood-borne) can reach lymphatic tissue; and immediately subjacent to it, germinal centers develop following antigenic stimulation.

3. The White Pulp

The white pulp consists of diffuse lymphoid tissue and lymphoid follicles. The diffuse tissue, which corresponds to the diffuse cortical tissue and paracortical nodules of lymph nodes is termed the periarteriolar lymphocyte sheath (PAL). It does not contain postcapillary venules. Secondary follicles are similar in all respects to those of lymph nodes. However, primary follicles are more difficult to recognize in the spleen. In fact, their presence can only be convincingly shown through techniques which utilize their remarkable antigen-trapping potential (see Chapter 7). The reticular cell cap of secondary follicles always faces toward the marginal sinus and marginal zone.

4. Marginal Zone (Fig. 5.7)

The marginal zone consists of rather loose reticular tissue with an abundant volume of extracellular plasmal spaces (Weiss, 1964). The reticular cells (Fig. 5.7) characteristically possess long, branching processes. The meshes of the reticulum contain moderate numbers of lymphocytes and macrophages, and soon after intensive antigenic stimulation, large numbers of pyroninophilic lymphoid cells transiently fill this region. The marginal zone is in free communication with the red pulp and it is sometimes not easy to define its outer limit.

5. Red Pulp

The red pulp cords usually develop around a readily identifiable blood vessel. After antigenic stimulation, they fill with plasma cells of progressively greater maturity. No anatomical barrier exists between cords and

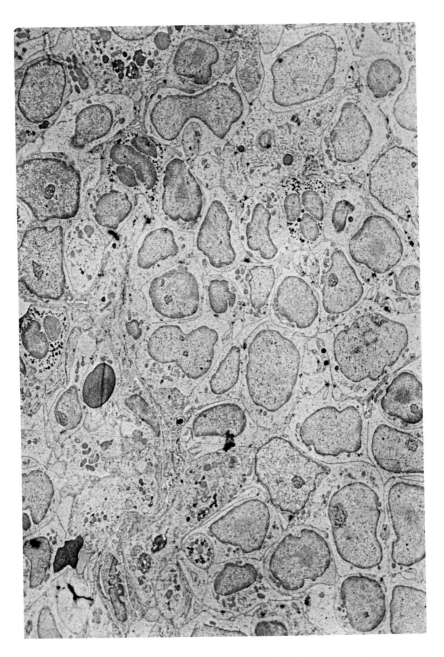

FIG. 5.7. An electron micrographic view of the spleen marginal zone.

sinuses. The sinuses are incompletely lined by rectangular reticular cells and contain a complex mixture of free cells engaged in erythropoiesis, myelopoiesis, and erythrophagocytosis.

D. PEYER'S PATCHES

Peyer's patches are lymphoid collections which drain submucosal spaces of the intestine. They are of interest as they have been regarded as possessing some features of primary lymphoid tissue. However, histological examination shows them to resemble secondary or peripheral lymphoid tissue much more closely than either the thymus or the avian bursa of Fabricius. In conventional animals, they possess large germinal centers with the reticular cell "cap" facing the intestinal lumen. The medullary tissue contains macrophages and plasma cells, and drainage is via lacteal lymphatic vessels toward the mesenteric lymph node. Diffuse lymphatic tissue with postcapillary venules can also be seen.

E. OMENTAL "MILKY SPOTS" OR NODES OF RANVIER

Organized lymphatic tissue can also be seen in connective tissue in a wide variety of sites. An excellent example, which has recently come into prominence through the work of Fischer and colleagues (Ax *et al.*, 1966; Kaboth *et al.*, 1966), is to be found in the omentum. Here, in an animal not antigenically stimulated, tiny collections of lymphocytes can be found between the two apposed layers of flattened omental cells. When an antigen is given intraperitoneally, these undergo extensive reactive hypertrophy. The special advantage is that, in the initial stages at least, these miniature lymph nodes are, for practical purposes, two-dimensional entities. Cell traffic, multiplication, and differentiation can be observed by time-lapse microcinematography. These so-called "milky spots" or "nodes of Ranvier" increase not only in size but also in number. This suggests that organized lymphatic tissue can arise *de novo* in a suitable environment. The chief feature which the remarkable films of Fischer and colleagues brings out is the great dynamism of the lymphoid system. This characteristic is further considered in the next chapter.

It is not our intention to review here the structure or ultrastructure of the thymus, bursa, or bone marrow, as this would take us too far from our central purpose. The interested reader is referred elsewhere (Smith, 1964; Clark, 1964a,b; Ackerman and Knouff, 1964).

IV. Summary

This chapter considers the lymphoid organs from those viewpoints that are especially relevant to the problem of how antigen causes its stimulatory effect on lymphocytes. In particular, we consider the genesis of lymphocytes and the functional anatomy of primary and secondary lymphoid organs.

The findings of Moore for the embryonic origin of lymphocytes are adopted, namely that lymphoid cells are ultimately derived from multipotent blast cells derived from the blood islets of the yolk sac. These cells seed out into various organs and become committed to differentiation toward lymphocytopoiesis through the action of locally produced inducers. The compartments of the lymphoid system are deemed to be threefold: bone marrow (and embryonic equivalents), primary lymphoid organs, and peripheral lymphoid system. The bone marrow is the source of self-perpetuating stem cells or lymphocyte precursors. The primary lymphoid organs, thymus and avian bursa of Fabricius, receive such stem cells via the circulation. They are the sites of extensive cell differentiation and multiplication, and finally of export of lymphoid cells to the peripheral compartment. A key feature of these organs is that lymphocyte proliferation is independent of antigenic stimulation. The peripheral lymphoid system comprises all the major organs of antibody formation, including the lymph nodes, spleen, and Peyer's patches. These constitute a dynamic whole, the cells comprising them possessing extensive capacities of movement both from region to region in one organ, and from organ to organ.

The structure of lymph nodes and spleen is considered in some detail. The view is supported that in mammals there exist thymus-dependent cells and regions, mainly in the diffuse lymphoid tissue of the lymph node cortex and the splenic white pulp; and a thymus-independent system of germinal centers and the plasma cell filled cords of the lymph node medulla and splenic red pulp. On classical views, the former universe is more concerned with cellular immunity and the latter with humoral immunity, but recent work is revealing that humoral immune responses depend on some type of collaboration between the two cell systems. Most, if not all, cell division in the peripheral compartment is dependent on the driving force of antigen.

Knowledge of the histological organization of lymphatic tissue will prove helpful to an understanding of antigen capture as given in Chapter 7.

CHAPTER 6

BEHAVIOR PATTERNS OF
LYMPHOID CELLS

The appearance of lymphocytes is most deceptive. An examination of a conventional smear of thoracic duct cells will reveal a population of cells, 95% of which are almost indistinguishable from each other. These cells, the small lymphocytes, in fact look so alike both on light and electron microscopic examination, that until a decade or so ago few investigators doubted the functional homogeneity of lymphocytes. Red cells transport oxygen, polymorphonuclear leukocytes phagocytose, platelets aid hemostatis, so why should not lymphocytes have a single, common job to perform? It required the combination of five elaborate technologies and an intense effort in many laboratories to arrive at our present appreciation of the extraordinary diversity in origin, behavior, and potential among these cells. The five approaches are (1) the cannulation of the thoracic duct and other lymphatic vessels, (2) various biophysical procedures for separating lymphocyte subpopulations, (3) isotopic labeling of lymphocytes for subsequent autoradiography, (4) techniques of adoptive transfer of lymphocytes into embryonic, young, and adult animals, and (5) selective extirpation of primary lymphoid organs. The summary of the nature of lymphoid cells which follows is dependent on results which use these methods, and as each approach is still evolving and continuing to yield surprising results, our total picture must of necessity be somewhat tentative.

In this chapter, we will consider the migration patterns of lymphoid cells, the various functions of lymphocytes, and the problem of heterogeneity within a group of lymphoid cells with a single function such as antibody formation.

I. Migration Patterns of Lymphoid Cells

A. Fate of Marked Lymphocytes

Lymphoid cells, contrary to early views on the question, are very mobile cells. In the body, the peripheral lymphoid systems must be regarded as a single, highly dynamic compartment with cells in constant motion between the various individual organs composing it. The great importance of this constant traffic was first clearly shown by Gowans (1959) in a classic study with demonstrated that an animal drained of its circulating lymphocyte pool by chronic thoracic duct cannulation could not establish a sufficient rate of lymphocyte production to make up for the loss, and developed progressive lymphatic tissue atrophy and immunodeficiency. Gowans (1962) also showed that small lymphocytes, on appropriate antigenic stimulation, can transform into large pyroninophilic blast cells and divide. Autoradiographic examination of lymph node sections from rats that had received isotopically marked thoracic duct lymphocytes demonstrated a special pathway which lymphocytes use to enter lymphatic tissue from the blood stream. This is via the postcapillary venules (PCV) of the diffuse cortex (Marchesi and Gowans, 1964). In fact, the lumen of PCV is always crowded with lymphocytes. These actually enter the cytoplasm of the cuboidal cells which line the PCV and exit on the other side, i.e., within the diffuse cortex. By contrast, monocytes exit through spaces between these cuboidal cells (Marchesi and Gowans, 1964). The diffuse cortex is the main "traffic area" of lymph nodes, in the sense that after the injection of labeled cells the highest concentration is found in this region. Labeled cells also reach the medulla of the node, probably by migration from the cortex, but always in smaller numbers. Sections also show scattered labeled cells in primary lymphoid follicles after an intravenous injection. Practically no cells appear to reach the inside of germinal centers, though there is appreciable traffic through the lymphocyte cuff which lies external to the center (Austin, 1968). It must be remembered that nothing is known of the rate of local traffic of cells within lymph nodes. If, for example, injected labeled cells were to enter follicles and were to leave them again very quickly, the local concentration could be low though the total number of cells that had passed through the follicle might be quite high.

It is clear that small lymphocytes can complete the migration cycle lymph node → lymphatic circulation → blood stream → postcapillary venule → lymph node → lymphatic circulation, etc., more than once, and in all probability the cycle is repeated dozens if not hundreds of times for many lymphocytes. Cells partaking in this migration constitute the recirculating lymphocyte pool. It must be clearly realized that this is not the only migration stream of importance in the lymphoid system. Migration of bone marrow stem cells to the thymus, of thymus lymphocytes to the peripheral compartment, or of germinal center cells to the lymph node medulla all play a role in lymphoid cell physiology.

The mode of entry of small lymphocytes into the periarteriolar lymphocyte sheath (PAL) of the spleen is not as completely established as for lymph nodes. It is clear that the PAL is the chief traffic area of the spleen in the sense described above. It seems altogether unlikely that lymphocytes could penetrate the thick wall of the central arteriole of the PAL, though there are some superficial similarities between this vessel and the lymph node PCV, notably the narrow lumen and the cuboidal endothelial cells. Probably the chief mode of entry of cells into the PAL is via the marginal sinus (Goldschneider and McGregor, 1968). Both lymphocytes and macrophages can frequently be seen in apparent transit across this space. The rate of appearance and concentration of migrant cells in the lymphoid follicle and red pulp regions of the spleen correspond to those found, respectively, in the medulla and follicles of lymph nodes. It is likely that lymphoid cells migrate freely from white pulp to red, especially after antigenic stimulation.

The constant traffic of cells through lymphoid organs is of importance in at least some types of immune responses. For example, perfusion experiments of spleens stimulated with the antigen sheep red blood cells have shown that the rate of traffic of lymphocytes through the spleen is far more important in determining the degree of stimulation than the number of lymphocytes present in the spleen at any given time (Ford and Gowans, 1967).

B. THYMUS-DEPENDENT LYMPHOCYTES

After neonatal thymectomy, the lymphoid areas that we have described as "diffuse" areas or "traffic zones" are found to be atrophic.

This implies that the diffuse cortex of lymph nodes and the PAL of the spleen are in some way dependent on the thymus (Parrott, 1967). The simplest view of this finding is to suppose that the lymphocytes which are found in these areas, and which constitute the bulk of the recirculating pool, are cells which have migrated from the thymus, or are descendants of such cells. Two findings lend support to this view: (1) direct isotopic labeling of thymic cells *in situ* is followed by the appearance of marked lymphocytes only in the thymus-dependent areas (Nossal, 1964; Weissman, 1967); (2) thymus cells, injected into a lethally irradiated host, have the capacity to home to the spleen PAL. There, they can be made to undergo blast cell transformation and the progeny can be shown to be capable of joining the recirculating pool (Miller and Mitchell, 1969). Whether the thymus influence is direct, as these studies seem to imply, or more indirect, the quantitative deficiency in the recirculating lymphocyte pool induced by thymectomy is a profound one. The rate of drainage of lymphocytes from the thoracic duct is 100-fold lower in neonatally thymectomized mice than in sham-operated controls (Miller and Mitchell, 1969).

It is also possible to approach the question of migration patterns of thymic cells by direct labeling experiments. One of us first studied this question in the guinea pig (Nossal, 1964), by injection of thymidine-³H directly into the thymic artery. This allowed specific labeling of dividing thymus lymphocytes and demonstration of export of such cells to the peripheral compartment, more extensive in newborn than adult animals. A more detailed study using direct labeling has been made by Weissman (1967), who labeled rat thymus cells *in situ* either by direct operative microinjections or by painting isotope on the surface of the organ. He showed an orderly movement pattern of thymus cells from near the capsule to deeper in the cortex, to the medulla, and finally to the thymus-dependent regions of the lymph nodes and spleen. Thymus-derived cells did not appear in follicles. All the exported cells were small lymphocytes and an orderly maturation sequence, lasting about 3 days in the thymus and followed by export, was suggested. Calculations showed that seeding from the thymus could account for a substantial proportion of all small lymphocytes in the peripheral compartment, provided their mean life-span was several weeks.

C. Thymus-Independent Lymphocytes

In contrast to the paucity of cells in the thymus dependent areas, the lymphoid follicles and medullary and red pulp cords of neonatally thymectomized animals develop normally. Indeed, they frequently exhibit intense activity, with abundant germinal center formation and plas-macytopoiesis, presumably as a result of the infections to which such animals are prone. In such animals, a functional relationship between the germinal centers and the plasma-cell rich cords seems especially plausible. Most of these mice have normal or heightened levels of circulating immunoglobulins (Humphrey *et al.*, 1964), and indeed their capacity to form antibodies against various types of test antigens remains unimpaired. This suggests that the universe of germinal center-medullary (or red pulp) cord cells is a thymus-independent (bone marrow-derived) system for humoral immunity, analogous to the bursal-dependent system of birds. However, unfortunately it is not yet possible to propose this as a universal rule, as humoral antibody formation against some test antigens is wholly or partially thymus-dependent. The nature of and reasons for the differences between various model systems is still obscure.

It has been observed that splenic germinal centers can be made to disintegrate following intensive antigenic stimulation (Hanna, 1965) and evidence has been presented that the pyroninophilic germinal center cells are caused to leave the center, transiently enter the marginal zone, and finally embark on plasmacytopoiesis in the red pulp cords. However, the specificity of such an effect is not clear. Moreover, many germinal centers exist in a steady state for long periods. They must export cells at a brisk rate, but the fate and function of these progeny cannot be charted by presently available techniques.

II. Functional Categories of Lymphoid Cells

Lymphoid cells are heterogeneous not only in their origins and migration patterns but also in their functions. In the absence of anything approaching a complete knowledge of the number and variety of functional categories, one is forced to describe them in terms of the various tests that have been used to delineate them. Table 6.I summarizes the situation at the present time.

Rather than commencing with the least differentiated compartment, as might be logical, we will begin with a description of the most differentiated cell, the antibody-forming cell, as we know far more about this category.

A. ANTIBODY-FORMING CELLS (FIG. 6.1)

Thanks to a variety of techniques which can detect antibody formation by single cells (Nossal and Lederberg, 1958; Jerne and Nordin, 1963;

Ingraham and Bussard, 1964), our knowledge of this category of cells is advanced, and one of us has discussed their properties at length elsewhere (Nossal and Mäkelä, 1962a). All antibody-forming cells appearing in a typical *in vivo* immune response are the results of antigen-induced mitotic division. If thymidine-^{3}H is given once (in sufficient quantity) at around the time of antigen injection, or repeatedly (in smaller amounts) between antigen injection and time of killing, all anti-

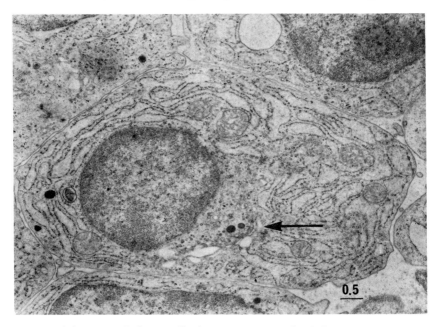

FIG. 6.1(a). A typical plasma cell. The arrow points to the Golgi region. Note extensive development of rough-surfaced endoplasmic reticulum and the eccentric nucleus.

body-forming cells formed in response to the antigen will be labeled. There exists a stage in the progressive maturation of antibody-forming cells where the cell can simultaneously prepare for division and secrete antibody. However, the fully differentiated, maximally synthesizing cells are end cells, incapable of further division (Mäkelä and Nossal, 1962). There is no agreement on the number of mitotic cycles involved in the development of an antibody-forming clone, estimates varying from 1 to 9 or 10. There is considerable variation in the ultrastructure of antibody-forming cells. One type, the plasma cell (Fig. 6.1a) is very characteristic, possessing an appearance similar to that of a secretory gland cell, including well-developed rough-surfaced endoplasmic reticulum and prominent Golgi apparatus. In addition, the nucleus occupies an eccentric position. Less mature variants of this cell are also readily recognized, being characterized by their larger size, larger nucleus with nucleoli, and less well-developed endoplasmic reticulum. However, there are also other types of antibody-forming cells which lack the features of the plasma cell family (Cunningham *et al.*, 1966; Hummeler *et al.*, 1966). (Fig. 6.1b); these are lymphocytes, but usually with a more

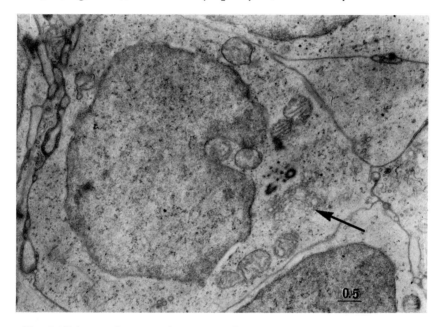

Fig. 6.1(b). Lymphocyte with numerous free polyribosomes, occasional profile of endoplasmic reticulum, also capable of antibody formation, particularly in primary antibody response. Arrow points to Golgi region.

abundant cytoplasm than the usual small lymphocyte. They possess abundant polyribosomes free in the cytoplasm. Many of these exhibit 5–7 or 15–18 ribosomes per polysome, probably representing the factories for the synthesis of the light and heavy chains of antibody, respectively (Williamson and Askonas, 1967; de Petris, 1967). The life-span of antibody-forming cells is highly variable. The median life-span of the antibody formers appearing during a typical intentional immunization is short—2 days or less for the rat (Nossal and Mäkelä, 1962b); that of plasma cells found in unimmunized animals, presumably representing cells forming antibody to natural antigenic stimuli is somewhat longer—

TABLE 6.I
CATEGORIES OF FUNCTION OF LYMPHOID CELLS

Type of cell	Test	Probable *in vivo* function
Antibody-forming cell	Hemolytic plaque tests[a]; immunocytoadherence[b]; immunofluorescence[c]; microdrop assays[d]; electron microscopic methods for detection of antibody complexes[e]	Release of humoral antibodies into circulation
Antigen-reactive cell (virgin or memory)	Hemolytic focus assay of Kennedy and Playfair[f]; other adoptive immunity tests	Cell not secreting antibody but capable of dividing on antigenic stimulation
Antibody-forming cell precursor	Complicated assays involving adoptive immunizations using mixtures of thymus-derived and bone marrow-derived cells[g]; not yet quantitative	Cell capable of dividing and yielding antibody-forming progeny, regarded by many authors as identical to antigen-reactive cell
Effector cell of cellular immunity	Macrophage migration inhibition test[h]; graft vs. host reactions[i]; including Simonsen-CAM test[j]; adoptive transfer of delayed hypersensitivity or graft rejection; *in vitro* damage to target cells[k]	Reaction with antigen leading directly or indirectly to tissue damage.
Colony-forming unit	Formation of colonies of erythroid and myeloid cells in irradiated spleens[l]	Precursor of normoblasts and myeloblasts; lymphocyte morphology inferred only.
Macrophage precursor	Chromosome analysis of dividing Kupffer cells in regenerating liver[m]	One type of precursor of macrophages
Bone marrow-derived precursors of thymus and lymph node cells	Parabiosis techniques[n]	True, self-perpetuating stem cell pool of the lymphoid system

[a] Jerne and Nordin, 1963; Ingraham and Bussard, 1964.
[b] Mäkelä and Nossal, 1961; Zaalberg, 1964; Biozzi *et al.*, 1966.
[c] Leduc *et al.*, 1955.
[d] Nossal and Lederberg, 1958; Attardi *et al.*, 1959.
[e] de Petris and Karlsbad, 1965.
[f] Kennedy *et al.*, 1966; Playfair *et al.*, 1965.
[g] Miller and Mitchell, 1969.
[h] David *et al.*, 1964.
[i] Simonsen, 1962.
[j] Boyer, 1960.
[k] Möller, 1968.
[l] Till *et al.*, 1964.
[m] Howard *et al.*, 1966.
[n] Moore and Owen, 1967b.

ca. 4 days; and a significant minority of antibody-forming cells is very long-lived. Such cells can maintain themselves and produce antibody for 6 months or more without division (Miller, 1964a). We know of no evidence that suggests that antibody-forming cells can cease to form antibody and commence to subserve another function, and for the moment feel that a reasonable hypothesis is to regard these as a highly specialized end stage of a particular line of differentiation, in principle not too different from a polymorphonuclear leukocyte, a macrophage, or even an erythrocyte.

The group of cells homogeneous in their function as antibody formers still displays great heterogeneity in a variety of measurable parameters, and we will consider this in Section III of this chapter.

B. Antigen-Reactive Cells (ARC)

1. Techniques for Enumeration

Populations of lymphocytes not synthesizing antibody in detectable amounts can be stimulated to form antibody by the action of antigen. The members of such a population which can be stimulated by a given antigen (be they frequent or infrequent) are termed antigen-reactive or antigen-sensitive cells. Considerable current research effort is being directed toward identifying such cells morphologically and obtaining them in pure suspension. Methods are now available which purport to be able to enumerate them with reasonable accuracy. The most important is the "hemolytic focus assay" of Kennedy et al. (1965) and Playfair et al. (1965), which has since been adapted to other antigens (Armstrong and Diener, 1969). This technique is as follows: The cell suspension to be tested for its content of antigen-reactive cells (ARC) is injected intravenously into a lethally irradiated mouse. A proportion of the cells reach the spleen, and this proportion can be measured by ways we will discuss shortly. The host animal is stimulated with an optimal dose of sheep red blood cells (SRBC). About 7–8 days later, it is killed and slices of the spleen are layered over agar containing SRBC and complement. After brief incubation at 37°C, areas of foci of lysis appear in the agar, and their number is linearly related to the number of cells injected. The number of such foci is believed to correspond to the number of cells in the original suspension which possess the power to interact with that particular antigen. It is also possible to take alternate spleens from a given experiment for assay of number of hemolytic foci, on the one hand, and number of antibody-forming cells (AFC), on the other, thus arriving at an estimate of the mean number of AFC per focus. With an inoculum of normal spleen cells, this is of the order of 100 AFC/focus.

A variation of this method, applicable to cells forming antibody against *Salmonella* flagellin, has been developed by Armstrong and Diener (1969). It depends on the inhibition of swarming motile bacteria in a semisolid medium by anti-H antibody. It has been used to show that the number of ARC is increased in a state of immunological memory and decreased in a state of specific tolerance.

Though the idea of this type of experiment is excellent, in practice its effectiveness is limited by both theoretical and technical problems. The hypothesis on which the technique rests demands an adjustment factor for the "homing efficiency" of the injected ARC. This can be measured by killing the first host at a fixed interval after injection of cells, e.g., 4 or 24 hr, and assessing the number of ARC in the first host's spleen by use of a second set of irradiated hosts. This experiment has yielded a "homing efficiency" of 5 to 10%. However, in fact, we know that ARC are in constant movement; it is by no means established that ARC present in the spleen 4 or 24 hr after injection will actually stay in that spleen and form a focus; and it seems highly probable that the final count of foci at 7–8 days after injection will represent a summation of highly asynchronous inductive events.

This difficulty is not as disturbing as the practical problem of confluence of foci. Unfortunately, the AFC presumed to be derived from a single ancestor do not stick together in a tight little clump. They disperse over a wide area, so that when a spleen is cut into, e.g., 25 slices, a focus may well be dispersed through four contiguous slices. In other words, when the number of foci exceeds 4, the whole spleen may give effects of confluent lysis. As the technique also has a certain "background," which may approach 1 focus/spleen, the range of effective readings is severely restricted, a difficulty not shared by the Armstrong variant. A further difficulty of the technique has been pointed out by Cunningham (1969a,b). When he performed adoptive transfers of numbers of cells capable of yielding 1–2 hemolytic foci per spleen, he obtained a poor correlation between the ability of spleen slices to form foci and the content of AFC in that focus. Using a somewhat different technique, he was able to show that the number of AFC in a focus varied enormously—from around 10 to 28,000 cells. Despite this variation, there was some evidence favoring the clonal nature of a focus. For example, the antibody specificity, size and appearance of plaques, and morphology of AFC at the center of the plaque were all more homogeneous among cells of a given focus than among AFC chosen at random.

With all its limitations, the technique can give reliable *relative* estimates of ARC content between different types of donor cell suspensions. It would appear on the basis of this type of test that in normal mouse spleen, ca. 1 cell in 50,000 is an ARC for those antigens on the surface of the SRBC, which are measured by the plaque test and the figure for flagellin-reactive cells is of the same order.

There are also many investigations which have sought to determine the antigen-reactivity of cell suspensions without attempting to place a number on their content of ARC. These are all the tests of adoptive immunization including diffusion chamber techniques (Nettesheim and Makinodan, 1965). The principle behind all these methods is similar. A population of cells currently making little or no antibody is placed into an "immunologically neutral" host and is antigenically stimulated. The response is studied by determining either the number of AFC appearing in, or the amount of antibody made by, the recipient animal.

2. "Virgin" ARC vs. "Memory" ARC

It is clear that the "antigen reactivity" of a population of lymphoid cells can rise after antigenic stimulation, i.e., that a second contact with antigen can elicit a greater reaction than the first. The details of the cellular basis on which this property of "immunological memory" rests are not established, but it is known that lymphoid cell populations from appropriately immunized animals possess an increased proportion of ARC for the antigen concerned. It has become customary to speak of these as "primed cells" or "memory cells," and of the ARC from an animal not intentionally preimmunized as "virgin" ARC. The question of whether there is any essential difference between these two categories of ARC is the subject of lively debate, and is not resolved. It is true that the secondary response *in vivo* is characterized by a number of features different from those of the primary, e.g., lower radiation and drug sensitivity, greater avidity of antibody formed, and lessened susceptibility to negative feedback by passive antibody or to tolerance induction by antigen excess. However, these *in vivo* differences do not prove a dependence of the secondary response on a special cell type. Many of them could be explained, as Siskind *et al.* (1966) have done, by postulating that the antigen given as a primary stimulus causes to proliferate a subset of antigen-reactive cells with surface receptors of high affinity for the antigen. In other words, the antigen selects out those cell clones capable of producing the most avid antibody. The "memory" cells, possessing extremely well-fitting receptors, might then appear to respond in a different fashion from the population of relatively poor mean affinity existing in a virgin animal. Only further research will resolve the issue.

An interesting set of experiments by Fazekas de St. Groth (1967) attest to the importance of memory cells. These relate to the phenomenon of "original antigenic sin." When an animal is primarily immunized with an antigen A and secondarily with a cross-reacting antigen B, the resulting antibody has far more specificity for A than for B. The simplest explanation of this seems to be that the population of memory cells (i.e., cells possessing anti-A specificity) outnumbers the population of virgin anti-B ARC, and that antigen B, through its cross-reactivity, can stimulate these memory cells to antibody formation.

3. Thymus–Bone Marrow Interactions

Until very recently, it has been universally assumed that the ARC was the immediate ancestor of all the AFC appearing in response to antigenic challenge. The first doubt was cast on this by experiments of Claman (Claman et al., 1966), who took two lymphoid tissues, thymus and bone marrow, each demonstrably low in its ability to transfer antibody-forming capacity against SRBC to irradiated hosts. Surprisingly, a mixture of thymus and bone marrow was much more active than would have been expected from a simple addition of the two individual response capacities. Much further light was shed on this apparent bone marrow-thymus interaction by the work of Miller and associates (Miller and Mitchell, 1968; Mitchell and Miller, 1968; Nossal et al., 1968c). Thoracic duct lymphocytes (TDL) had been regarded as the classical source of ARC. Miller et al. showed that while TDL were rich in their ability to cause the production of hemolytic foci of the Kennedy type, these foci were always small when compared with those induced with a splenic inoculum. An average TDL-derived focus possessed only 10 AFC. When TDL were mixed with bone marrow cells (BMC), the number of foci did not increase, but their average size rose by a factor of about 10, i.e., to 100 AFC per focus. Thus a collaboration had taken place between TDL and BMC, and chromosome marker studies showed that the majority of antibody-forming cells were in fact of bone marrow origin. Another interesting model involved the use of neonatally thymectomized hosts. At age 6–8 weeks, such animals give a much poorer response to the antigen SRBC than do sham-thymectomized mice. Their response capacity can be restored to normal not only by TDL but also by suspensions of thymus cells.

Analysis of the actual origin of the AFC in experiments using chromosomal markers or isoantisera showed that most, if not all, the AFC were derived from some cell type present *not* in the restorative inoculum but in the host. Presumably an interaction or collaboration had occurred between the donated thymus cells (or the thymus-derived TDL) and a lymphoid cell of host origin, probably a bone marrow-derived lymphoid cell. A variety of ingenious experiments showed : (1) that thymus cells multiplied in the spleen following antigen stimulation of the host; (2) that resultant progeny cells could enter the recirculating lymphocyte pool; (3) that the collaborative effect was antigen-specific and could not be due to some trephocytic function of the thymus cells; and (4) that the collaboration could be mimicked, at least in part, in a simple *in vitro* system.

Important work from a number of laboratories has substantiated the reality of the bone marrow–thymus collaborative effect for a variety of antigens (Davies *et al.*, 1967; Strober and Law, 1969; Taylor, 1969; Claman, 1970; Weigle, 1970). One important question which remains controversial is in which cell lines the immunological information for antibody synthesis rests. There appears to be consensus that the thymus-derived cell line is information-bearing, in as much as thymus-derived cells from tolerant animals fail to collaborate with bone marrow cells (Miller and Mitchell, 1969; Taylor, 1969; Weigle, 1970), and those from preimmunized animals are more effective than those from unimmunized donors (Cunningham, 1970). What is more controversial is whether the bone marrow-derived cell is similarly immunologically specific, perhaps with reactivity to a different set of antigenic determinants. Some experiments suggest that this is so (Weigle, 1970) but the possibility that information is passed from the thymus line to the bone marrow line has not been formally excluded. Operationally, for the SRBC system Miller has proposed that the thymus-derived cell can be termed the ARC and that the bone-marrow-derived cell which is the direct precursor of the AFC receive the name of antibody-forming cell precursor or AFCP. In this system, Miller believes that thymus is the chief source of ARC, bone marrow of AFCP, and TDL are a mixture of both types with a predominance of ARC. Another view which has been put forward by Mitchison (1970) is that the thymus-derived cell, though itself not secreting antibody, possesses antibody receptors on its surface which help in the correct "focusing" of antigen prior to stimulation of the bone marrow-derived cell. This "helper" function of the thymus-derived cell is conceived of as a specialized example of the well-known "carrier effect" in antigenic stimulation, which we must now consider.

4. Effects of the Carrier Portion of the Antigen Molecule in Immunogenicity

It has long been known that when one considers the formation of antibodies against a haptenic determinant, the nature of the carrier portion of the antigen is important in immunogenicity. In general, immunization proceeds much better if the carrier is a strong antigen. This "carrier effect" has been the subject of a number of detailed recent studies, all of which point to the conclusion that recognition of the foreignness of the carrier is vital for maximal antibody production against the hapten. For example, in quantitative studies of the effectiveness of antigens for *in vitro* stimulation of antibody production, Mitchison (1967) has shown that homologous hapten–protein conjugates are one-thousandfold more effective in stimulating antihapten antibody than conjugates of the hapten with some protein unrelated to the original carrier, even though the new carrier be a highly immunogenic molecule. If an animal is rendered tolerant to a carrier (Rajewsky *et al.*, 1967) or is genetically incapable of recognizing its foreignness (Benacerraf *et al.*, 1967), antibody production against a hapten associated with this carrier is hampered or abolished. In the description of many of these experiments, the term hapten has been used somewhat loosely. It is, in fact, more correct to refer to an antigenic determinant which is part of some larger antigen molecule. It is evident that a determinant regarded as the hapten in a particular experiment utilizing a particular antibody titration technique may serve as the carrier when the same complex antigenic molecule is used in a different experimental protocol. The key point is that the efficiency of antibody production to a particular determinant of the molecule may be influenced by the immunological status of the animal toward other determinants on the same molecule.

The most interesting aspect of this "carrier effect" that has recently come to light is that it may depend on thymus–bone marrow collaborations. The arguments leading to this conclusion are complex and, as yet, incomplete. The chief architect of this viewpoint has been Mitchison. First, he has shown the antibody production against a hapten can be aided by the presence of "helper cells" with immunological reactivity to the carrier (Mitchison, 1970). It is vital that such cells be antigenically stimulated, and the helper effect cannot be simulated by passively administered anticarrier antibody. Irradiated animals reconstructed with bone marrow can be "helped" to form antibody to a hapten by carrier-primed thymus-derived cells. Figure 6.2 gives the speculative interpretation favored by Mitchison (1970) He considers that the thymus-derived cell may have on its surface an antibody, perhaps of some unknown immunoglobulin class, which he has termed IgX. This is seen as uniting with the carrier portion of the antigenic molecule, leaving the haptenic group uncombined with antibody, but now linked to the thymus-derived cell. The migration pattern of this thymus-derived cell is seen as favoring the transport of the haptenic determinant to

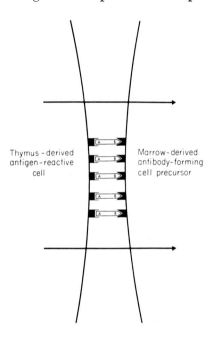

Thymus - derived antigen-reactive cell

Marrow-derived antibody-forming cell precursor

FIG. 6.2. The Mitchison-Taylor hypothesis to explain thymus–marrow collaboration in antibody formation. An antigen is pictured as having carrier determinant A and "immunodominant tip" B. The investigator monitors the production of anti-B antibody. The thymus-derived antigen-reactive cells, through its anti-A determinants, focuses B determinants onto the anti-B receptors of a marrow-derived, thymus-independent antibody-forming cell precursor. The arrows, not a necessary part of the scheme, indicate the possibility of added, nonspecific stimulatory factors. (After Taylor, 1969.)

the vicinity of the bone marrow-derived cell. In other words, the thymus collaborative effect is one of "antigen-focusing." On this view, both thymus and bone marrow cell lines are clonally individuated with respect to their surface receptors. The hypothesis demands that meetings between the two rare cell types (antihapten and anticarrier) be reasonably frequent, and Mitchison postulates that this is achieved through the specific movement patterns of the two lymphoid cell lines. One of the attractions of this hypothesis is that it brings together two obscure but important phenomena: the carrier effect and bone marrow–thymus collaboration. Further exploitation of the idea is awaited with interest.

C. OTHER CATEGORIES OF FUNCTION OF THE LYMPHOCYTE

This book will make no attempt to deal with the basis of delayed hypersensitivity, yet it is clear the effector cell which reacts with antigen and, probably by a complex chain reaction, causes tissue damage, is also a lymphocyte. Its formation is also the result of antigenic stimulation of certain lymphocytes, and the relationship of this type of ARC with those involved in antibody production is entirely speculative. It is by no means impossible that the one ARC can subserve both functions: to interact with antigen and BMC, promoting antibody formation by the latter; and, through blast cell transformation and division to produce a brood of progeny which are the effector cells of delayed hypersensitivity. In fact ARC, effectors of delayed hypersensitivity, and "memory cells," may all represent the same functional category, i.e., a small lymphocyte with a specific antibody on its surface, simply measured by a variety of distinct techniques. However, without further data, such speculation can hardly be very fruitful.

Table 6.I also lists some other cellular functions which we will not consider in detail. In each case, the morphology of the cell responsible is not known, but the presumption that one is dealing with a lymphocyte is strong. The table makes no pretence at completeness. It seems inevitable that as our knowledge of the lymphoid system increases, new functional categories will be defined. The small lymphocyte is, after all, little more than a nucleus with the most slender of cytoplasmic factories. Little wonder that its appearance gives no clue to its potential. For the same reason, biophysical separation of the various functional categories will be a most difficult task. Nevertheless, some progress has already been made. A number of authors have described means for fractionating lymphoid cell populations into morphologically or functionally distinct populations (reviewed in Gerritsen, 1969), but we will confine our attention to two methods devised by Shortman of our Institute (Shortman, 1966; 1968; Haskill, 1969) as they have been accomplished by a careful assessment of many functional parameters of the resulting cell fractions. The first method separates cells purely on the basis of size. It yields a population of "small lymphocytes" essentially free of cells capable of thymidine-^{3}H incorporation. The method involves passage of cell suspensions through columns of glass beads of defined size under carefully controlled conditions (Shortman, 1969a). The small lymphocytes obtained are active in the following functional tests: graft vs. host reactivity; capacity to transform into blasts following exposure to phytohemagglutinin; content of ARC cells, SRBC system in mice; production of proliferative foci on allogeneic transfer to chorioallantoic membrane in chickens. Interestingly, the small lymphocyte population is severely depleted in its ability to transfer adoptive immune capacity to the flagellar antigen of *Salmonella* bacteria, both as regards primary and secondary reactivity (Lewis *et al.*, 1969).

The second technique is probably of more general interest. It separates cells on the basis of their buoyant density in bovine serum albumin gradients (Shortman, 1969b). This technique has been applied to a search for the ARC in the SRBC system, and has shown the existence of multiple density peaks capable of transferring antibody-forming capacity adoptively. Ten hours after antigenic stimulation of the animal giving the cell suspension, the ARC are found mainly in two peaks of low density, one of which fails to appear if mitotic poisons are given (Haskill, 1969). This suggests that the ARC have transformed into blasts and have commenced to divide, the light density peaks corresponding to a pre- and a postmitotic phase. The existence of multiple peaks of ARC may be due to some degree of prestimulation of normal adult animals with antigens cross-reacting with SRBC. In general, the method has shown unexpectedly complex density profiles which further annotate the extreme heterogeneity of the lymphoid system. In general terms, it can be stated that biophysical techniques for the fractionation of lymphocytes into functionally more homogeneous subpopulations is a formidable task, not only because of the morphological similarities existing between cells with differing potential but also because of the tedious and complex nature of the bioassays needed to test the fractions. Yet it is only through painstaking work of this type that the various metabolic steps involved in induction of immunity will eventually be unraveled.

III. Heterogeneity among Antibody-Forming and Antigen-Reactive Cells

So far we have limited our attention to heterogeneities in the kind of physiological function with lymphoid cells subserve. We must now turn to another type of heterogeneity, dealing with differences within a single functional group, e.g., AFC or ARC. The most clear-cut information is available for AFC.

A. Heterogeneity among Antibody-Forming Cells

Shortly after Burnet published his clonal selection theory of antibody formation (Burnet, 1957, 1959), intense interest developed in the question of whether a single AFC cell could simultaneously manufacture more than one type of antibody. Nossal and Lederberg (1958) immunized rats with flagellar antigens of two serologically unrelated strains of *Salmonella* bacteria, incubated single lymph node cells in microdroplets, and studied the capacity of the nutrient medium to immobilize bacteria of the two serotypes. They found that all cells studied could immobilize only one type of bacterium and suggested that a single cell could make only one type of antibody. There followed a period of controversy (reviewed in Nossal and Mäkelä, 1962a) during which this problem was approached by many different techniques, but consensus now appears to have been reached that the great majority of cells form only one serological specificity at one time. Most investigators found a small minority of cells (usually less than 2%) that did not adhere to this rule, apparently making or containing two antibodies simultaneously. In our hands, these "double-producers" were always a little suspicious, in that they appeared to form standard amounts of one antibody and only trace quantities of the second. It is our impression that many of these apparent double-producers were methodological artifacts and it is possible that this was true also for many double-producers reported by other workers. It is of interest that no one has ever reported a cell seeming to make three antibody specificities simultaneously.

We now have many more markers available for assessment of homogeneity of antibody produced by a single cell that could be applied to the problem in our original studies of 1957. These include definition of the immunoglobulin class (Chiappino and Pernis, 1964), light chain type (Bernier and Cebra, 1964), allotype (Pernis and Chiappino, 1964), and electrophoretic mobility (Marchalonis and Nossal, 1968) of the antibody contained in or produced by a single cell. All of these studies have strengthened the notion of an extreme phenotypic restriction of synthetic capacity among single AFC. Thus, while each individual of a species can manufacture antibodies belonging to all the different classes and subclasses made by that species, most single cells make only one class. Within each class, light chains of kappa and lambda type can be found, but single cells make either kappa or lambda light chains and not both. Most interestingly, animals heterozygous for a given allotypic marker yield single AFC each making only one of the two allotypes, suggesting that only one of the two chromosomes of the cell is expressing its potential. Finally, when the electrophoretic mobility of antibody made by a single cell is examined, it is found to be just as homogeneous as a myeloma protein. At present time it thus seems reasonable to accept the probability that each antibody-forming cell makes a single, homogeneous population of protein molecules and that the great heterogeneity of antibodies made against a simple antigen mirrors a heterogeneity among the AFC producing them.

Interesting examples supporting this general concept come from the work of Mäkelä (1965, 1967). He studied antibody formation by single cells in microdroplets against bacteriophage antigens. First, he immunized animals against a phage serotype A, antisera against which cross-reacted to an approximately equal extent with the two related phages B and C. Then, he examined single cells from anti-A immune animals for their ability to produce anti-B and anti-C neutralizing antibody. Though the anti-B and anti-C antibody content of the serum was comparable, individual cells varied greatly in their relative abilities to neutralize B or C. Some produced high-titered anti-B antibody with little anti-C activity and some the reverse. Each cell had its characteristic anti-B:anti-C ratio, and only when all these were summed, did the ratio appear as 1. In a second study, Mäkelä showed the existence of a minority of cells which produced "heteroclitic" antibody, or antibody with a greater affinity for a cross-reacting phage than for the phage used as immunogen. This result strongly suggests that the cells concerned were expressing some preexisting potential, and is difficult to reconcile with any instructional theories of antibody formation.

One apparent exception to the rule that single cells form antibody of only one class deserves mention. In many primary immune responses, the first antibody produced is IgM and the synthesis of IgG follows somewhat later. In 1963, we examined the question of whether single cells can simultaneously manufacture IgM and IgG with identical serological specificity (Nossal et al., 1964c). We obtained results consistent with the possibility that a significant minority of cells taken from animals at the stage of immunization where the switch from IgM to IgG synthesis was occurring actually made both classes of antibody at one time. The idea was advanced that some cells switched from IgM to IgG synthesis. The methodology of this study was subject to certain limitations of which we were fully aware: it utilized 0.1 M 2-mercaptoethanol as a "specific"destroyer of IgM, and rabbit anti-rat 7 S globulin antisera of lesser specificity than would now be acceptable. Nevertheless, the results were very clear-cut and, to our knowledge, have not been specifically refuted though many authors have pointed to the theoretical difficulties posed by the hypothesis. This question deserves reexamination with currently available reagents. Some degree of support for the idea that a single cell can simultaneously produce two classes of immunoglobulin is given by studies of cloned lines of lymphocytes in tissue culture (Takahashi *et al.*, 1969a,b), although antibody specificity has not been claimed for such products. Oudin and Michel (1969) have shown that IgM and IgG antibodies from a single rabbit can share idiotypic specificities, this observation being consistent with the derivation of both cell lines from a single cell.

It is frequently asked whether a cell found to be producing a given antibody at one point in time might not be capable of forming a totally different one at a later stage in its life-span. In general, single, isolated AFC are difficult to maintain in a healthy state *in vitro* for more than a few hours, and thus the question has not been subjected to study. Even if the nature of the antibody made by the cell did not change, it could always be argued that events *in vivo* might have been different. In the absence of direct evidence, one must resort to indirect arguments. If such switching were a frequent event, perhaps "double-producers" ought to be found more frequently. Also, it seems part of the design of the normal immune response that certain cells are caused to proliferate and form a clone of progeny AFC. If switching of production from one type of antibody to another were possible and frequent at the single cell level, this design seems slow and clumsy. However, the question cannot be answered dogmatically at this time.

B. Heterogeneity among Antigen-Reactive Cells

Accepting that single cells synthesize only one type antibody at one time, the next problem to consider is whether the ARC and/or AFCP, the original stimulation of which led to the creation of the AFC, are likewise phenotypically restricted. Is there an inherent variation among ARC which makes one reactive to antigen A, another to B, and so forth? Putting this another way, is Burnet's clonal selection theory basically correct or not? This question is still debated in immunology, though clonal selection certainly has far more advocates at the time of writing than it did a decade earlier. The reason the question is so difficult to answer is because one does not know whether "commitment" of a given cell clone to a given pathway of synthesis precedes or follows antigenic stimulation. Cells might be "predestined" to react to a given antigen and to fail to react to others. Alternatively, cells might be inherently capable of reacting to all antigens, but might be preempted by their first antigenic contact, being incapable of subsequently reacting to other antigens.

One group of experiments is easier to explain on the former of the above two ideas. The same type of experiment has been done *in vivo* and *in vitro*, and involves the stimulation of ARC in limiting dilutions. *In vivo*, Playfair *et al.* (1965) and Cunningham (1969a,b) have taken two types of red blood cells as antigens, and have injected them into lethally irradiated mice together with sufficient numbers of lymphoid cells to cause the formation of hemolytic foci in the recipient's spleens. They were able to show that the distribution of foci of the two types (anti-RBC-A and anti-RBC-B) was independent, suggesting that different antigens "spoke to" different cells. The *in vitro* studies have been reported by Jerne (1969) and Osoba (1969). Normal mouse spleen cells were placed in tissue cultures of small volumes, ca. 250,000 cells per tube. The cultures were stimulated by either one or two types of RBC, and some days later, the number of AFC in each culture was determined. It was found that only about one-third of the cultures had responded to a given antigen, and the number of cultures responding to both antigens was no greater than could be expected by random chance. Moreover, when the cultures were exposed to only one antigen, there resulted two distinct populations of cultures—those in which there had been no response at all (i.e., no AFC found on harvest) and those in which 20–50 AFC appeared (suggesting development of a single clone analogous to the *in vivo* hemolytic foci). The results can be readily reconciled with the idea that some of the cultures had contained an appropriate ARC before antigenic stimulation, while others had not. Of course, other interpretations are tenable, and it would be most desirable to perform a classic Luria-Delbrück fluctuation test using the above sort of design. This would be possible only if a way could be found for ARC to be made to divide (and preserve their functional characteristics) without antigenic stimulation. There are reasons to believe that ARC do not divide without antigen, and thus proof of the above type may never be feasible. Finally, if antibody formation depends on a collaboration between two cell lineages, the arithmetic pertaining to the "number of different clones" in an animal becomes more complex. It is perhaps too easy to presume that an average of 1 hemolytic focus for every 50,000 cells that reach the spleen means that 1 in 50,000 of the cells is correctly "preadapted" to the antigens of SRBC. More probably, the number of foci depends on the frequency with which the correct type of bone marrow-derived cell lodges sufficiently close to the correct thymus-derived cell; and on the concomitant availability in the vicinity of an antigen depot adequate for proper stimulation of the clone. One can but hope that the gradual development of tissue culture methods for the study of antibody production will shed more light on this issue. All in all, however, experiments available at present point to at least some degree of heterogeneity of potential amongst the functional group of antigen-reactive cells. A key experiment difficult to reconcile with any theory except clonal selection will be described in detail in Chapter 9.

IV. Summary

This chapter considers some of the functions of lymphocytes. The great migratory power of these cells is described. It is shown that thymus-derived cells obey a particular migration pattern, tending to home to the diffuse cortical tissue of lymph nodes and the periarteriolar lymphocyte sheath region of the splenic white pulp. Bone marrow-derived (? bursal analog) lymphocytes are associated with germinal centers and plasma cell cords.

Turning to the different categories of lymphoid cells, it is becoming recognized that quite a variety of functions can be measured quantitatively. Most easily dealt with is the antibody-forming cell, thanks largely to the hemolytic plaque technique. A clearly separable function is that of antigen reactivity or the capacity of a cell to react specifically to antigen by proliferation, the events finally leading to antibody production. In some systems, it is becoming clear that a full immune response depends on a collaboration between antigen-reactive cells and a second category that has been termed antibody-forming cell precursor. These three functions of lymphoid cells are considered in detail, and several others are dealt with more briefly.

Within the groups of antibody-forming cells and antigen-reactive cells, residual heterogeneity is to be found. Each antibody-forming cell is highly specialized to the production of an extremely homogeneous protein, restricted with respect to electrophoretic mobility, antigen-combining specificity, immunoglobulin class, light chain type, and allotype. The heterogeneity of most antibody populations raised against even simple antigens reflects a heterogeneity in the antibody-forming cell population. There are some indications that the antigen-reactive cells are similarly restricted and heterogeneous, but these are, as yet not so firmly based.

It is inevitable that this chapter, which attempts to give an outline of the physiology of the whole lymphoid apparatus, will overlap to a certain extent with material to be presented in Chapters 7 and 9, and the problem of heterogeneity in antigen-reactive cells will certainly engage us again.

CHAPTER 7

MICROSCOPIC AND ELECTRON MICROSCOPIC DISTRIBUTION OF ANTIGEN IN LYMPHOID ORGANS

I. Background Information

While antibody formation of classic type occurs only in vertebrates, entry of antigens from the environment must have posed a threat to bodily integrity in even the most primitive of life forms. Thus means for disposal of foreign organisms and molecules have evolved over a much longer period than the means by which these same foreign entities cause stimulation of lymphocytes to antibody formation. The latter should, in the broadest sense, be regarded as a by-product of phylogenetically more primitive disposal mechanisms. This is the reason why the systematic study of where and how antigen exerts its immune inductive effect is so difficult. As has already been discussed in Chapter 4, it is probable that the great majority of the antigen molecules which enter the body are degraded and disposed of without ever impinging on the immune apparatus. The job of stimulation is left to the minority of molecules which find themselves in the "right" place at the "right" time, possibly after the "right" processing. To inject antigen, to detect it later in the body by some sensitive technique, and to study its histological distribution is no great feat; to arrive at a knowledge of what this antigen is doing to lymphoid cells by the same methods is much more difficult.

Before 1963, when we began our series of studies on the fate of antigens after injection, considerable background knowledge was available on the histological distribution of antigens in lymphoid tissues, obtained almost exclusively by histochemical techniques and especially by fluorescent antibody methods (Kaplan et al., 1950). These had revealed the great antigen-capturing power of the macrophages present, especially in the lymph node medulla. This capacity of macrophages to trap and retain antigens was so striking that the notion that the same macrophages must also be the cells which subsequently formed antibody appears to have gone unchallenged until the 1940's when attention was directed toward plasma cells (Fagraeus, 1948).

In contrast, the question of an association between antigen and lymphoid cells (either antibody-forming cells or their precursors) after injection of antigen in vivo had received scant attention. The sole article of major relevance was one by Roberts and Haurowitz (1962). They had immunized mice by four injections of ^{3}H-labeled aniline azoporcine γ-globulin, or arsanilazo porcine γ-globulin, and studied the cellular distribution of these antigens by radioautography. This particular antigen was found to be spread widely through lymphoid tissues, and label was found associated with many cells including antibody-forming cells. The wide distribution of the antigen and the protocol involving several successive antigen injections prevent one from ascribing any inductive function to the antigen in or on antibody-forming cells. There was also brief reference in the work of Coons' group to antigen present in lymph node follicles, which they believed to be in small lymphocytes (Kaplan et al., 1950). In all, the questions of where antigen-reactive cells encountered antigen, of how much became attached to or entered them, and how much remained associated with the eventual antibody-forming cells at the various stages of their progressive maturation remained entirely open. In contrast, in our work on the fate of antigens and in a large body of other work published concomitantly since 1963, these questions became the primary object of study. We consider it helpful to begin our detailed description of this work with a brief summary of the most important findings.

II. Chief Features of Antigen Capture in the Mammalian Lymphoid System

(1) All materials injected subcutaneously and traveling to a draining lymph node, enter medullary macrophages of lymph nodes. The rate of elimination of ingested materials from macrophages varies greatly, but the degree of trapping and rate of degradation show no consistent relationship with the inherent immunogenicity of the materials.

(2) The degree to which injected materials permeate diffusely into the extracellular fluid bathing lymphocytes in the cortex of lymph nodes or white pulp of spleen also varies greatly. It is minimal or nonexistent with particulate antigens, and less extensive with soluble molecules that are immunogenic than with less potent antigens of equivalent molecular weight. Foreign serum protein antigens permeate particularly extensively before the commencement of antibody formation.

(3) There are two sites in lymph nodes where long-term antigen retention may occur: the medullary macrophages and the lymphoid follicles; there are also two in the spleen: the marginal zone and the lymphoid follicles.

(4) Retention of antigens in macrophages as opposed to follicles depends on different mechanisms. Retained antigen in macrophages is mainly in phagocytic vacuoles though some may remain at or near the cell surface; that in follicles is extracellular and membrane-associated, lying chiefly attached to the surface of dendritic reticular cells with long, thin processes.

(5) Follicular antigen trapping, but not medullary antigen capture, is dependent on the presence of antibody. Many antigens are specifically localized in follicles only after antibody formation has been induced, or if passive antibody has been administered. Other antigens are localized rapidly in follicles even following their first injection; this is probably due to the presence of "natural" antibody in the animal. The association probably depends on some attachment site situated on the Fc portion of the globulin molecule linked to antigen (see Chapter 3).

(6) In lymphoid tissues, cells engaged in antibody production are found in areas which are not sites of antigen concentration; and conversely antigen depots may be found where no antibody-forming cells exist.

(7) In ontogeny, the capacity for antigens to be localized in follicles precedes the appearance of germinal centers. In phylogeny, antigen-retaining mechanisms characterized by membrane-binding of antigen antedate the appearance of germinal centers.

Key information relative to antigen content of antibody-forming cells will be dealt with in Chapter 9, and to questions of immunological tolerance in Chapter 10.

III. Design of Experiments to Study Antigen Action *in Vivo*

The ideal method for the study of antigen distribution after injection would be one in which the fate of every single antigenic determinant could be charted. Clearly the only methodology of relevance involves radiolabeled antigens and radioautographic detection methods. Though reasonably high specific activities of labeling of antigens can be achieved with isotopes such as ^{3}H and ^{35}S, the labeling method which most closely approaches the desired goal is radioiodination of antigens with carrier-free preparations of ^{131}I or ^{125}I, most conveniently by the direct chloramine-T oxidation technique of Greenwood *et al.* (1963), or one of its modifications (McConahey and Dixon 1966). This method is of particular value when the labeled iodine atom is actually a part of the antigenic determinant under study. In fact, specific activities of labeling high enough to approach the ideal level can be reached (Humphrey and Keller, 1970), but unfortunately such preparations are not immunogenic, presumably because they induce radiation damage in lymphocytes exposed for long periods to the isotope (see also Chapter 9), and so there would be little point in studying their fate. In practice, most studies in this field have used degrees of labeling such that between one per hundred and one per thousand of the amino acids of the marked antigen was a radioactively labeled tyrosine or histidine residue.

A second feature of importance in experimental design is the dose and nature of antigen used. Unfortunately, most of the antigens commonly used in immunological experiments, such as hapten–protein conjugates, serum proteins, or synthetic polypeptides, are of rather low inherent immunogenicity. Thus, to achieve significant antibody formation, the investigator must usually administer milligram quantities of antigen, and frequently on several occasions and with adjuvants. As a sufficient degree of labeling of such antigens would involve the administration of several Curies of radioactivity, it is scarcely possible from a practical point of view to proceed. A different category of antigens is that of natural bacterial or viral products. Proteins such as bacterial flagellin or phage tail fiber protein and carbohydrates such as bacterial wall polysaccharides are immunogenic in picogram amounts. They thus present attractive practical and theoretical features for antigen-tracing work. Whatever the antigen used, it is important that the investigator chooses the smallest dose that can achieve the desired immunological result, be this antibody formation in a primary response, the triggering of a secondary response, or the induction of immunological tolerance. Even when very small doses are used, it is clear that much of the antigen eventually found in radioautographs is "waste," essentially irrelevant to the inductive process (Dixon and McConahey, 1970). Naturally, this problem is exaggerated when supraoptimal antigen doses are used. When this is necessary because of some limitation of isotope detection methodology, great care must be used in interpretation of results.

In much of our work, we have used as model antigens the various flagellar preparations of *Salmonella adelaide*, usually labeled so that between 1 and 10 molecules of flagellin contained 1 atom of radioactive iodide. Animals were killed at intervals of 3 min to 32 weeks after injection of a single dose of labeled antigen, usually given in saline without adjuvants. For the study of lymph node localization of antigen, injections were given subcutaneously into the hind footpads and the popliteal node was the chief organ examined. For experiments involving splenic antigen trapping, intravenous immunization was used. Experiments in which light microscopic radioautography only was intended, formolsaline fixed specimens were processed by usual techniques for paraffin embedding except that radioactivity measurements were routinely made at the beginning and end of processing; and sections (cut at 5μ) were dipped in Kodak NTB-2 emulsion for radioautography, usually for an exposure period of one half-life, i.e., 60 days. Electron microscopic experiments were performed on specimens half of which were fixed in glutaraldehyde with osmic postfixation and half with osmium tetroxide. Radioautography was by the method of Salpeter and Bachmann (1964) using Kodak NTE emulsion. Details of the radioautographic techniques are given in Appendix II. Special care was taken to ensure that electron microscopic fields could be accurately oriented with respect to matching thick sections so that at all times one knew the area of lymphatic tissue under study.

Humphrey and collaborators (McDevitt *et al.*, 1966; Humphrey and Frank, 1967; Humphrey *et al.*, 1967; Humphrey 1969; Janeway and Humphrey, 1969) have performed an extensive series of investigations using as antigen a branched multichain polypeptide synthesized from l-lysine, l-tyrosine, l-glutamic acid, and tritium-labeled DL-alanine ([3]HTGAL). They have compared the distribution of this substance to that of ^{125}I-labeled TGAL. Both radioactively labeled antigens localized in qualitatively similar manner. Gross retention studies showed a somewhat faster rate of disappearance of ^{125}I than of ^{3}H, probably because of a greater susceptibility to peptidase activity of the L-tyrosine residues (at the ends of side chains) than that of the underlying polymeric DL-alanine. In general, the similarity of labeling patterns has been cited as encouraging evidence in favor of the basic validity of studies using external labeling with iodine.

Labeled antigens have been used extensively by Askonas and colleagues (Argyris and Askonas, 1968; Askonas et al., 1968; Askonas, 1970) in essentially biochemical studies of the role of macrophages in immune induction. These findings are considered chiefly in Chapter 8 but some most interesting work with ^{125}I-labeled hemocyanin will concern us here. Other model systems to which we shall refer have used ^{125}I-human γ-globulin, horse ferritin, human and bovine serum albumin, various immunoglobulin fragments and chains, and a variety of synthetic products.

It is important to know the exact sensitivity of the radioautographic method used in antigen tracing work, and thus in collaboration with Dr. Humphrey's group we performed a series of model experiments in which silver grain counts in a radioautographic emulsion were calibrated against known isotope amounts in an underlying protein film (Ada et al., 1966). Important variables included the nature of the isotope, the thickness of the labeled specimen, and the emulsion used. Armed with such calibrations, reasonably accurate antigen concentrations in certain cells and regions could be established for most experiments.

IV. Antigen Capture in the Lymph Node Medulla

A. MEDULLARY MACROPHAGES

In the flagellar system, transport of antigens from the hind footpad to the medulla of the popliteal node was remarkably rapid. Three minutes after the injection, even when minute volumes only of fluid had been injected, isotope had reached the node and was prominently visible in radioautographs of the afferent lymphatics and circular sinus. Some medullary sinuses filled directly from the circular sinus, especially near the hilum of the node where the efferent lymphatic vessel leaves. These hilar medullary areas or "poles" of the node were the first to be labeled, macrophages here being found to contain antigen about 5 min after injection. Both the number of labeled macrophages and the mean intensity of labeling of macrophages increased rapidly, reaching maximal intensity 1–2 hr after antigen injection. After this, antigen left the medulla very slowly, the biological half-life being 2 to 3 weeks with a suggestion that the half-life might be even longer after the first week had elapsed.

The electron microscopic radioautographs gave a detailed picture of the sequence of events in macrophages (Nossal et al., 1968a). As these are of some general biological interest apart from their possible significance to immunology, they are described in some detail (Figs. 7.1 and 7.2). Two basic mechanisms of entry of labeled material into the cell seemed to be at work: pinocytosis, and a more controversial phenomenon, namely direct penetration of the plasma membrane of the cell without detectable vacuole formation. The pinocytosis followed the classic sequence of plasma membrane indentation, formation of caveolae, and pinching off of the inverted plasma membrane resulting in the formation of a pinocytic vacuole. The size of vacuole formed at the cell surface varied within the wide limits of approximately 40 to 500 mμ. The other mechanism of entry, direct penetration of antigen through the plasma membrane, was thought to occur because of the frequent finding, at 10 to 60 min after antigen injection, of significant label in areas of cytoplasm where there was no visible vesicle or granule. This finding might have been due to rupture of certain vesicles during fixation or failure to identify unit membrane components because of tangential sections. We felt it was important to know whether antigens ever enjoyed a period of lying free in the cytoplasm of macrophages; if so, one could imagine that three-dimensional antigenic configurations could come in contact with some sterically complimentary macromolecule, e.g., RNA. If, on the other hand, antigen were, from the moment of its initial entry into the cell, separated from the actual cytoplasm and sequestered in a digestive vacuole, it is more difficult to imagine how the original antigenic configurations could interact with macrophage macromolecules, as proteolysis would soon begin to destroy tertiary structure. The question of membrane penetration and free sojourn in the cytoplasm of entering antigen could not be answered unequivocally with radioautographic techniques, so we turned to another marker antigen, ferritin. This is a protein molecule with high iron content (up to 23%) which endows it with good marker qualities for electron microscopy. Investigations with this antigen again revealed a proportion of phagocytic cells with aggregates of antigen molecules apparently lying free, i.e., without surrounding membrane, in the cytoplasm. However, current studies involving serial sections appear to support the view that the appearance

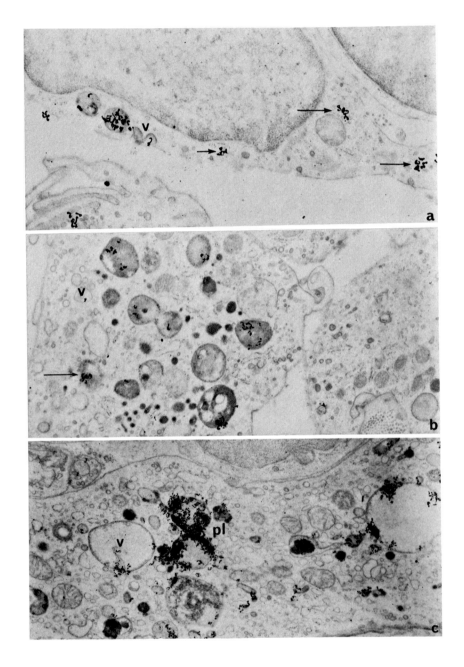

See facing page for legend→

of such accumulations is dependent on the plane of section. Succeeding sections through a "free" aggregate eventually display a tangentially sectioned membrane indicating immurement of the conglomerate antigen molecules. Nevertheless, the concept of plasmalemmal penetration cannot yet be dismissed in view of the not infrequent finding of an inclusion-laden cell which also exhibits individual ferritin molecules diffusely spread throughout the ground substance of the cytoplasm, yet with the mitochondria and nucleus remaining completely free of marker. There is, as yet, no explanation for this phenomenon but the possibility of some other type of artifact cannot be ignored.

Returning to antigen that enters cells by pinocytosis, it is clear that this is soon subjected to lysosomal action. A frequent appearance between 30 min and 4 hr after antigen injection was a cluster of small, electron-opaque vesicles (protolysosomes) around an antigen-containing pinocytic vacuole. Areas of fusion became progressively more frequent, the result being the formation of a more electron-opaque granule resembling in all details the acid hydrolase-containing lysosomes described by other authors (Gordon et al., 1965; Cohn et al., 1966). This activation of the lysosome-generating mechanism of the cell, and the rapidity of specific morphological changes around and within the pinocytic inclusion represent fascinating phenomena. By what mechanisms does the cell sense the presence of antigen within it?

The original "phagolysosomes" having been formed, the subsequent morphologically observable history of the cell is a story of progressive vacuolar fusion. This process resulted in the formation of larger and

---

FIG. 7.1. Examples of ingestion of flagellar antigens by lymph node medullary macrophages. Technique of electron microscopic radioautography using ^{125}I-labeled flagella and electron microscopic radioautography of ultrathin sections. (a) Thirty minutes after antigen injection. The arrows point to areas where antigen appears to be lying free in the cytoplasm, but serial sections would be needed to show whether these were inclusions or not. V, represents pinocytic caveolae and vesicles. ×16,000. (b) Thirty minutes after antigen injection; this is to show commencement of fusion of pinocytic vacuoles. The arrow points to an area where serial sectioning would probably show membrane profiles. Note the way that small vesicles are clustering around larger inclusions, probably prior to fusing with them. ×13,000. (c) Twenty-four hours after antigen injection. The vacuoles (v) contain an electron-opaque layer just inside their limiting membrane; most of the antigen is attached to or close to the wall. In the region marked pl, we appear to be watching the imminent fusion of at least eight inclusions, including two large ones, into a phagolysosome. Note that discrete, rounded electron-opaque entities are still visible within the larger vacuoles. The cytoplasm also includes numerous smaller labeled inclusions of varying sizes and degrees of electron opacity. The appearance is most characteristic of the 1-day time point. ×13,000.

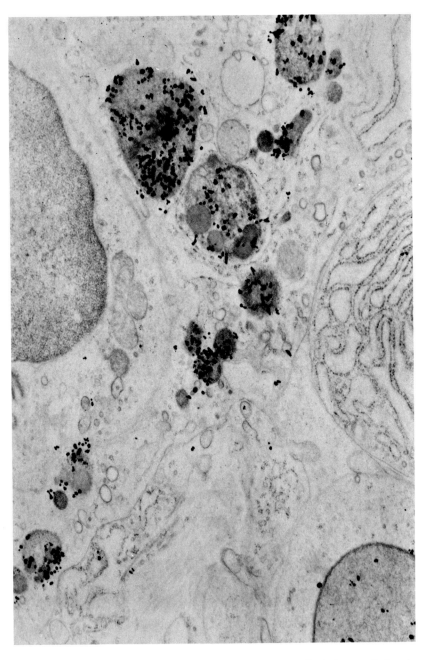

See facing page for legend→

more complex inclusions (phagolysosomes) displaying great variety in size and detailed ultrastructure. In many cases (Figs. 7.1c and 7.2) the appearances suggested temporary preservation of the integrity of smaller dense bodies even though they had fused with larger vacuoles. Flagella must be rather difficult for the cell to digest, because even 6 weeks after injection, electron micrographs showed persisting large inclusions which at times exceeded 5 μ in diameter and which were filled with a variegated, inhomogeneous electron-opaque material of flagellar origin. The digestive inclusions formed after injection of ferritin showed basic similarities to the above picture. At early time points, much ferritin is seen free in the sinus lumen and many examples of early stages of endocytosis are evident. As early as 10 min after injection, examples of fusion of dense bodies and ferritin-laden vesicles can be encountered. Our electron microscopic studies with ^{125}I-monomeric flagellin have been much less extensive, but strongly suggest that the basic sequence of events in macrophages is not very different from that seen with flagella. From the limited material we have examined, it appears that the late inclusions are not of as great a degree of size and complexity as with the carbohydrate-containing, particulate flagella.

We must turn now to a phenomenon not yet noted in lymph node macrophages but of great potential importance. It involves peritoneal macrophages fed ^{125}I-labeled proteins *in vivo* and subsequently observed in tissue culture (Unanue and Askonas, 1968b; Unanue and Cerottini, 1970). Peritoneal macrophages take up antigen and rapidly catabolize 80 to 90% of the foreign proteins by the lysosome mechanism which we have already discussed. However, a small proportion of the foreign material is maintained in and on the cell in what appears to be a bound form, protected from rapid catabolism. It appears to be this portion which allows an interaction between macrophage and lymphoid cell to be followed by antibody production. Electron microscopic radioautographs have shown that much of this fraction was present in close association with the cell membrane, and could be removed by trypsinization. Such treatment did not affect lysosome-located antigen, but did reduce the immunogenic potency of the antigen-containing macrophages. This

---

Fig. 7.2. Radioautograph of section of lymph node medulla 3 days after antigen injection. The broad process of a heavily labeled macrophage protrudes between a plasma cell at right and a lymphocyte with distinct centriole at left, and continues on to bottom left. At bottom right is portion of another macrophage with a somewhat unusual inclusion. Note the varied size, shape, and ultrastructural features of the labeled inclusions. A few single grains are also present, including one in the plasma cells; these may well represent background or isotope scatter. ×21,125.

striking observation, made using hemocyanin-^{125}I is in complete contrast to the situation with flagellar antigens and ferritin in lymph node (rather than peritoneal) macrophages. It is clear that surface-located nondenatured antigen in or on macrophages could play a vital role in stimulating lymphocytes which it might contact. The further development of this work is awaited with interest.

B. Anatomical Relationships between Macrophage and Lymphoid Cells

In both sinuses and cords, medullary macrophages come into close contact with lymphoid cells of various sorts. We have tried to see if there is any systematic sequence of changes in the relationship between these two cell types in the medulla during the early, inductive stages of the immune response. Examples of phenomena which could have pointed to a special role of macrophages in induction of antibody formation include: (1) presence of lymphocytes around macrophages forming a "rosette;" (2) blast cell transformation specifically in those lymphocytes which were close to macrophages; (3) formation of cytoplasmic bridges between macrophages and plasma cells or lymphocytes. No evidence for any event of this type was obtained. Occasionally, an antigen-containing macrophage was seen surrounded on all sides by plasma cells, but more characteristically, large numbers of unlabeled plasma cells were seen without a macrophage profile in the vicinity. Inversely, contiguous sheets of heavily labeled macrophages could be seen on some sections without any significant crowding of lymphoid cells around them. For a variety of reasons, such negative observations cannot be considered as too compelling. In even the most extensive series of electron microscopic experiments, the sampling problem is serious. Moreover, details of cell proximity could only be judged on the basis of extensive serial section work, which has not been performed. Finally, it is not excluded that fragmented antigen or antigen-RNA complexes could leave macrophages and travel long distances extracellularly to reach and to stimulate lymphoid cells. Thus one can by no means eliminate an important role for macrophage-processed antigen. However, the lack of detailed anatomical correlation between antigen deposition and subsequent lymphoid proliferation in the medulla stands in obvious contrast to the situation in the cortical lymphoid follicles which we will shortly describe.

Some studies have found extensive antigen localization in eosinophils in lymph nodes (Roberts, 1966a). We have occasionally seen some label over tiny vesicles in eosinophils, always less intense than that over macrophages, and never involving the characteristic eosinophilic granule. In all, radioautographic studies have not shed much light on the role of the eosinophil in the induction of antibody formation. Neutrophils also play a definite, though transient role in antigen capture, particularly in the spleen. Neither type of polymorph, however, displays the long-term antigen retaining powers of either follicles or macrophages (see Chapter 8).

C. Antibody-Forming Cells

In Chapter 9, we will be dealing extensively with the question of entry of antigen into antibody-forming cells and their precursors. Here we need only consider the question of antigen distribution to those areas and cells in which antibody formation is known or believed to occur. The chief of these are the medullary cords of lymph nodes and the red pulp cords of the spleen. In these areas, pyroninophilic cells that are probably antibodyformers can be seen in great numbers in both light and electron microscopic sections. Radioautographs occasionally show isolated grains over such cells, but the numbers and distribution of the grains suggest that this is not a specific phenomenon in most cases. After injection of some labeled antigens (serum albumins, ferritin) the grains can be seen diffused extremely widely at early time points after injection. Label is found in and on antibody-forming cells, but not at a higher concentration than with any other cell type. With particulate antigens, the scarcity of label over plasma cells is a notable feature. In fact, the only cells having grains over them are those which lie close to a labeled macrophage. In these cases, label is most likely due to electrons taking an oblique path from the macrophage, giving "false" labeling of the adjacent cell. This whole question is more appropriately attacked by single cell methods, as we shall see in Chapter 9.

An elegant portion of the work of Humphrey's group (McDevitt et al., 1966) was to combine radioautographic study of antigen localization with immunofluorescent study of antibody synthesis. Unfortunately, the latter was possible only for the secondary response to the antigen ^{125}I-TGAL. It was found that antibody-forming cells had, in fact, slightly less than the average background level of grains over them, just as was the case in the flagellar system. Wellensiek and Coons (1964) found scattered ferritin molecules in plasma cells presumed to be forming anti-ferritin antibody, though other authors (de Petris and Karlsbad, 1965; Buyukozer et al., 1965) have failed to note this after the use of ferritin

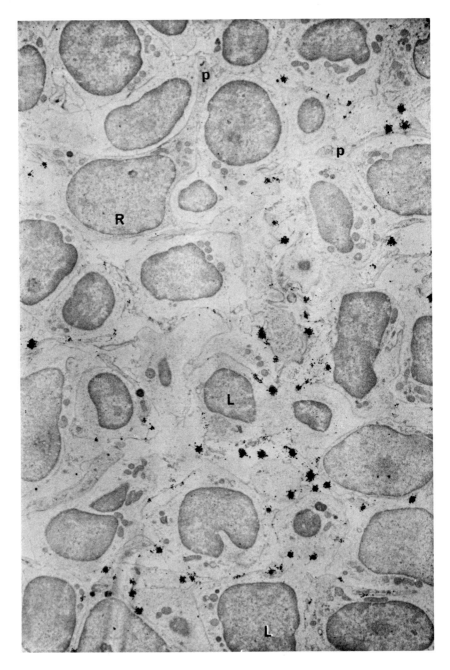

See facing page for legend→

as antigen. In view of the large ferritin doses used and the slow clearance rate of this antigen after first injection, a diffuse spread is not surprising and cannot be taken to indicate a role of intracellular antigen in immune induction. Similar arguments apply to the work of Roberts (Roberts and Haurowitz, 1962; Roberts, 1966b) who used tritiated azoprotein antigens.

V. Antigen Capture by the Lymph Node Follicle

A. GENERAL CONSIDERATIONS

We have already dealt with the structure of lymphoid follicles in Chapter 5, but considerable further information on these complex entities can be obtained by the use of labeled antigens. Examples illustrating the role of follicles in antigen capture are given in Figs. 7.3 to 7.5.

The first mention of localization of antigens in lymphoid follicles came from Coons' group (Kaplan et al., 1950). Mellors and Brzosko (1962) were the first to note the trapping of injected antigen–antibody complexes in germinal centers. White (1963; White et al., 1967) not only described the retention of antigen by cells in germinal centers but also drew attention to the fact that the pattern of localization differed from that exhibited by normal macrophages in that the injected material appeared to be in long fine dendritic cell processes. All these three studies had been conducted using immunofluorescent staining techniques. Using radioautographic methods and radioiodinated antigens, we independently confirmed the chief anatomic features reported by White, and added the observation that antigens become localized in primary follicles as well as germinal centers (Nossal et al., 1964b,c). However, by far the best delineation of the nature of the antigen-retaining structures in follicles can be obtained by electron microscopic radioautography, and the anatomical descriptions which follow depend largely upon the use of this technique (Nossal et al., 1968a,b).

The rate of entry of antigens into follicles depends on the antigen used and on the level of antibody against it which exists in the serum

FIG. 7.3. A typical pattern of localization of antigen in a primary lymphoid follicle. Even at low power, reticular cells (R) and their processes (p) can be distinguished. Numerous small lymphocytes (L) are present, but there are no blasts, mitotic figures, or "tingible body" macrophages. Note that the heavy clumps of label are located between cells and that there is an absence of heavy deposits within lymphocytes. ×5280.

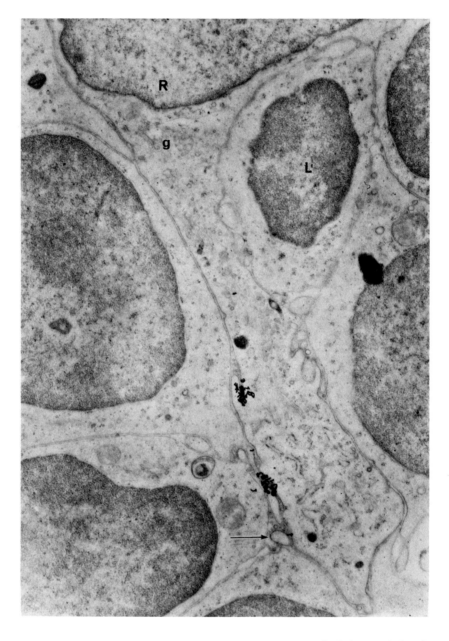

See facing page for legend→

(vide infra). There are circumstances, such as the injection of flagellar antigens into preimmunized animals, when the process is essentially complete within 2 to 4 hr (Nossal *et al.*, 1965b). This allows detailed examination of the sequence of events leading to localization. The antigen which arrives in the node via the afferent lymphatics is mainly unassociated with phagocytic cells. It enters the circular sinus and, if complexed with antibody, very rapidly begins to penetrate the lymph node cortex. A small proportion enters the phagocytic sinus lining cells (see Chapter 5) but much more percolates between the cells and, 15 min or so after antigen injection, can be found in the intercellular spaces between the lymphocytes lying superficial to the lymphoid follicles. This region is usually only two to six cells deep, yet antigen can be significantly retarded here. It is not till 1 hr or so after injection that significant amounts of label can be found in the follicle itself. The detailed pattern of movement from the perifollicular region into the follicle involved a progressive penetration not only from the overlying sinus region but also an encroachment from the sides. Radioautographs of lymph node sections taken about 1 hr after injection of labeled flagella into preimmunized animals frequently showed a ring of label around the follicle, with a small portion beginning to penetrate the follicle. Electron micrographs revealed that at such times the antigen was lying between the lymphocytes bordering the follicle.

At later time points, a difference in labeling pattern between primary and secondary follicles became manifest. This difference was more readily apparent in light than in electron microscopic radioautographs. Primary follicles showed uniform labeling over the whole of their extent; in secondary follicles, though antigen did penetrate diffusely, the highest concentration was usually reached in the caplike region rich in reticular cells which lies at the surface of the follicle. Germinal centers were not grossly more active in antigen capture than the smaller, less prominent primary follicles. Considerable quantitative variation existed in the

FIG. 7.4. Higher power view of portion of a primary follicle includes a reticular cell (R) and several lymphocytes (L). The cytoplasmic process of the reticular cell extends from its source at top, where there is a prominent Golgi region (g) in the paranuclear zone, to bottom right where the terminal region displays the characteristic hyaloplasm so frequently observed when the ends of fine processes are viewed in transverse section: several of these fine processes ranging in size down to less than 100 mμ diameter, can be seen (arrow). Note the two heavy clumps of label on or near the plasma membrane at surface invaginations. Even where it is widest, the process contains only occasional dense granules in contrast to medullary macrophages and it makes close contact with at least five lymphocytes in this short extent of its length. ×17,500.

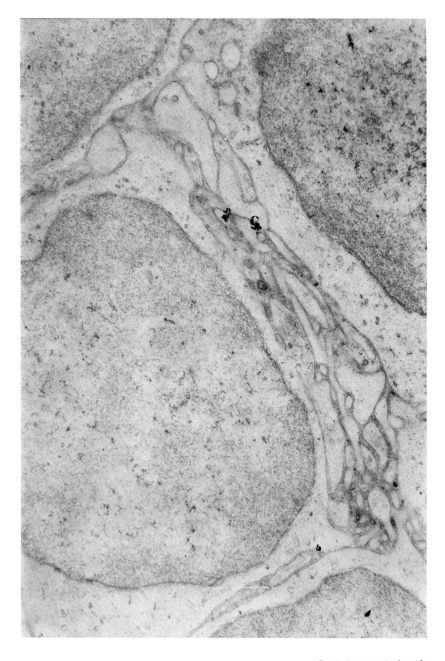

See facing page for legend→

intensity of labeling between different follicles. However, with adequate antigen doses and labeling intensities it soon became apparent that every follicle in a node could trap some of the injected antigen. We showed that radioautographic methods were about 10,000 times more sensitive in their ability to demonstrate follicular antigen retention than were immunofluorescent methods (Miller and Nossal, 1964), so it is not surprising that this fundamental point was missed by earlier workers who used the latter technique. It is difficult to escape the conclusion that the antigen-trapping mechanism of follicles shows no antigen specificity.

Injection either of labeled antigen into specifically immunized animals or of antigen-antibody complexes into unimmunized animals has shed considerable light on the nature of primary follicles. Germinal centers are obvious structures; every immunologist interested in cells knows their characteristics. Primary follicles are much less obvious. Usually an experienced histologist can recognize their presence in a section, either because they appear as a spherical aggregation of lymphocytes somewhat more dense than the surrounding cortex, or because of a slight bulging of the overlying sinus region. Sometimes, as in the spleen, the follicle is literally indistinguishable on standard histological examination. We have read claims in the literature that a particular strain of animal "does not exhibit the type of structure termed primary lymphoid follicle." Some of these authors have become convinced of the universal existence of these structures when they have viewed radioautographs of antigen capture particularly if antigen-antibody complexes had been injected.

B. The Antigen-Retaining Dendritic Cells

1. Ultrastructure

Both primary and secondary follicles demonstrate unexpected ultrastructural complexity. Primary follicles contain basically two types of cells, lymphocytes and dendritic cells. The lymphocytes are mainly small and medium in size. The dendritic cells are characterized by a profusion

---

Fig. 7.5. A view of portion of a secondary lymphoid follicle exhibiting the presence of a homogeneous electron-opaque material between a complex, characteristic pattern of cell processes cut tangentially and in cross section. This rat had received rat IgG iodinated with ^{125}I and injected into the footpad 24 hr before killing. Note two small clumps of label and one single grain close to the surface of various processes. Some free polyribosomes are present in the otherwise clear cytoplasm of adjacent lymphocytes. ×20,000.

of cytoplasmic processes. These cytoplasmic extensions are so long, convoluted, and profuse that substantial areas of follicle are encountered which consist of little else *but* interdigitating processes and cytoplasmic infoldings (Fig 7.5). In such cases, it is not possible to state from which cell the bulk of the processes emanated. On occasion, the origin of a process from a dendritic cell body could be seen clearly (Fig. 7.4); more usually, it had to be surmised. Also, cells which were obviously lymphocytes engendered delicate cytoplasmic extensions which, when examined in transverse section, were not distinguishable from dendritic cell processes. This profusion of intertwining processes made a veritable labyrinth out of the extracellular space in the follicles.

Antigen in follicles was found predominantly in association with these processes, on and between cells rather than inside them. This contrasted sharply with the situation in medullary macrophages where antigen was rapidly taken into cells. The interdigitating dendritic cell processes created a weblike structure (Miller and Nossal, 1964) displaying the capacity to hold antigen extracellularly. Little penetrated into the dendritic cell cytoplasm. Also, only occasional silver grains could be seen over adjacent lymphocytes.

The technique of electron microscopic radioautography has been employed by Hanna and colleagues (Hanna *et al.*, 1967, 1968, 1969a,b), in a thorough study of the distribution of ^{125}I-human γ-globulin, chiefly in the spleen, after injection into mice. A remarkable series of changes was noted in the specialized antigen-retaining dendritic cells of the follicles. The cells developed progressively deeper and more convoluted plasma membrane infoldings, similar to, but even more extensive than, those shown in Fig. 7.5. In the secondary response, these characteristic regions underwent a rapid and specific degradation. This process was observed in all germinal centers examined later than 1 day after secondary antigen injection, and was associated with a loss of label from the area. It was believed that these results could be due to complement fixation, as undoubtedly during the secondary response the bulk of the follicular antigen is present as antigen–antibody complexes. This destructive phenomenon resulted in a rather brief, 8-day retention only of the antigen during the secondary response, in contrast to very long range persistence in follicles during the primary response. The authors speculated that this failure of prolonged retention could be part of a regulatory mechanism to prevent excessive stimulation by one antigen, and to "clear" the center for their later reaction against other, unrelated antigens.

On reviewing our own electron micrographs after reading this group's work, we also noted some areas of apparent cytotoxic damage in follicles that had taken up labeled flagellar antigens. In general, this was not prominent and did not correlate with the time after antigen injection. However, doses of antigen used by us were much smaller, and not sufficient to induce the germinal center dissociation previously described by this group. Larger doses might well have been capable of showing a more dramatic effect.

Another aspect of Hanna's studies, and one which closely parallels our own experience, is the intimate association of the plasma membranes of the antigen-retaining reticular cells with cytoplasmic processes of immunoblasts in germinal centers. The possibilities for a stimulatory action of the retained antigen is obvious.

One interesting difference between our observations and that of Hanna's group is that the latter found no tendency for isologous mouse 7 S γ-globulin to localize in follicles, while we obtained intense localization of our rat 7 S γ-globulin in rats, and the reasons for this discrepancy are obscure.

Hanna et al. (1969a) have had the opportunity to perform extensive studies on germfree mice. Whereas we had found that follicular localization of flagellar antigens was reduced and delayed in germfree rats (Miller, et al., 1968), these workers noted that the overall pattern of HGG-^{125}I-localization during the first 10 days after injection was similar in germfree as opposed to conventional mice. The major difference was that the germfree animals contained no preformed germinal centers, and localization of antigen was in the poorly defined spleen *primary* follicles. However, between 10 and 20 days after antigen injection, germinal centers developed in relation to the primary follicle antigen depots of the germfree mice. This finding is in happy agreement with the view of germinal center development expressed earlier in this chapter.

Hanna et al. (1969b) have extended some of our observations (Jaroslow and Nossal, 1966; Williams, 1966b) on the radiosensitivity of the follicular antigen-trapping mechanism. We found that when antigen was given 1 day after whole body X-irradiation, the anatomical entity representing the follicle web was much more radioresistant than the follicle lymphocytes. In fact, it took 8000 r to destroy it completely. However, much smaller doses, e.g., 450 r, interfered with the functional integrity of the follicle as measured by its capacity to retain antigen for long intervals. Damage appeared to be progressive over the first 8 days after X-irradiation. Medullary macrophages were not affected by any of the doses used. Nettesheim and Hanna showed that 7 to 14 days after 400 r, the capacity of follicles to retain antigen fell markedly, and this in spite of the presence of either 7 S or 19 S antibody to the antigen concerned. Repair of the X-ray damage took 4 to 8 weeks, and was not complete. Electron micrographs showed that the antigen-retaining dendritic cells were damaged by as little as 400 r of X-irradia-tion. Cytoplasmic vacuolation, nuclear pyknosis, and disappearance of the characteristic plasma membrane infoldings developed over the first 7 days after irradiation. This somewhat unexpected degree of radiosensi-tivity of a cell type believed to be of long life-span naturally raises the question of whether impaired antigen retention is one of the causes of diminished immune responsiveness of X-irradiated animals. However, the capacity of irradiated animals to act as hosts in adoptive immune responses suggests that damage to follicle cells is unlikely to be of central importance in irradiation damage of the immune response.

In summary, the structure of the specialized antigen-retaining den-dritic cells of lymphoid follicles is such as to provide a mechanism whereby antigen can accumulate progressively and can rise to concen-trations much higher than those prevailing in serum or extracellular fluid. The antigen is maintained extracellularly for long periods, and in concentrated, undenatured form. Thus, a unique opportunity exists for the surface of lymphocytes which move past to encounter extracellu-lar antigen. It seems likely that this represents one inductive mechanism in the immune response.

2. Cell Membrane and Antigen

Given that the follicle represents an antigen-trapping structure of great efficiency, what is the actual mechanism of association between indi-vidual antigen molecules and the plasma membranes of follicle cells and their processes? This question is rendered more complex by the strong probability that antigen will be specifically trapped by follicles only if coupled to antibody or if specific antibody is already present in the follicle. The experiments which lead to this conclusion are the following. (1) Many antigens begin to be localized specifically in folli-cles only after antibody production has started or can be presumed to have started (White, 1963; Humphrey and Frank, 1967). (2) Follicu-lar localization of all antigens can be accelerated by prior immunization of the animal, be this active or passive (Nossal et al., 1965b). (3) Treat-ments which are known to lower the immunoglobulin levels of serum and lymph very substantially, such as chronic thoracic duct drainage (Williams, 1966a), impair follicular localization of those antigens which normally localize rapidly in follicles on primary injection. This defect can be corrected by passive injections of specific antibody or, less readily, of normal serum. The presumption is strong that the constituent of normal serum involved is a natural antibody or "opsonin." (4) Germfree rats, which presumably possess lowered levels of natural antibody against bacterial antigens, show impaired follicular localization of flagellar antigens (Miller et al., 1968). (5) Isologous, labeled immunoglobulins can themselves lodge in follicles (Ada et al., 1964c). (6) Immunofluorescent studies have shown deposition of immunoglobulins in germinal centers in a distribution identical to that described for antigens (Mellors and Korngold, 1963). We will thus adopt as a working hypothesis the idea that an antigenic molecule or particle must be linked to at least one immunoglobulin molecule to be retained in a follicle.

In this case, the next issue is whether some specific molecular interaction occurs between an antigen–antibody complex and a dendritic follicle cell. Are there receptors on the dendritic cell plasma membrane for certain site(s) on the Fc portion of immunoglobulins? If so, the long-term retention of antibody-linked antigen would be easy to understand. The resolution of radioautographic procedures is not sufficiently good to determine whether the follicle antigen is firmly adherent to or embedded in the dendritic cell plasma membrane rather than simply trapped between two opposing membranes, and thus the electron microscopic approach cannot yield a final answer. However, immunochemical studies of relevance have been performed and will be reported in Chapter 8.

C. Differences between Primary and Secondary Follicles

The problem of the exact relationship between dendritic cell process and antigen depot becomes even more complex when one considers secondary follicles with germinal centers rather than primary follicles. In germinal centers, the dendritic cell processes are even more prominent than in primary follicles. It has been shown that dendritic cells, after specific antigen deposition on them, develop highly convoluted plasma membrane infoldings which entrap and retain antigen (Hanna et al., 1969b). A typical example of the result of such infoldings and intertwinings of processes is seen in Fig. 7.5, and still more complex areas can readily be found. A characteristic feature of such areas is the gradual accumulation of an electron-dense, homogeneous material between the cell processes. This becomes more prominent with increasing stimulation of the follicles. In an active germinal center, this accretion is very obvious. Its distribution corresponds exactly to the distribution of labeled antigen. It seems probable that this electron-opaque layer between processes consists of antigen-antibody complexes. Newly arriving antigen entering a preformed germinal center thus percolates into this layer. Using ferritin as antigen, we have noted molecules some 100 Å or more from the nearest apparent plasma membrane. Here it seems likely that many antigen molecules are entrapped in an expanded intercellular space containing a viscous deposit without themselves necessarily making contact with receptor sites on plasma membranes. It can be presumed that such antigen could still subserve inductive functions so long as *all* the antigenic determinants were not complexed with antibody. (See Fig. 8.1, where this concept is elaborated more fully.)

The characteristic tingible body macrophages (TBM) of germinal centers (Chapter 5) appear to play only a secondary role in antigen capture. They contain variable amounts of label, usually inside a well-defined phagocytic inclusion. Antigen localization was equally efficient in follicles containing few, if any, TBM. One gained the impression that TBM labeling represented little more than the inevitable consequence of the presence of a highly phagocytic cell in a region of heavy concentration of extracellular antigen. It has recently been shown by Hanna and Szakal (1968) that follicle reticular cell processes can be severely damaged during a secondary reaction, possibly through complement fixation. In this case, it would be logical to expect that TBM would engulf the damaged cellular material and any associated antigen.

D. Comparison of Different Antigens

The ultrastructural features of antigen localization appear to be similar for all antigens so far studied. The chief differences are in the timing of follicular localization relative to time of injection. We have ourselves studied five materials with electron microscopic techniques: four radio-iodinated proteins, i.e., intact flagella, monomeric flagellin, human serum albumin complexed with antibody, and rat 7 S immunoglobulin, and the electron-dense horse ferritin. All these showed the extracellular, membrane-associated localization already described. The work of Hanna and colleagues (Hanna *et al.*, 1969a,b) adds a sixth antigen, namely iodinated human γ-globulin. Moreover, at least a dozen other antigens have been shown to localize in follicles by means of either light microscopic radioautographic or immunofluorescent techniques, and though the weblike pattern of retention is not shown with as exact a resolution it is nevertheless clearly evident.

The rate of entry of antigen into follicles no doubt is influenced by many factors, but the level of serum (and therefore lymph) antibody is by far the most important. With high antibody levels, follicular localization can be prominent 1 hr after injection. In the absence of antibody present at the time of injection, follicular localization may be delayed until an active immune response has been induced. In fact, follicular localization may serve as the most sensitive known index of the presence of antibody in many cases (Humphrey and Frank, 1967). These considerations may prompt the conclusion that follicular localization is solely the end result (rather than the cause) of the events of immune induction. We feel this conclusion is not warranted but will postpone discussion of this important issue to Chapter 12.

Another variable in follicular localization of antigen is the concentration of antigen achieved in follicles. This must be considered relative to the amount of antigen injected, the serum antigen level, and the degree of medullary phagocytosis. The question has not been studied in great detail, but it seems that some antigens are inherently likely to achieve a higher ratio of follicular to medullary concentration than others. For example, fragment A of *Salmonella adelaide* flagellin (see Chapter 2) shows relatively much greater follicular than medullary localization (Ada and Parish, 1968), whereas ferritin, even on injection into preimmunized rats, shows much higher medullary than follicular trapping. This problem is complex for several reasons, and above all because both follicular and medullary antigen levels are the results of dynamic equilibria. The level in each region at any time depends on rate of arrival of antigen via the lymph and circulation, rate of specific trapping (be it by phago- or pinocytosis or by the special mechanism of the follicles), rate of degradation by intracellular or extracellular enzymes, and finally rate of departure of intact or degraded antigen by active or passive processes. Thus in considering the possible roles of the two paramount antigen-capturing mechanisms of lymph nodes, the medullary macrophages and the follicular dendritic cell web, in immune inductive mechanisms, these variable factors must be borne in mind and the exact experimental conditions must be clearly defined.

The group of Humphrey *et al.* have used a variety of antigens to study follicular localization, including TGAL-^{125}I, hemocyanin and human serum albumin, and TGAL-^{3}H. With the synthetic polypeptide injected in saline into normal adult mice, labeling was initially most prominent over the circular sinus and the medullary macrophages. By 8 days after injection, however, quite definite follicular localization, similar in general pattern to that observed in our experiments, was noted.

Even though the injection in saline caused no antibody formation measurable by routine serological methods, the most likely explanation of this late follicular localization is that a feeble primary response had indeed been induced, and that antibody had caused residual, free antigen to go to follicles. If this explanation is correct, it emphasizes that the occurrence of follicular localization is a most sensitive index of the presence of antibody in an animal. Injection of labeled antigen into mice that had previously been primed with antigen in Freund's adjuvant showed greatly enhanced and accelerated follicular localization.

The use of ^{3}H as a label for TGAL allowed more precise histological localization of antigen than was possible with ^{125}I. With this advantage, this group was able to show the existence of minute channels, filled with antigen at early times after its injection in saline into unprimed mice. These channels ran from the circular sinus to germinal centers or across the lymph node cortex to the medulla. Serial sections showed no evidence of antigen permeating laterally from these sinuses. In our electron micrographic studies, we have not observed channels lined by any definable cell type in this region. However, our studies were in rats and not in mice. While a species difference is not ruled out, it seems more probable that the spaces noted by Humphrey et al. were dilated intercellular spaces between the closely packed lymphocytes of the cortex.

An important extension of the Humphrey group's work involved the use of hemocyanin or human serum albumin injected into rabbits. Small, single doses of ^{125}I-labeled material were given to animals that had been (1) rendered tolerant, (2) been preimmunized, or (3) previously untreated. Medullary macrophage localization did not differ significantly in the three groups, as is also true in the flagellar system. Fully tolerant animals never showed follicular localization. Primed animals showed rapid and intense follicular localization. Virgin animals localized the labeled materials in follicles only when antibody, albeit in very small amounts, appeared in the serum. This study reemphasizes the key role played by antibody in follicular localization.

VI. Special Features of Antigen Capture in the Spleen

We have already mentioned follicular localization in spleen germinal centers and must now consider specialized features of antigen capture in the spleen. Our studies on the localization of antigen in the spleen were performed largely with *Salmonella* flagellar antigens (Nossal *et al.*, 1966). In the lymphoid follicles, the pattern of localization resembled that seen in lymph nodes. Antigen entry was via the marginal zone and marginal sinus (see Chapter 5) and both the rate and detailed entry pattern were comparable to those already described. Primary follicles were frequently difficult to identify until their striking antigen-retaining power was shown by radioautography. Secondary follicles showed heavy intercellular labeling especially in the reticular cell cap region which faced toward the antigen-entry portals at the border of the white pulp. The most noteworthy difference between lymph nodes and spleen in antigen-retention patterns was the absence in the spleen of a region corresponding to the medullary sinuses. Spleen red pulp sinuses do contain macrophages, which can be marked by an injection of carbon. However, these seem to play a minimal role in antigen retention as the red pulp of the spleen was almost unlabeled 24 hr or more after the injection of radioiodinated flagellar antigens or a variety of other proteins. However, cells at the border of red pulp and marginal zone remained labeled after injection of flagella (though not of the more readily digested flagellin or polymerized flagellin). The consistent placing of these antigen-retaining cells was noteworthy. The marginal zone itself played an interesting role in antigen capture. During the first day after intravenous antigen, it was prominently labeled. Electron microscopic radioautographs showed the label to be extracellular, sometimes associated with dendritic cell processes. With soluble protein antigens, labeling of the marginal zone was transient, being quite light 2 days after antigen and negligible thereafter. With flagella, it was of longer duration. On examination of radioautographs of spleens from animals killed at progressively longer intervals after a single intravenous injection, one gained the impression of a continuous flow of antigen from marginal zone across the marginal sinus and into the white pulp, with long-term retention in the follicles. However, the capillary circulation in the spleen is complex and, with the limitations inherent in the interpretation of static histological sections, one cannot formally distinguish between active transport of antigen in the manner indicated, and differential rates of deposition and degradation of antigen in the various regions. Whatever the detailed mechanism, the end result is very clear. For many antigens, the lymphoid follicles represent the sole sites of significant antigen retention in the spleen; and the marginal zone an important site of transient concentration of extracellular antigen.

The minor role played by macrophages in antigen capture in the spleen is of considerable theoretical interest. The overall pattern of multiplication and differentiation of antibody-forming cells in the red pulp cords is very similar to that in lymph node medullary cords; yet the latter lie close to antigen-laden macrophages while the former do not. Taken at face value, these differences suggest that if macrophage-processed antigen is of importance in the induction of antibody formation, then spatial proximity to the developing clones of antibody-forming cells is not an essential prerequisite.

VII. Antigen Distribution in the Thymus

In general terms, the thymus is far less a site of antigen trapping than are other lymphoid organs. In fact, the thymus shows so little propensity for antigen capture that the concept of a "blood–thymus" barrier for antigens came into being (Marshall and White, 1961; Clark, 1964b). We have discussed this problem extensively elsewhere (Nossal and Mitchell, 1966) and it now appears that the term blood–thymus barrier is a misnomer or, at least, an oversimplification (Horiuchi *et al.*, 1968). In adult animals, particulate radiolabeled antigens injected intravenously can be found in the adventitia of thymic blood vessels, where occasional marked histiocytes are found. In contrast, soluble protein antigens do permeate into the thymic cortex, and can even enter thymic lymphocytes (Clark, 1966). In newborn animals, even particulate antigens can be shown briefly to leak into the extracellular fluid of the thymic parenchyma. In all these three situations, the time for which antigen persists in the thymus is much shorter than that during which it remains in lymph nodes or spleen. We believe the relatively low antigen retention in the thymus can be explained simply by the absence in it of structures specifically designed to trap antigen. There is no afferent lymphatic stream, no follicular mechanism, no structure even vaguely comparable to lymph node sinuses or spleen marginal zone. There is thus no reason for lymph-borne antigen to enter the thymus; as regards blood-borne antigens, if these are particulate they are so rapidly removed by active reticuloendothelial elements, including those mentioned, that there appears to be hardly any need for an anatomical shield to prevent their entry into the thymic cortex. The normal integrity of the capillary wall seems sufficient. If the blood-borne antigens are soluble, they may transiently enter the thymic cortex, but in the absence of specific trapping mechanisms, they are rapidly diluted out and catabolized.

The question of transient entry of antigens into the thymus is of some importance in tolerance induction (Staples *et al.*, 1966; Horiuchi and

Waksman, 1968). Clearly, if the thymus were completely shielded from antigen, it would represent a depot of lymphoid cells unmodified by the tolerance-inducing antigen, and tolerance would rapidly break down once these were seeded out to peripheral lymphoid organs. This may be a contributory factor to the generally poor tolerance-inducing properties of particulate antigens. It has also been postulated (Burnet, 1965) that thymic lymphocytes are in a metabolic state particularly susceptible to tolerance induction, perhaps to allow the local elimination or suppression of lymphoid clones with reactivity to "self" antigens. This viewpoint remains speculative.

VIII. Effects of Adjuvants on Antigen Localization

As adjuvants can increase the amount of antibody appearing after the injection of a given dose of antigen, we have examined the effects of adjuvants on antigen localization as one possibly important factor. The first model system (Ada *et al.*, 1968) used was an endotoxin adjuvant from *Escherichia coli* injected together with labeled flagellin or human serum albumin (HSA); the latter was used unmodified, heat-aggregated, or as an HSA-antibody complex. In no case did endotoxin injection modify localization or retention of antigens. Unmodified HSA was retained rather poorly in lymph nodes; aggregated HSA was retained better, chiefly in medullary macrophages; and HSA-antibody complexes localized mainly in follicles.

Heated HSA caused no detectable antibody production when injected by itself, but significant antibody production when accompanied by endotoxin; yet the antigen localization patterns were identical. The same set of statements was true for HSA-antibody complexes except that antibody levels were much lower. Clearly the endotoxin effect was aimed at some mechanism other than antigen localization.

An interesting set of experiments has been carried out by our colleague Lind (1968) on antigen localization following its injection incorporated in Freund's complete adjuvant (Fig. 7.6). Using *Salmonella adelaide* flagellin, she found the expected increase in both magnitude and duration of the primary response of rats to this antigen. On this occasion, antigen localization patterns in the draining lymph node were very different from those observed after injection of antigen in saline. The extent of both medullary and follicular localization was diminished. Instead two new patterns of localization were noted. During the first 2–3 days after antigen injection into the rat hind footpads, large amounts of label

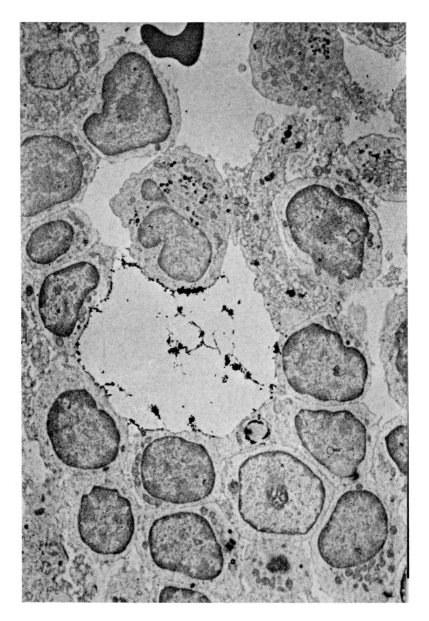

FIG. 7.6. Electron microscopic radioautograph of the cortical region of the popliteal node three days after the injection of ^{125}I-labeled flagellin in complete
Freund's adjuvant. A lipoid droplet containing labeled antigen appears to be entering the lymph node from the circular sinus. ×4000.

were found attached to the inner lining of the circular sinus of the popliteal lymph nodes. Second, antigen present in the lymph node substance was mainly present in microscopic droplets, presumably containing adjuvant and antigen, which penetrated into the substance of the lymph node cortex. These droplets constituted local depots of antigen apparently available to the surrounding lymphocytes. Three days or so after antigen injection, there were occasional antigen droplets which were surrounded by pyroninophilic blast cells. The appearance was consistent with the hypothesis that contact between the antigen-filled droplet and lymphocytes had caused blast cell transformation, resulting in the formation of a structure somewhat analogous to a small germinal center. Without pressing the analogy too far, there appeared to be similarities in principle between the trapping of antigen on the surface of dendritic cells in lymphoid follicles, and the display of large surfaces containing antigen caused by the permeation of adjuvant droplets into the lymph node cortex.

Lamoureux and colleagues (1968) studied the fate of a ^{125}I-bovine encephalitogenic peptide after injection into rats. Material injected without adjuvants left the draining lymph node very rapidly. Material incorporated in Freund's adjuvant showed a distribution pattern almost identical with that described for flagellin.

Simultaneously but independently of these two studied from the Hall Institute, the distribution of adjuvant-incorporated TGAL in mouse lymph nodes was studied (Humphrey et al., 1967) and again the antigen-laden droplets permeating the lymph node cortex were the key feature. In fact, the published photomicrographs of these three articles are practically interchangeable, so it seems reasonable to conclude that the basic localization pattern of all antigens incorporated in Freund's adjuvant will be similar.

IX. Ontogeny of Antigen-Capturing Structures

At birth, the peripheral lymphoid organs of the rat and mouse are very small. The spleen is essentially alymphoid and the lymph nodes are little more than condensations of fibrous and reticular tissue. While the newborn rat possesses phagocytic cells, as evidenced by its ability to clear bacteria and inert particles from the blood, the antigen-trapping components characteristic of adult lymphatic tissue, namely medullary macrophages and lymphoid follicles, are not present. We have studied the progressive development of these antigen-capturing areas over the first 6 weeks of life (Williams and Nossal, 1966). The most interesting result pertained to the development of the follicle mechanism. Between days 8 and 16 after birth, the popliteal and aortic nodes underwent differentiation into cortex and medulla, the aortic node being 4 to 6 days more advanced in differentiation, and the mesenteric node being a day or two further advanced yet. This suggested that higher levels of antigenic stimulation might accelerate differentiation, a conclusion also reached by Silverstein (1970) for the fetal lamb. Over this interval, the area subjacent to the cortical sinus developed antigen-capturing properties. At 10–14 days, radioautographs taken a day after the injection of ^{125}I-labeled polymerized flagellin displayed label in a continuous rim at the surface of the cortex, varying from 5 to 35 cells in width. Rats injected at age 16 days showed this cortical rim becoming occasionally segmented. In radioautographs of lymph node sections, heavily labeled thick cortical areas alternated with thinner, less labeled areas near the surface of the node. This pattern was already suggestive of the more mature, classical follicular localization; however, inspection of sections not covered with radioactive emulsion failed to reveal any grouping of dendritic cells or lymphocytes into a definable pattern. In fact, the histological appearance gave no clue to the antigen-capturing power of these alternating zones. By 3 weeks of age, the antigen distribution in the lymph node cortex revealed a series of ovoid antigen-capturing areas reminiscent of, but much smaller than, adult primary follicles. Over the next 3 weeks, the follicles grew to almost adult size, the 6-week old rat popliteal node possessing excellent primary follicles with great antigen-retaining power, yet very few germinal centers. The study showed that some functional change in the lymph node cortex, endowing certain areas with antigen-retaining power, preceded the development of follicles. In fact, some of the earliest antigen-capturing areas, or follicle anlagen, contained very few lymphocytes. The implication seems to be that development of antigen-capturing capacity by dendritic cells is a primary event in the ontogeny of the lymph node cortex.

In the spleen, the "cortical rim" phenomenon took the form of continuous labeling in the marginal zone, first seen around 2 weeks of age. Later than this, progressively more clear-cut follicular localization was seen. Even at early ages and in the absence of obvious germinal center formation, this took the form of a caplike area of heavy label over the external aspect of the follicle.

In the medulla of the lymph nodes, a continuous evolution of antigen retention could also be noted between 10 days and 6 weeks. At 0–2 days of life, only occasional, scattered macrophages were encountered in the very undifferentiated node. By 2 weeks of age, the medulla could be distinguished as a definite structure and over the next 4 weeks it came to contain progressively more macrophages, organized into increasingly recognizable sinus regions. Not only did initial antigen localization (as measured by radioactivity content 1 day after injection) improve over the first 6 weeks of life, but *retention* of localized antigen also increased. Thus, the rate of drop of radioactivity between day 1 and day 6 was progressively lower over this interval. Between 2 and 6 weeks of age, the antigen-retaining power of the nodes, expressed per unit weight of lymphoid tissue, increased fivefold. This may well have represented one factor of importance in the progressive increase in antibody-forming power which occurred over this time. It is likely that an optimal development of an antibody-forming clone requires more than one contact with antigen, and poor antigen retention could militate against this. In this connection, it was of interest that antibody production could be stimulated in rats over the first 2 weeks of life by three injections of polymerized flagellin, though a single injection, of no matter how high a dose, did not cause significant antibody production at this age (Williams, 1966c).

X. Phylogeny of Antigen-Capturing Structures

Effective study of the phylogeny of antigen-capturing mechanisms in relation to antibody formation is rendered difficult by virtue of the fact that the lowest forms of antibody-producing animals do not contain lymph nodes. The spleen is a much more complex structure, with diverse functions other than immunological ones, and thus not as attractive for this kind of study. The most primitive type of lymph node is found in the Amphibia. It is termed the jugular body, and in the marine toad, *Bufo marinus*, this is a prime site of synthesis of antibodies against flagellar antigens. We have studied antigen localization patterns in this organ, and also in the toad spleen (Diener and Nossal, 1966). The jugular bodies trap antigen reasonably efficiently. Light microscopic radioautographs show a very diffuse labeling pattern. The organ is not differentiated into cortex and medulla, and no structures comparable to lymphoid follicles can be recognized. Antibody-forming cells appear to develop in a diffuse manner throughout the organ, without the appearance of medullary cords. Electron microscopic radioautographs proved very revealing. There was a striking paucity of macrophages in the jugular bodies. The few macrophages found showed little intracellular label and only a small number of lysosomelike inclusions. The great majority of the labeled antigen in the jugular body was extracellular, lying on and between cell membranes. The overall pattern of localization, right throughout the jugular body, was reminiscent of the rat lymph node follicle. The serum antibody titers and the numbers of antibody-forming cells found in the toad during the primary response to flagellar antigens, were comparable to those previously observed in mice or rats. The absence of macrophages speaks against their obligatory role in the induction of antibody formation. In contrast, the prominence of cell-surface localization mechanisms stresses the possible importance of contact between native antigenic determinants and lymphocyte surface receptors in induction.

A curious byway of evolution led to the egg-laying marsupial mammals, the monotremes. Two examples of this primitive type of animal remain available for study, the echidna and the platypus. Our group has investigated antibody formation and antigen localization in these species and particularly in the echidna (Diener et al., 1967). The lymph nodes are tiny and extremely numerous. Antigen localization patterns are intermediate between the highly organized follicle-medulla pattern of the adult placental mammal and the very random distribution found in the amphibia. While classic germinal centers are not found, a primitive variant can be seen, with antigen concentrated in an elongated or crescentic manner toward the exterior aspect. The localization pattern somewhat resembles that of 2 to 3-week-old rats, providing an example of the principle that ontogeny recapitulates phylogeny. Of course, monotremes are not on the pathway of evolution that led to the placental mammals, but it is believed that they are reasonably close to the primitive amphibia, now extinct, which were common ancestors to both types.

It would be of great interest to examine antigen-capturing patterns in the hagfish or the lamprey, the most primitive known antibody formers, particularly with a view to comparing the fate of antigen with that in higher fishes or amphibia with a more developed lymphoid system. No such information is available at present.

XI. Summary

This chapter has dealt with the distribution of antigen in lymphoid organs, especially as revealed by radioautographic study of histologic or ultrathin sections taken at varying times after the injection of labeled antigens. While over twenty different antigens are considered, the fate of our model flagellar antigens is described in most detail.

There are two predominant and quite different sites of long-term antigen retention in the lymph nodes: the medullary macrophages, and the lymphoid follicles. In the former region, the bulk of the antigen is sequestered in lysosomal inclusions and rapidly degraded, though a significant minority remains stably trapped and perhaps immunogenically intact. In the latter areas, the antigen is retained extracellularly on and between apposing cell membranes. Dendritic follicle cells with complex processes and plasma membrane infoldings are chiefly responsible for this retention, and insults to these cells result in rapid loss of antigen from the region. The capture and retention of antigen by medullary macrophages is surprisingly affected little by the presence of antibody in the animal under study. On the other hand, follicular localization appears to depend entirely on the presence of antibody, be this "natural" or immune, actively or passively acquired.

In the spleen, the marginal zone plays an important, though usually transient, role in antigen capture. In this area also, extracellular membrane-associated labeling is the rule. Macrophages are less prominent in the spleen than in lymph nodes, and no structure analogous to the lymph node medullary sinuses exists. It seems likely that extracellular membrane-bound antigen is responsible for the bulk of immune induction in this organ.

Surface trapping mechanisms appear to be of fundamental importance since they appear early in both phylogeny and ontogeny. In the young rat, an interesting series of changes in the antigen-retaining web of the lymph node cortex, culminating in the adult follicle mechanism, can be studied over the first 6 weeks of life.

One of the most important questions which we wished to answer in these studies was whether antigen became associated with and entered the precursors of antibody-forming cells, and if so, whether, and in what amounts, it persisted in their antibody-forming progeny. This type of question is best attacked with the use of cell smears prepared from isolated, washed, suspended cells. It will form a major part of Chapter 9. However, histological studies summarized in this chapter lend no support to the idea that antibody-forming cells contain large amounts of antigen.

Fleeting reference has been made to the fate of antigen in tolerant animals, but this question will concern us more fully in Chapter 10.

CHAPTER 8

INTERACTION OF ANTIGENS WITH CELLS
OF THE RETICULOENDOTHELIAL SYSTEM

There is no agreed definition of the cells which comprise the reticulo-endothelial system. Three major criteria have been used to delineate the system (e.g., Heller, 1958). The first criterion is morphological identification and relies on their histological appearance. The second criterion is based on embryonal origin and tends to include cells which are derived from primitive mesenchyme. The third criterion depends upon some demonstrable activity of the cells and is thus more functional. For the purpose of this monograph, the function of the cell is the matter of prime interest. Heller has listed several functions of cells in the reticuloendothelial system of which two are particularly important in this chapter: phagocytosis of particles or molecules, and intracellular destruction or metabolism of the phagocytosed substance. The two types of cells mainly involved in these processes are microphages and macrophages. The microphages are the polymorphonuclear leukocytes of which there are three types—the neutrophils, the eosinophils, and the basophils. At least two of these types have been shown to be active in phagocytosis of antigen or of antigen–antibody complexes.

I. Antigens and Polymorphonuclear Leukocytes

Polymorphonuclear leukocytes are known to play an important role in combating infection but whether they play a role in the induction of the antibody response is uncertain. They form a major part of the early cellular responses to antigens. Typically, neutrophils are considered to be the first cells to arrive at a site of tissue damage. Eosinophils often arrive at the site somewhat later and it is currently believed that they are attracted to a site where antigen–antibody complexes are formed (Litt, 1964) where they phagocytose such complexes and then lyse (Archer and Hirsch, 1963; Archer, 1968). It has been suggested that polymorphonuclear leukocytes might play an indirect role in the immune response. Speirs and Speirs (1963) reported that neutrophils in mice previously injected with tetanus toxoid took up labeled tetanus toxin. Some of these cells subsequently became phagocytosed by macrophages. Roberts (1966a) demonstrated the rapid uptake of labeled antigen by eosinophils in draining lymph nodes within 4 hr of primary antigenic stimulation and considered it unlikely that antibody would have been formed and been present extracellularly in such a short time. However, these reservations do not take into account the possible presence of natural antibody, nor the possibility of extremely rapid antibody synthesis. Recent work of Litt (1967) suggests, in fact, a much shorter delay in antibody synthesis. He injected chick red blood cells into the footpads of guinea pigs and studied their distribution and fate in a draining lymph node (the popliteal node). Some cells were found in the medulla of the node and lysis of these cells occurred as early as $7\frac{1}{2}$ min after their injection. As red cells are lysed in the presence of antibody and complement, the data was interpreted as indicating production of antibodies to chick red blood cells within this very short time interval. Again, antigen-triggered release of some preformed antibody cannot be excluded.

The possibility that antigen in polymorphonuclear leukocytes plays a role in the antibody response is doubtful because of reports (Walsh and Smith, 1961; Cohn, 1962, 1964) that after uptake of bacteria by either macrophages or polymorphonuclear leukocytes, the macrophages, but not polymorphonuclear leukocytes, retained immunogenic material. This agrees with our observations that polymorphonuclear leukocytes in lymph nodes from animals injected with labeled antigen did not retain the antigen for long periods. This was in contrast to the long-term retention of some antigens in macrophages.

II. Antigens and Macrophages

Macrophages have been studied in rather more detail than polymorphonuclear leukocytes as there is more evidence for their involvement in the process of induction of antibody formation. Most of this chapter will be concerned with the properties of macrophages and the interaction of antigens with macrophages.

A classification of reticuloendothelial cells is presented in Table 8.I (see also Humphrey and White, 1964). Three of these classes will be

TABLE 8.I
RETICULOENDOTHELIAL CELLS IN THE BODY

Peripheral lymphoid tissue (lymph nodes, spleen, etc.)	Thymus	Liver, bone marrow	Serous cavities	Blood	Central nervous system	Connective tissue
Sinus macrophages	Perivascular histiocytes	Sinus lining macrophages	Macrophages	Monocytes	Microglia	Histiocytes
Dendritic follicle cells	Tingible body macrophages (cortex)					
Tingible body macrophages (germinal centers)						

discussed. They are the macrophages of sinus cavities, e.g., the peritoneal cavity, the sinus macrophages of peripheral lymphoid tissues, and the antigen-retaining dendritic follicle cells of the lymphoid follicles.

Macrophages are frequently obtained from the peritoneal cavity. When this space is irrigated, a suspension of cells is readily recovered. The prior injection of foreign particles or substances into the peritoneal cavity causes a sequential series of changes in the cell population with, frequently, a great increase in the number of macrophages. Another source of large numbers of macrophages is the lungs, but these alveolar macrophages differ from peritoneal macrophages.

As discussed in Chapter 3, macrophages may be coated with cytophilic antibody. It is generally believed that macrophages do not themselves synthesize antibodies, although there are two reports which suggest they may (Hannoun and Bussard, 1966; Holub et al., 1970).

It is convenient to discuss separately the biochemical and immunological aspects of antigen handling by macrophages, although the two aspects are very relevant to each other. Biochemical studies have been carried out on isolated phagocytic cells and these have usually been obtained from the peritoneal cavity.

A. BIOCHEMICAL STUDIES ON ISOLATED PHAGOCYTIC CELLS

Early studies on the mechanism of phagocytosis have been reviewed by Karnovsky (1962). It is convenient arbitrarily to separate phagocytosis into two aspects—pinocytosis (drinking) and phagocytosis (eating)—although this is an oversimplification. Based partially on the earlier experiences of Holter and colleagues with ameba at the Carlsberg laboratories (Holter, 1959), Cohn and colleagues (Cohn and Benson, 1965a,b,c, and d; Cohn, 1966) studied pinocytosis in mononuclear phagocytes, obtained from the unstimulated mouse peritoneal cavity. Cytoplasmic vesicle formation was used as the index of pinocytic activity. Early work established that vesicle formation could be controlled by the concentration of newborn calf serum present in the medium and for the purposes of comparing various inhibitors a final concentration of 50% was chosen. Reagents or conditions which inhibited both glycolysis and respiration (particularly cyanide, antimycin A, and anaerobiosis) greatly reduced vesicle formation. A central role for ATP as the energy source was implicated by the finding that low concentrations of 2,4-dinitrophenol or of oligomycin were inhibitory. Puromycin and p-fluorophenylalanine, which inhibit protein synthesis, were also inhibitory. Cohn and Parks (1967a,b,c) proceeded to study the pinocytosis-inducing effect of a number of molecular species (amino acids, proteins, synthetic polypeptides, and acid mucopolysaccharides). In general, anionic molecules were better stimulators than were neutral or cationic species. The minimum effective dose of a macroanion was found to be a function of its molecular weight.

Following uptake of a foreign substance, the pinocytic or phagocytic vacuole acquires hydrolytic enzymes by a special mechanism. Preformed lysosomes (primary lysosomes or protolysosomes) fuse with the vacuole, converting it into a so called "secondary lysosome" in which catabolism of the foreign substance occurs. Ehrenreich and Cohn (1968b) studied the digestion of albumin-^{131}I by macrophages isolated from mouse peritoneal cavity. This protein became localized in secondary lysosomes and within 5 hours 50% of the intracellular isotope was lost. In contrast to the process of pinocytosis, this loss of isotope from the secondary lysosome was not inhibited by p-fluorophenylalanine, 2,4-dinitrophenol or by a reduction in the serum concentration in the medium. The lost isotope was recovered mainly as iodotyrosine. Earlier, Mego and McQueen (1965) had injected formalin-treated albumin-^{131}I into rats and studied the distribution of the protein between cell fractions. up within small pinocytic vesicles devoid of proteolytic enzymes and The results supported the view that the labeled albumin was first taken these were converted into larger vesicles of a lysosomal character, probably by fusion of the pinocytic vesicles with preexisting lysosomes. If, after this fusion, the vesicles were isolated carefully in an intact form, extensive degradation of the labeled albumin within them took place and monoiodotyrosine was liberated into the medium (Mego et al., 1967). Coffey and de Duve (1968) isolated liver lysosomes in a highly purified state, prepared lysosome extracts, and studied the ability of such extracts to degrade different proteins at pH values between 4.4 and 5.6. The susceptibility to degradation of a protein by the lysosome extract varied according to the degree of denaturation which occurred if the protein was exposed to acid. Proteins which were reported to persist intact within liver lysosomes in vivo were found to resist denaturation by acid. Thus, horse ferritin and invertase were relatively unaffected by lysosome extracts, whereas acid-denatured human and bovine globulins were rapidly degraded. After exhaustive dialysis of degraded proteins, 70% of the theoretically maximum amount of ninhydrin-positive material was recovered in the diffusate, mainly as free amino acids and dipeptides.

The possibility that similar enzymes are present in phagocytic cells from lymphoid tissues has also been investigated although not in as much detail. Bowers, de Duve, and co-workers (Bowers et al., 1967; Bowers and de Duve, 1967a,b) studied the enzymes present in lysosomes isolated from lymphoid tissues, particularly spleen. Spleen particles were found to be very sensitive to mechanical injury (cf. Conchie et al., 1961; Williams and Ada, 1967). Some thirteen different hydrolytic enzymes in spleen were studied, including three cathepsins, and all were shown to be associated to some extent with particles having the typical latent properties of lysosomes. With few exceptions, enzyme levels found by these authors were similar to those obtained by other workers (e.g., Bouma and Gruber, 1964, 1966). When compared (activity per gram wet weight of tissue), spleen and thymus had similar levels of cathepsins B and D but thymus was less active than spleen in cathepsin C and in some other hydrolases. If a splenic extract was subjected to differential centrifugation and isopycnic centrifugation, some hydrolases showed either a broad band or more than a single peak of activity (e.g., Levvy and Conchie, 1964). It was suggested that spleen contained two or more distinct populations of lysosomes, each of which might be homogeneous. Further experiments led Bowers and de Duve to suggest that one population of lysosomes (the L_{19} group, having a modal buoyant density of 1.19 and characterized by their content of N-acetyl-β-glucosaminidase and acyl sulfatase) was derived from macrophages. On the other hand it was suggested that the L_{15} lysosomes might be found to be "dormant and functionally inactive" until an appropriate stimulus triggered off the synthesis of a more comprehensive set of enzymes. Extension of this type of experiment will depend upon the isolation of particular cell populations.

Kolsch and Mitchison (1968) have recently described the distribution of two enzymes, acid phosphatase and β-glucuronidase, in subcellular fractions obtained from extracts of peritoneal exudate cells (obtained from mice injected earlier with thioglycolate). When examined on a sucrose density gradient, acid phosphatase was consistently found in two density fractions, 1.15 and 1.19, and variably (though always to a minor extent) in a fraction of density 1.26. The enzyme, β-glucuronidase, was consistently found only in the density fraction 1.15 and occasionally in the density fraction 1.26. This distribution pattern for β-glucuronidase was not found in rat lymph node extracts (Williams and Ada, 1967) or in rat spleen homogenates (Bowers and de Duve, 1967a).

Apart from this last evidence, there is no reason as yet to doubt that the enzymic complement of sinus lining phagocytic cells of lymphoid tissues is similar to that of liver Kupffer cells or the macrophages in the peritoneal cavity. It is now clear that the majority of reticuloendothelial cells do not represent a stationary population. In fact studies on the origin and migration of macrophages (Volkman and Gowans, 1965a,b; Roser, 1965; Spector et al., 1965) suggest that cells found in different locations may all have been derived from a common precursor cell pool in the bone marrow. Thus, quantitative enzymic differences, when detected, may reflect simply an effect of local environmental influences rather than a qualitative difference.

B. The Fate of Antigen in Macrophages

1. Peritoneal Cells

Peritoneal washings contain a variety of cells some of which are extraordinarily difficult to classify. Frequently, macrophages make up a considerable proportion of the cells present. If animals are injected intra-peritoneally with certain agents (commonly glycogen, peptone, thiogly-colate) a gross change in the number and type of cells recovered from the peritoneum occurs. Within a few days of injection, there is an in-crease in the number of cells present and between 70–90% of these are clearly recognizable as macrophages. These macrophages readily take up antigens, and recent work (Rhodes and Lind, 1968) indicates that there is little evidence of selectivity in this reaction. It is important to realize, however, that cells other than macrophages may avidly bind antigen (Chapter 9). Many authors assume that antigen associated with peritoneal cells must be inside macrophages. Though this is probably a valid assumption for the majority of antigens in most situations, a small proportion of antigen bound to the surface of macrophages and/or lymphocytes may be of critical importance in some immune phenomena.

Several studies on the fate of labeled antigen in mouse peritoneal ex-udate cells have recently been reported. Askonas et al., (1968) studied the persistence and degradation of protein antigens in cells from mice previously injected with peptone. After intraperitoneal injection of 1 μg of ^{131}I-labeled hemocyanin (M. squinado, sedimentation constant = 26 S) a maximum of about 0.4% was taken up by the cells, and this occurred within 2 hr. Of this amount 90% was degraded and lost from the cells within 3–4 hr. The residual 10% had a much longer half-life, some persisting for weeks. The size of this hemocyanin molecule is such that any process which resulted in a breakdown of the protein could be readily followed by sedimentation studies of cell extracts on sucrose gradients. Extracts of the cells examined in this way showed that within 5 hr after antigen injection, only a small proportion of material of the original size was recovered. Most of the material was degraded to a size which was no longer acid-precipitable.

Kolsch and Mitchison (1968) also studied in some detail the intracellu-lar distribution of labeled antigens (heat-denatured bovine serum al-bumin and synthetic polypeptides) in peritoneal cells from mice earlier injected with thioglycolate. Antigen was labeled with either ^{131}I or ^{125}I and this enabled "pulse and chase" experiments to be carried out. Both in vitro and in vivo experiments were performed. At various times after exposure to antigen, the cells were homogenized, subcellular fractions isolated, and then analyzed by isopycnic centrifugation in sucrose gradi-ents. Cells from normal and from X-irradiated animals were equally effective in taking up labeled antigens. Some 90% of cell-associated anti-gen was degraded within 3 hr and when cells from normal animals were used, the residual 10% of radioactivity was retained for at least 8 hr. Newly phagocytosed antigen was mainly located in a fraction with a density of 1.10 gm cm^{-3}, and "pulse and chase" experiments indicated that this was a compartment with a rapid turnover rate. In contrast, retained antigen was in a fraction banding at a density of 1.26 gm cm^{-3}, and called the *storage compartment*. Cells from X-irradiated animals appeared to be deficient in their ability to retain antigen in the storage compartment.

There has been considerable interest in the nature of the retained protein in macrophages exposed to hemocyanin or other antigens. In further experiments, macrophages were either exposed to labeled antigen *in vitro* for varying lengths of time or labeled antigen injected into the peritoneum, cells recovered from this cavity after a limited time period and maintained in tissue culture. Some of the persisting antigen was found to be retained on the plasma membrane of the cells (Unanue *et al.*, 1969a; Askonas and Jaroskova, 1970; Unanue and Cerottini, 1970) and could be removed by appropriate techniques. Unanue and colleagues demonstrated antigen to be in this position by (1) electron microscopic radioautography; (2) the ability to release antigen from the cell by brief treatment with trypsin. The material so released was 66–80% precipitable by trichloracetic acid. (3) Cells containing antigen were found to be capable of adsorbing either the Fab[1] or F(ab[1])$_2$ fragment prepared from purified preparations of specific antibody. Askonas and Jaroskova removed cell-associated antigen (hemocyanin) by exposing such cells to EDTA. When examined by polyacrylamide gel electrophoresis, the removed protein was present largely as the monomer, with only small amounts of degradation products.

Both groups showed that essentially undegraded antigen was also present inside the cell, and Askonas and Jaroskova showed that cells containing antigen would slowly release antigen possibly by a process such as exocytosis or because of membrane turnover (Wiener and Levanon, 1968; Heise and Myrvik, 1967; de Duve and Wattiaux, 1966). The role which such retained antigen might play in immune processes is discussed later in this chapter.

2. Lymph Node Cells

Ada and colleagues (Ada and Lang, 1966; Ada and Williams, 1966) studied the distribution of labeled (^{131}I or ^{125}I) antigens in the draining lymph nodes (popliteal and iliac) of rats after footpad injection. The antigens used were flagella and flagellin (*S. adelaide*), hemocyanin (*M.*

squinado), and human serum albumin. The finding that a considerable proportion of the antigen became associated with certain cellular components (called for convenience the "large granule" fraction) which sedimented at 165,000 g min was most interesting. When antigens which were well phagocytosed were used, up to 70% of the label in the tissue extract was recovered in this fraction. Compared to albumin injected alone, injection of albumin with rat anti-albumin antibody resulted in 100-fold more label being recovered in this fraction from the lymph node extracts. This fraction contained enzymes, the levels of three of which, acid phosphatase, acid ribonuclease, and succinic dehydrogenase, were measured. Techniques which liberated these enzymes from this fraction left most of the radioactivity associated with a residue (see also Askonas *et al.*, 1968; Kolsch and Mitchison, 1968). This bound radioactivity could be obtained in solution only by "solubilizing" procedures, suggesting a process of firm binding. Some radioactivity was always associated with low molecular weight material, and when ^{125}I-flagella was injected, this reached a peak value of about 11% of the total radioactivity between 1 and 2 days after antigen injection, and then rapidly decreased. A greater proportion of the total radioactivity in the nodes was recovered associated with low molecular weight substances when labeled flagellin, hemocyanin, or human serum albumin was injected. In all cases, much of this degraded material could be released from the "large granule" fraction.

When either labeled flagella or flagellin was injected, a high proportion of the label present in the nodes was shown to be associated with material of demonstrable antigenic specificity, even 2 months after the injection. After injection of hemocyanin or albumin, a much lower proportion of the radioactivity (5–10%) was shown to be associated with material of particular antigenic specificity. The proportion increased to as much as 50% if antibody was formed after the injection of the antigen or if an antigen–antibody complex was injected. Because a major effect of the presence of antibody was to cause or to augment the localization of antigen in the lymphoid follicles (Chapter 7), it seemed reasonable to conclude that antigen present in the lymphoid follicles was intact and possibly undegraded.

Askonas *et al.*, (1968) also studied the breakdown pattern of hemocyanin-^{125}I in mouse lymph nodes with results similar to those described above.

The "large granule" fraction from lymph nodes of rats injected with a variety of labeled antigens was submitted to equilibrium centrifugation in gradients of Urografin (Williams and Ada, 1967). Two or more peaks of radioactivity were found. It appeared that localized medullary macrophages banded in a region of the gradient rich in lysosomal enzymes and this antigen was considered to be present in vesicles. It also appeared that antigen which derived from the lymphoid follicles of lymph nodes or of spleen white pulp banded at a sufficiently high density to suggest that it might be present as an antigen–antibody complex, possibly associated with membranous material. No antigen was found in a region of the gradient rich in a mitochondrial enzyme.

Uhr and Weismann (1968) have studied the distribution of bacterial viruses in homogenates of liver cells. Forty-eight hours after the injection of ϕX174 or T2 bacterial virus into rabbits, the livers were excised and the "large granule" fraction isolated. When submitted to isopycnic centrifugation in a sucrose gradient, infectious virus banded at the same level as did two enzymes characteristic of lysosomal particles but differently to an enzyme known to occur in mitochondria. If the rabbits were, in addition, injected with Thorotrast, both the lysomal enzymes and infectious virus banded at a higher density than previously, suggesting that the bulk of the virus was in fact associated with vesiclelike particles.

C. The Mechanism of Antigen Localization on Dendritic Cells in Lymphoid Follicles

Peritoneal exudates can be obtained in which 70–90% of the cells are macrophages. In contrast, there is at present no known way of isolating reticular cells from lymphoid tissue for chemical studies. The most convenient and sensitive method of detecting follicular localization of antigens is radioautography of sections of lymphoid tissues. Antigen in this region can also be detected by immunofluorescence, but with less sensitivity (Chapter 2). The evidence presented earlier (Chapter 7) suggested strongly that antigen became localized in follicles because of the presence of antibody. In fact, immunoglobulins themselves (either IgG or IgM) were able to localize in this region. Two possible explanations for this behavior of immunoglobulins are: (1) The globulins localized either because they contained antibody which would specifically react with antigen which was already present in the follicle, or (2) because there was a reaction between the reticular cell membrane and the globulin molecule. To decide between these possibilities, Herd and Ada (1969b) fractionated IgG from normal rabbit serum into light and heavy chains and into the Fc and Fab fragments. The Fab fragment was also isolated from rat IgG. Each globulin fragment was labeled with ^{125}I and injected into the hind footpads of rats. Rabbit IgG, heavy chains, and the Fc fragment localized both in the medulla and in the follicles of the rat popliteal and iliac lymph nodes whereas the light chains and the Fab fragment localized only in the medullary macrophages. As the Fc fragment is present in both the heavy chain and the IgG molecule, this finding favored the view that the globulin molecule reacted with the reticulum cell membrane through groupings present in the Fc portion. If this view is correct, there might be a possibility of determining the responsible groupings on the Fc fragment. Three peptides, C_3, C_4, and C_5, isolated from the heavy chain of rabbit IgG (Cebra, 1967) by cyanogen bromide treatment, were labeled and tested. The C-terminal peptide was C_3 (18 residues) followed by C_4 (60 residues) and C_3 (ca. 97 residues). Peptide C_3 localized strongly in the lymphoid follicles. Heimer et al. (1967) described the isolation of Fc-like fragments from peptic digests of a variety of human IgG preparations. On starch gel electrophoresis these were heterogeneous and existed as dimers of non-covalently linked peptide chains, with an approximate molecular weight of 25,000. These fragments reacted with anti-Fc but not anti-Fab sera, failed to react with rheumatoid factor or with serum complement, and were Gm (a⁺) but Gm (y⁻) (Heimer and Schnoll, 1968). This material was also found to localize in lymphoid follicles of rat lymph nodes (Ada, unpublished).

Direct reaction of the Fc portion of the globulin molecule with the reticular cell menbrane may not be the only mechanism involved. Herd and Ada (1969a) also found that rabbit Fab localized in rabbit follicles and rat Fab localized in rat follicles. That is, there was an apparent discrepancy between the behavior of heterologous vs. homologous Fab in lymph nodes. A possible explanation lies in the finding of a normal antibody (called *homoreactant*) to homologous Fab in rabbits (Mandy et al., 1966). Thus, homologous Fab may have no intrinsic ability to localize in follicles but is held there by species-specific antibodies to the Fab fragments. If this is the correct interpretation, either or both of two mechanisms may operate to effect follicular localization of antigens. It may be speculated that the process of follicular localization of antigen is sufficiently important in the immune response and that a double or "fail-safe" mechanism has been developed by evolution. The different mechanisms are schematically represented in Fig. 8.1.

III. Antigen–Macrophage Interaction and the Immune Response

We now turn to a consideration of the effects which interaction between antigen and reticuloendothelial cells may have on the subsequent immune response to that antigen. Antigen taken up by macrophages may be handled in two ways. Quantitatively, the most important occurrence is rapid and extensive degradation of the antigen. The second possibility is that some of the antigen is restrained in a more or less intact form. Factors which may affect the latter possibility are: (1) the resistance of the antigen to degradation, even if present within secondary lysosomes (e.g., bacterial flagella, D-amino acid polypeptides, pneumococcal polysaccharides); (2) the geographical location of the antigen, whether within the cytoplasm or at the cell surface; and (3) the degree of metabolic activity of the macrophage.

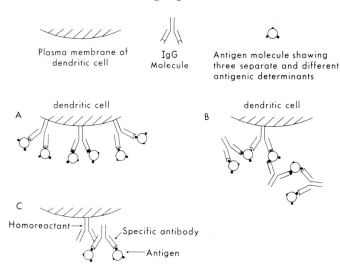

FIG. 8.1. The diagrams demonstrate three ways in which molecules of antigen may be localized at the surface of the follicle dendritic cell. (A) A simple mechanism in which the antigen is coupled via one antigenic determinant to the antibody molecule (IgG) which in turn is linked to the cell membrane via the Fc portion of the molecule. If the antigen in question contained n antigenic determinants, $n - 1$ would remain exposed. Different patterns of antigenic determinants would be exposed according to the specificity of each antibody molecule. It also follows that free hapten molecules, if bound in this way, would be "immunologically silent." (B) The "build up" mechanism which would occur if large amounts of antigen and antibody were present. Electron micrographs of germinal centers frequently show a homogeneous, electron-dense material between dendritic cell processes which may represent layers of antigen–antibody complexes. (C) An additional mechanism of antigen fixation which invokes the presence of "homoreactant" and so allows the trapping of Ig or an Ig–antigen complex via the Fab portion of the molecule in syngeneic situations. These mechanisms may constitute a "fail-safe" approach by the body to ensure follicular localization of antigen. Similar but rather more complex diagrams could be drawn for antibodies of other classes than IgG.

What role does antigen–macrophage interaction have on the antibody response? Perhaps the simplest concept is that this interaction is no more than a mechanism for the convenient removal of unwanted antigen from the body. Two operations achieve this—degradation followed by excretion, like a kitchen sink disposal unit. In experimental situations, the consequence of this might be either the restriction of the antibody response because the macrophage competed with other cells for the antigen or even the prevention of tolerance for a similar reason. On the other hand, the interaction might have a more positive effect, either as a step in the inductive process of antibody formation or as a means of enhancing or facilitating this process. Thus, macrophages might not only handle antigen and retain it in an immunogenic form, but this activity might also be augmented by the ability of macrophages to keep antigen in an appropriate location within lymphoid tissues or to transport antigen throughout the body. Other work suggests that macrophages may take up antigen and the slow release of this antigen may be an important mechanism for the maintenance of tolerance or for antibody formation. Results which have given rise to these concepts will be presented in the next section. The concepts will be discussed in more detail in later chapters.

A. INHIBITION OF THE ANTIBODY RESPONSE

Perkins and Makinodan (1965) studied the effect of adding mouse peritoneal macrophages to spleen cells on the production of antibody to sheep red blood cells. They found no evidence for the storage or release of immunogens or immunogenlike substances from macrophages actively engaged in phagocytosis under either *in vitro* or *in vivo* conditions. The macrophages acted as destructive competitors, as shown most clearly when opsonized red blood cells were used. Parkhouse and Dutton (1966) reported an inhibition in spleen cell DNA synthesis by autologous alveolar or peritoneal macrophages but not by autologous polymorphs. Dutton and Eady (1964) had previously shown that *in vitro* exposure of sensitized rabbit spleen or lymph node cells to antigen caused cell proliferation (uptake of thymidine-^{3}H into DNA) and antibody synthesis. The inhibition caused by macrophages did not appear to depend upon the release of a soluble factor, was independent of the presence of serum, and was not due to the consumption or degradation of essential medium ingredients. Inhibition only occurred when both cell types were in intimate contact. Macrophage extracts were neither inhibitory nor stimulatory. Destruction of macrophages by silica resulted in a small stimulation, possibly because of the liberation of nutrient material into the culture fluid.

B. Stimulation of the Antibody Response

In many other experimental situations, however, antigen-containing macrophages or extracts of such macrophages have stimulated the induction of antibody formation. As most work indicated that macrophages did not themselves produce antibody, it was a short step to the consideration of a two-cell phenomenon. It had been thought unlikely by many early workers that large particulate antigens would interact directly with the precursors of antibody-forming cells, especially as the "instructive" theory of antibody formation which was then in favor stipulated the presence of many antigen molecules inside the antibody-forming cell. Processing of particulate antigens in phagocytic cells to form soluble antigenic substances might be a prerequisite to the stimulation of the precursor lymphocyte. One who actively espoused this notion was Marvin Fishman and the present strong evidence in favor of a two-cell phenomenon is in part a result of his early work which stimulated much interest and some controversy. At present, a major argument in favor of a multicell system is that although most if not all workers agree that the precursor of the antibody-forming cell is a lymphocyte, there has been only an occasional report of antibody production by isolated lymphocytes directly exposed to antigen and when the intervention of other cell types is ruled out. For example, Unanue (1968; and quoted by Humphrey, 1968) found that low titers of antibody are produced when keyhole limpet hemocyanin is incubated with lymphocytes without "macrophages," in diffusion chambers in the peritoneal cavity of X-irradiated mice. Mitchison (1969) has also referred to experiments of this type. Shortman et al. (1970) have found that mouse spleen cell suspensions from which phagocytic cells had been removed, can be stimulated in vitro by exposure to polymerized flagellin to form specific antibody (see Chapter 11).

There are four experimental techniques, in particular, which have greatly contributed to the analysis of the role of different cell types in the immune response. One is the sequestering of cells in the peritoneal cavity of animals by their inclusion in diffusion chambers fitted with appropriate filters which allow transfer of macromolecules but prevent the passage of cells. A second procedure is the use of irradiated, syngeneic animals as hosts of the particular cellular preparation under study.

The third procedure is the use of cells in tissue culture, a technique which has only recently been completely successful in demonstrating the antibody response (Chapter 11). It may be that the use of this technique will bring advantages which will relegate this monograph into an historical account of the pioneer days in this field. Finally, the introduction by Jerne and Nordin (1963) and by Ingraham and Bussard (1964) and more recently by others of several techniques for the easy detection and enumeration of antibody-forming cells. These are further discussed in Chapter 9.

One of the most convincing experiments implicating a physiological role for macrophages in the antibody response is that of Ford *et al.* (1966) who reacted rat peritoneal macrophages with lysed sheep red blood cells. The macrophages were then allowed to interact with thoracic duct lymphocytes for several hours before the lymphocyte preparation, freed from macrophages, was injected into irradiated hosts. The host rats produced antibody within a few days of the cell transfer. Antibody was not produced if macrophages were omitted from the procedure. An experiment showing similar results has been reported by Mosier (1967) except that all steps were carried out in tissue culture (Chapter 11). Shortman *et al.* (1970) have confirmed that the presence of phagocytic cells appear to be necessary in mouse spleen cell suspensions in order to obtain *in vitro* antibody production to sheep intact red blood cells.

An increasingly popular alternative approach is to use cell fractions enriched with macrophages and usually obtained from the peritoneal cavity. These are exposed to the antigen, and then injected into irradiated syngeneic hosts. Antibody titers are determined some days later. Mitchison (1967) showed that live peritoneal macrophages which had been previously exposed to labeled bovine serum albumin were able to prime normal syngeneic hosts for a secondary antibody response more efficiently than did equivalent amounts of bovine serum albumin itself, if given as a single injection. In a series of papers, Askonas, Unanue, and others have looked more closely at this reaction. Argyris and Askonas (1968) showed that cell preparations from the unstimulated adult mouse peritoneal cavity, if reacted with antigen (Type III pneumococcal antigen), transferred immunity to irradiated recipients. This ability was associated with cells which did *not* adhere to glass surfaces after maintenance in tissue culture and which contained lymphocytes. These results of Argyris and Askonas confirmed those of other workers who provided evidence for immunocompetent cells in the peritoneum. Bussard (1966) and Bendinelli (1968) have shown that a high proportion of cells in peritoneal exudates were capable of secreting and probably synthesizing antibody to foreign red blood cells. Others have produced evidence of a comparable nature (Weiler and Weiler, 1965; Granger and Weiser, 1966; Cole and Garver, 1961). The properties of these cells have recently been examined in much greater detail by Nossal and Bussard (Chapter 11).

The peritoneal cavity of mice injected 3 days earlier with protease peptone contains 80–90% macrophages and only a small proportion of lymphocytes. Such preparations did not contain sufficient, immunocompetent cells to give an antibody response in irradiated, syngeneic mice unless lymph node cells from normal donors were also injected (Unanue and Askonas, 1968a). Using this test system, these workers compared the ability of free antigen (*M. squinado* hemocyanin) or macrophage-bound antigen (from mice injected intraperitoneally 45 min earlier with antigen) to prime mice for a subsequent challenge with soluble hemocyanin. The type and kinetics of the antibody response in the recipient mice were the same in each case, but there were marked quantitative differences, the macrophage-bound antigen being three to forty times more effective than free antigen. Small amounts of antigen were found to prime for IgM synthesis, while larger amounts primed for increasing amounts of both IgM and IgG. Similarly, macrophage-bound antigen was effective in inducing a secondary immune response in mice primed earlier with free antigen.

The immunogenicity of antigen carried by macrophages could be attributed either to the rapidly catabolized antigen—the degraded material— or to persisting, intact antigen. A considerable proportion of the macrophage-associated antigen has been shown to persist either on the cell membrane or adjacent to it in the cytoplasm (Unanue and Askonas, 1968b; Unanue *et al.*, 1969a; Askonas and Jaroskova, 1970; Unanue and Cerottini, 1970) and much of this could be released either by trypsin or by EDTA (see p. 149). The results of the two types of experiments caused Unanue and Cerottini to conclude that the surface-bound antigen (key hole limpet hemocyanin) was largely, if not completely, responsible for the immunogenicity of the antigen-containing macrophages. (1) Transfer of such cells into mice which had received specific antibody $3\frac{1}{2}$ hr earlier abrogated the antibody response. If the antigen-containing macrophages were incubated *in vitro* at 2°C with antibody before transfer, the resulting antibody response was less than half of the usual response. (2) Trypsinization, which removed most of the surface-bound antigen, decreased by about 70% the immunogenicity of the macrophage preparations. Macrophages, treated in this way, still migrated to the spleen as did untreated macrophages (see below).

In contrast to the results of Unanue and Cerottini, Askonas and Jaroskova found that if macrophages which had been first exposed to *Maia squinado* hemocyanin, were incubated with rabbit anti-MSA *in vitro* for 2 hr at 37°C, washed free of antibody, and then injected into syngeneic recipients, the resulting antibody response was the same as that given by cells not exposed to antibody. The same antibody preparations, injected into mice 4 hr before the transfer of antigen-containing macrophages did depress the antibody response though not to the same extent as reported by Unanue and Cerottini. With this antigen, then, the surface-bound portion did not account for all the immunogenicity, suggesting that internal antigen could also be immunogenic. Askonas and Jaroskova likened the antigen-containing macrophage to an "antigen pump" in that the cell might gradually release antigen over a considerable period of time.

The different results obtained by these two groups may be a reflection of the different antigens used. Humphrey (1969), Mitchison (1969), and Unanue and Cerottini (1970) have drawn attention to the different behavior of different antigens. Humphrey has referred to work of Askonas and colleagues in which two hemocyanins—*Maia squinado,* sedimentation constant of 26 S, and key hole limpet, sedimentation constant of 93—were compared. In brief, it was found that MSH associated with macrophages was *more* immunogenic than was unbound MSH, whereas KLH associated with macrophages was *less* immunogenic than unbound KLH. Mitchison has placed antigens in a hierarchy according to the potency of the macrophage-bound antigen relative to the free form. The greatest effect is shown with serum albumin, the least with KLH, and it is predicted that flagellar antigens would behave like KLH. Because of this relationship, antigens such as KLH and flagella proteins are sometimes referred to as "sticky," though there is little evidence as yet to justify this terminology. In fact, preliminary results (Parish, personal communication) suggest that flagellar antigens, associated with macrophages and injected into rats, are considerably more immunogenic than the antigen in free form.

A second finding which further clouds the present picture is that some antigens which are rapidly phagocytosed and yet are relatively insusceptible to digestion by macrophages are powerful inducers of tolerance. Examples are pneumococcal polysaccharides (Felton *et al.,* 1955) and synthetic D-amino acid polymers (Janeway and Humphrey, 1968). Antigen-containing macrophages can also, in this situation, be envisaged as "antigen pumps" but why tolerance rather than antibody production ensues is at present obscure.

1. The Susceptibility of Macrophages to X-Irradiation

Macrophages appear to be more radiation resistant than are lymphocytes. This is probably because (1) the frequency of cell division of this population is low so that their numbers are not greatly decreased after exposure to radiation; (2) this type of cell, unlike lymphocytes, does not need to divide in order to carry out its normal functions. Even large doses of X-irradiation do not greatly depress their phagocytic function. For example, Perkins et al. (1965) exposed peritoneal macrophages to as much as 50,000 r of X-irradiation and found a decrease of only 20% in the cells' ability to phagocytose foreign red blood cells (see also, Jaroslow and Nossal, p. 47). Muramatsu et al. (1966) found that, though the frequency of cell division of macrophages was decreased after irradiation, there was a transient enhancement of their ability to phagocytose substances. However, Gallily and Feldman (1967) have described a more subtle effect of X-irradiation on macrophages. These authors obtained macrophages from normal mice, exposed them to Shigella antigen, and transferred them to sublethally irradiated (550 r) mice. The residual lymphoid cells in the host animal were stimulated and antibody production occurred. If the macrophages were derived from mice irradiated 2 days previously with 550 r, incubated with antigen, and injected into irradiated mice, little antibody was formed and the authors concluded that radiation damaged the capacity of the macrophages to process the antigen to an "immunogenic" state. Kolsch and Mitchison (1968) also found that irradiated macrophages do not respond to antigen in the same way as normal macrophages (see p. 148). In contrast, Unanue and Askonas (1968a) found that if mice received 750 r of whole body irradiation 24 or 48 hr before intraperitoneal injection of hemocyanin, the immunogenicity of antigen-containing macrophages derived from them was of the same order as antigen-containing macrophages obtained from nonirradiated donors. The reasons for these different results remain to be elucidated. Mitchison (1969) suggests that the Gallily and Feldman effect may only be found with those antigens that manifest a drastic macrophage requirement (see p. 158).

2. Immaturity of Macrophages of Young Animals

Neonatal or very young animals are frequently unable to mount an antibody response to some antigens. The results outlined above suggest that this might be due to the immunological immaturity of macrophages in such animals and this is reinforced by the finding that macrophages in young rats did not phagocytose some antigens (Mitchell and Nossal,

1966). Braun and Lasky (1967) and Argyris (1968) have found that if a certain number of macrophages from adult mice were transferred to 1 to 3-day-old mice, injection of the recipients with sheep red blood cells resulted in an enhanced antibody response. Such results may be best demonstrated in some animals as it has been shown that the fetus in other animals, e.g., the sheep (Silverstein and Kramer, 1965) can respond to a variety of antigens.

3. Antimacrophage Serum and Its Effect on the Antibody Response

The preparation of antiserum which has a specific action against a chosen cell line promises to become a tool of increasing importance. Panijel and colleagues (Panijel and Cayeux, 1965; Cayeux et al., 1966; Panijel and Cayeux, 1968) showed that injection of heterologous antimacrophage serum (AMS) into mice reduced their resistance to infection by certain group A streptococci. A series of injections of AMS greatly inhibited the secondary response to phage ϕX174. Unanue (1968) found that AMS injected intraperitoneally into mice caused aberrant nuclear changes in peritoneal exudate macrophages; when injected intravenously, AMS caused changes in the spleen red pulp but not in the white pulp. Injection of high, nonlethal amounts of AMS did not impair the antibody response to key hole limpet hemocyanin, but the quantitative effect on tissue macrophages by AMS is not known. Unanue also used AMS to obtain a "pure" preparation of lymphocytes which were capable of synthesizing specific antibody when incubated with key hole limpet hemocyanin in diffusion chambers implanted in mouse peritoneal cavities.

Much of the work quoted above presents a convincing case for a role for macrophages in the inductive phase of antibody formation in many test systems. They may also play a role in the priming of cells. Some evidence indicated that this effect was mediated by antigen remaining at or near the cell membrane. There is a substantial amount of other evidence which suggests that fractions of macrophages which have phagocytosed antigen are active in inducing an antibody response.

IV. Immunogenicity of Isolated Constituents from Antigen-Fed Macrophages

A. Cell Fractions

As a further step in the elucidation of the suggested role played in immune processes by antigen in macrophages, many workers have studied the immunogenicity of fractions or of suitable extracts made from antigen-containing cells.

Franzl (1962) isolated subcellular fractions from the spleens of mice injected 4 to 8 days earlier with sheep red blood cells. These fractions were injected intraperitoneally into recipient mice which had been sensitized by a prior injection of sheep red blood cells. The mice were then bled at intervals and hemolysin titers were determined. Spleen "lysosomal" fractions consistently elicited high hemolysin titers in the recipient mice and the activity of spleen fractions was higher at 1 and 3 days than at 2 days after injection of the sheep red blood cells. Liver cell fractions from antigen-treated donors were ineffective. Uhr and Weismann (1965) followed the fate of two bacterial viruses, T2 and ϕX174, in guinea pigs and rabbits. The viruses rapidly became associated with the "large granule" fractions of tissues such as liver which contains many phagocytic cells, but the recovery of plaque-forming units from such fractions decreased with time. At 48 hr however, the immunogenicity of this fraction was high and this suggested that some catabolism of these viruses preceded antibody formation. Askonas and Auzins (reported Askonas et al., 1968) found that a cell homogenate supernatant obtained by high-speed centrifugation of a lymph node homogenate from mice injected less than 24 hr previously with soluble hemocyanin-^{125}I was more immunogenic (per unit of radioactivity) than were sedimented fractions of a sample of the original inoculum.

Results of this type suggested to many that the antigen in cells may be in a special state. Early work of Campbell and colleagues led to the notion that this special state may have involved the participation of nucleic acid fractions.

B. RNA-RICH FRACTIONS

Garvey and Campbell (1957) originally reported that after administration of ^{35}S-labeled BSA to normal or immunized rabbits, liver fractions could be isolated in which at least some of the label was still associated with material specifically related to the original antigen. Furthermore, there was some evidence for an association between retained antigen or antigen fragments and nucleic acid. This was later confirmed (Saha et al., 1964; Garvey, 1968) and extended to a more detailed investigation of the association of RNA with antigen fragments. Some of the peptide-RNA complexes isolated were found to contain between one and seven amino acids.

The work of Fishman and colleagues (Fishman, 1959, 1961; Fishman and Adler, 1963; Fishman *et al.*, 1965) provided a necessary impetus to this field. The essence of their experimental procedure was to incubate a particulate antigen, T2 bacterial virus, with a population of cells rich in macrophages. After about 30 min, the antigen-containing macrophages were treated with phenol to yield an extract rich in RNA. This extract was added to a preparation of lymphocytes either in an *in vitro* culture system or in diffusion chambers in X-irradiated hosts. Virus-neutralizing factors with the properties of antibodies were elaborated in either situation. Treatment of the phenol extract with ribonuclease destroyed the activity which appeared to be associated with an RNA fraction of low molecular weight. The addition of virus alone to lymphocytes did not result in antibody production. Fishman and Adler did not discount the possibility that the RNA-rich phenol extract might contain fragments of the antigen and Friedman *et al.* (1965) using similar procedures, showed the presence of head, tail, and internal protein antigens of the virus in the active phenol extract. These authors found that treatment of the phenol extract with ribonuclease reduced, but did not abolish the biological activity. Askonas and Rhodes (1965) independently studied the behavior of labeled hemocyanin (*M. squinado*) in mouse peritoneal macrophages. Upon extraction with phenol, an RNA-rich extract was obtained which was incubated with normal mouse spleen cells and the mixture then transferred to mice primed by a previous injection of hemocyanin. When compared on a radioactivity basis, phenol extracts made in this way were found to be more immunogenic than the original antigen preparation; they were also found to contain antigen as indicated by the presence of radioactivity in the phenol extract. Furthermore, RNA preparations made from peritoneal cells immediately after the addition of labeled antigen were also immunogenic, showing that this activity could not be due to the *de novo* formation of informational RNA. In each case, the activity of the extract was reduced but not abolished by treatment with ribonuclease.

Fishman *et al.* (1965) studied the effect in their system of varying the ratio of antigen (T2 virus) to macrophages on the production of "active RNA," as tested by subsequent reaction with lymph node cells form normal rats. When high ratios, i.e., an excess of antigen, were used, an "RNA preparation" was obtained which elicited two waves of antibody production, the first consisting of IgM and the second consisting mainly of IgG. Furthermore, a study of the susceptibility of the "RNA preparation" to ribonuclease showed that the early IgM response was more readily abrogated than was the IgG response. This suggested that two types of "RNA" were involved, the type responsible for the formation of IgM being more susceptible to ribonuclease than was the second type. This observation was extended by Adler *et al.*, (1966). Rabbits were chosen so that the peritoneal exudate and lymph node cells came from animals of different allotypes. The rabbits were homologous at the *b* locus (Ab^4/Ab^4 and Ab^5/Ab^5) which determined the antigenic markers on the light chains which in turn are common to the several classes of rabbit immunoglobulins. It was reported that the IgM formed (i.e., the first peak of antibody) contained the allotypic markers characteristic of the donor of the *macrophages*. In contrast, the IgG formed (i.e., the second peak of antibody) was found to possess the allotypic specificity of the donor of the *lymph node cells*. Further it was found that the RNA responsible for the formation of IgM was free of demonstrable viral antigen whereas the RNA responsible for the formation of the IgG was precipitable by antiviral serum, indicating the presence of antigen in this latter fraction. Fishman *et al.* (1968) have summarized the results of experiments which show that the competent cells in their peritoneal exudate preparations are in fact macrophages. They believe that peritoneal macrophages play a unique role in the formation of specific IgM. This cell, they suggest, has the potential for immunoglobulin (and thus antibody) production. This would explain the ability of such cells to form a messenger type RNA, which in favorable circumstances, could transfer information to a suitable cell. If their interpretation of these results is correct, the findings form a very important advance in our knowledge of cell-to-cell interaction. However confirmation of these results is lacking to date.

Gottlieb *et al.* (1967) studied the properties of immunogenic RNA preparations isolated by a procedure involving detergent and phenol treatment of cell suspensions rich in macrophages which had phagocytosed bacterial viruses. Their findings can be summarized as follows: (1) The immunogenic RNA was found to hybridize with macrophage DNA. Furthermore, two different antigens (T2 and T17 bacterial viruses) produced antigen–RNA complexes of which the RNA portions were shown to compete for the same coding site on the macrophage DNA. Thus, in these experiments, the macrophages did not produce a unique RNA in response to a particular antigen so that the immunogenic "RNA" was unlikely to be a specific, informational RNA. (2) In the presence of labeled precursors, the immunogenic RNA was slowly labeled; the degree of labeling could not be distinguished from RNA isolated from "unexposed" macrophages. (3) Isopycnic centrifugation of RNA extracts in cesium sulfate gradients revealed two bands, repre-

senting, respectively, a major one containing only RNA and a minor
one containing RNA–protein complexes. Of these two bands, only the
one containing RNA–protein complexes could be shown to be immunogenic. Incubation of the RNA extract with pronase eliminated both
the immunogenic activity and the minor band in the gradient. Furthermore, the immunogenic activity could also be diminished by treatment
with RNase, though not so readily. These findings have since been extended by Gottlieb (Gottlieb, 1968; Gottlieb and Straus, 1969; Gottlieb,
1969a,b). The RNA protein complex was found to contain about 5%
of the total extracted RNA. Its formation was not inhibited by actinomycin D. When T2 bacterial virus, labeled with ^{125}I was used as the antigen,
there was a peak of radioactivity at the density where the complex
was found. This RNA–protein complex could also be recovered from
spleen but not from several other tissues examined. Gottlieb and Straus
showed that it was an RNA–protein complex, rather than free RNA,
which became associated with antigenic fragments. The complex had a
molecular weight of about 12,000 and was found to be homogeneous by
polyacrylamide gel electrophoresis.

Bishop et al. (1967) have also studied the synthesis of "immunogenic"
RNA. In their system sheep red blood cells were mixed with rat peritoneal cells, an RNA extract was made by treatment with detergent
and phenol, and this was added to normal rat spleen cells. Specific
hemagglutinating antibody was formed. Much of the biologically active
RNA was 6–10 S in size, and was synthesized more rapidly in cells
exposed to antigen than in control cells. Both the antibody response
and the synthesis of the active RNA were inhibited by actinomycin
D although the active RNA was found to be stable for at least $2\frac{1}{2}$ hours
after formation. Subsequently, Bishop and Abramoff (1967) confirmed
the presence of a minor band of macrophage RNA in cesium sulfate
gradients. This minor band had a lower density than the major RNA
band and probably contained the "immunogenic" RNA.

Work being carried out by Roelants and Goodman (1968) promises
to clarify some of the mystery which still surrounds the antigen-RNA
complex. They used a "hapten–carrier" system in which the hapten, poly-
γ-D-glutamic acid (average molecular weight about 33,500), was non-
immunogenic but elicited anti-polypeptide antibodies when complexed
with methylated bovine serum albumin (see Chapter 4). In either form,
the tritiated polypeptide was taken up to an equal extent by rabbit
peritoneal macrophages, in vivo or in vitro. In both cases the polypeptide
was very firmly bound by RNA which had been prepared by exhaustive
phenol treatment of the macrophages. This firm association could also

occur in cell-free extracts. *In vivo*, the associated RNA was in the 4–5 S fraction and was the only type perceptibly synthesized after the introduction of polypeptide. This finding differed from Gottlieb's work (see above). Many tests suggested that the binding of polypeptide to RNA was an active biological process but one which did not appear to distinguish between antigens on the basis of immunogenicity. The small size of the RNA suggested to these authors that, if it was to act in an informational capacity, the mechanism might involve *insertion* into a larger messenger in the lymphocyte, rather than separate translation. It was pointed out there was precedent for such an event in DNA, but not in RNA.

Gottlieb (1969a) criticized the work of Roelants and Goodman on the ground that the specific activity of their preparations were so low (50 μCi/mg) that a ribonucleic acid–protein complex banding at 1.588 gm/ml might have been overlooked. Gottlieb reinvestigated his system using as antigen, a synthetic polypeptide (poly-GAT; L-glutamic acid, L-alanine, and L-tyrosine). Using material of high specific activity (18.5 μCi/μg), he found that the polypeptide complexed exclusively to the ribonucleoprotein complex (density, 1.588 gm/ml) of the macrophages. In solutions of high ionic strength, the polypeptide was partially released from the complex.

How big is the antigenic fragment of an immunogen which becomes associated with the ribonucleoprotein complex of the macrophage? Gottlieb (1969b), using T2 bacterial virus as an immunogen, showed that the maximum size was 31 amino acids. Even after treatment with alkali, this fragment retained the ability to react with specific antiserum so it is most likely that the complete tertiary structure of the T2 virus tail antigen was not required for immunogenicity. The extent of alteration of the tertiary structure is not known.

Cohen and colleagues have described the preparation of an RNA fraction from spleen cells or from lymphocyte-enriched preparations of peritoneal exudate cells after incubation with antigen (red blood cells of different species). The RNA, which had a sedimentation coefficient of 8–12 S, caused some spleen cells from nonimmunized mice to form specific antibody, and it was suggested that the few competent, recipient cells which responded by producing antibody possessed specific recognition sites for the RNA (Cohen, 1967a,b). The active RNA hybridized with a large proportion of the DNA from the spleen of nonimmunized mice (Cohen and Raska, 1968). Addition of this RNA to peritoneal or spleen cells from nonimmunized mice caused the secretion of specific antibody, within 3 hr, as shown by plaque-forming cells. The process appeared to require both protein synthesis and cellular respiration (Mosier and Cohen, 1968).

The relationship between this type of RNA and the "informational" RNA claimed to exist by Adler et al. (1966) is not known. Cohen and Raska (1968) provided some evidence for specificity of the RNA formed in their system and Pinchuck et al. (1968) have recently further documented such a specificity. They used two different synthetic polypeptides, $Glu^{60}.Ala^{30}.Tyr^{10}$ (GAT) and $Glu^{36}.Lys^{24}.Ala^{40}$ (GLA) and inbred strains of mice. The "RNA" extracted from normal peritoneal macrophages (mouse, rat or rabbit) after exposure to GAT initiated a good antibody response in $C_{57}BL/6J$ mice, although GAT injected alone caused little response. The RNA contained 0.02% of its weight as the polypeptide and the activity of the complex was destroyed by ribonuclease. The RNA obtained from cells incubated with GLA caused the formation of antibody specific for GLA but even when preincubated with GAT, failed to initiate the formation of antibody specific to GAT.

V. The Carriage of Antigen by Macrophages

Whether intact antigen at or near the macrophage membrane or processed antigen within the macrophage or both is an active inducer of antibody formation, it is obviously necessary for the inducer to be at the right place and at the right time for this to happen. Is a major role of the macrophage to transport and hold the antigen in an appropriate place? There is some evidence for this. Roser (Roser, 1965; Russell and Roser, 1966) labeled peritoneal and alveolar macrophages with radioactive, colloidal gold. Upon intravenous injection into mice, the macrophages localized almost exclusively in liver, where they were similar in appearance to Kuppfer cells, and in the red pulp of spleen. After injection of peritoneal macrophages, the spleen contained five times as many of these cells per milligram of tissue than did the liver and by 10 hr, as much as 10% of the injected cells. Thus, the higher efficiency of macrophage-bound antigen found by Unanue and Askonas (1968a) might well have been a reflection of the high proportion of antigen which was carried to and held in the spleen in this way, compared to the amount present in the spleen after injection of free antigen (cf. Chapter 4). This could perhaps be further tested by using splenectomized mice. Antigen in killed macrophages, though more immunogenic than antigen itself, was considerably less immunogenic than antigen in live macrophages (Unanue and Askonas, 1968a). Colloidal gold in killed macrophages is also found in spleen after intravenous injection, though to a lesser extent than when live macrophages are used (Roser, 1965).

Unanue and Cerottini (1970) injected peritoneal macrophages containing hemocyanin-^{125}I (key hole limpet) either intravenously or intraperitoneally into mice. Radioautography of spleen and lymph node sections revealed the presence of labeled cells in the periarterial sheath and marginal zone of spleen and in the paracortical areas and medulla of lymph nodes, i.e., well-recognized areas of cell circulation. Labeled antigen was not seen in the germinal centers.

VI. Nonspecific Enhancement of the Antibody Response by Macrophages

In addition to their role as helper cells in the carriage of antigen, macrophages may provide a nonspecific stimulus for the proliferation and differentiation of lymphoid cells. Unanue et al. (1969b) found that *Bordetella pertussis* vaccine or beryllium sulfate were potent adjuvants and increased the antibody response to *Maia squinado* hemocyanin in mice. Many factors might play a role, but one was the effect of the adjuvant taken up by macrophages. Antigen-containing macrophages treated with adjuvant *in vitro* and injected into mice elicited higher antibody titers than did macrophages not treated with adjuvant. The same was not true of lymph node cells. This adjuvant action did not require the presence of antigen and adjuvant in the same macrophage. The presence of adjuvant did not change the catabolism and retention of the antigen in macrophages. A known action of adjuvants such as these is to labelize lysosomal membranes and this could result in the release of nonspecific stimulators such as oligonucleotides. Askonas and Jaroskova (1970) point out that a nonspecific stimulus of this nature might account for the increase in "nonspecific" immunoglobulin production which occurs after adjuvant treatment (Askonas and Humphrey, 1958).

VII. Summary

Three types of cells of the RES have been discussed. Polymorphonuclear leukocytes appear in tissues, particularly after damage, and it is clear that after antigen is present in a particular system, they play a role in the uptake and removal of antigen–antibody complexes. No convincing evidence for their participation in immune induction has as yet been presented.

Two types of antigen-trapping cells present in lymphoid tissue have been considered. One type is the classical macrophage, for example, that present in the peritoneum, especially after nonspecific stimulation, any by the sinus lining cells of lymphoid organs. The other type is the antigen-retaining, dendritic cell of lymphoid follicles.

Antigen is found associated with dendritic follicle cells when antibody, either "natural" or "specific," is present. Studies on localization patterns in lymph nodes indicate two possible methods of antigen localization. Our studies indicated that the Fc fragment isolated from syngeneic or xenogeneic IgG preparations, became attached to dendritic cells, and from this it followed that an IgG molecule would attach to the cell wall by the Fc portion of the molecule, leaving the Fab portions free to bind antigen. In allogeneic, but not xenogeneic, situations, the Fab fragments also localized in the dendritic cell surface and this may be due to the presence of an isoantibody.

Our knowledge of the biochemical and phagocytic properties of macrophages is more extensive. Pinocytosis of substances with vesicle formation is an energy-dependent process and is reduced by inhibitors of protein synthesis. Vesicles formed in this way fuse with lysosomes which contain a broad range of enzymes including several cathepsins. The stability of various proteins to lysosomal extracts paralleled their reported ability to persist *in vivo*. The enzyme profile of lysosomes isolated from lymphoid tissues was very heterogeneous but could be explained in part by postulating two or more separate populations, presumably present in different cell types.

The reaction of several labeled proteins, used as antigens, with peritoneal macrophages has been studied in considerable detail. In most cases, the greater portion of the phagocytosed antigen is degraded and the breakdown products excreted. With some substances, e.g., polymers of D-amino acids, degradation is a slow process. A minor portion of the antigen may be retained in undegraded form on or near the plasma membrane and can be released by trypsin or EDTA. Antigen bound in this way is immunogenic.

When it was realized that macrophages did not synthesize antibody, the possibility of a "two-cell" interaction in some antibody responses was examined. Though some work showed that macrophages might act simply as competitors for antigen, there is now considerable evidence that macrophages may play an enhancing, if not obligatory, role in some antibody responses. In one type of experiment, the antigen (often red blood cells) is mixed with macrophages; these are then mixed with lymphocytes, which, after injection into X-irradiated recipients, produced specific antibody. In another type of experiment, macrophages, exposed *in vivo* or *in vitro* to antigen are transferred to syngeneic recipients. Antigen associated with macrophages in this way was found to be up to forty times more efficient than free antigen in inducing an immune response. A possible explanation of this finding was that peritoneal macrophages, injected intravenously into mice, localized in the spleen to a greater extent than did free antigen. The effect is far more striking with some antigens than with others. Some workers claimed than X-irradiation of macrophages interfered with their "antigen-handling" ability but others found no evidence for this. Again the type of antigen used may be important. Macrophages in young animals can be deficient in antigen-handling ability as the transfer of adult macrophages to 1 to 3-day-old mice resulted, upon antigenic stimulation, in an enhanced antibody response. The recent availability of antimacrophage serum may lead to a greater understanding of the role of macrophages.

Ever since the original discovery that RNA-rich (phenol) extracts of macrophages which have phagocytosed antigen could induce lymphocytes to synthesize specific antibody, this topic has aroused great interest. There is now much evidence that cellular RNA can become very firmly associated with antigen or antigenic fragment. Such complexes may be more immunogenic than the original antigen per se and cause an IgG response. In some respects, however, the effect is nonspecific, e.g., immunogenic and nonimmunogenic substances are found complexed in this way and the RNA is of a preexisting species. More intriguing are the several recent reports of different sorts of RNA, still of low molecular weight but claimed to be specifically informational in nature. For example, it is reported that this type of RNA may cause the production of IgM antibody and the transfer of specific information between animals of different allotypic specificity. Only further work will delineate the role of such phenomena in immune responses.

An additional role for macrophages may be the release, by stimulated macrophages (antigen or adjuvant treated) of nonspecific factors which enhance cell division and immunoglobulin production by lymphocytes.

CHAPTER 9

THE INTERACTION OF ANTIGEN WITH LYMPHOID CELLS

It is now almost universally assumed that the first event in the stimulation of a cell toward antibody formation is an encounter between antigen (be this macrophage-processed or not) and a naturally occurring antibodylike determinant on the surface of the lymphocyte. This assumption has gained credence in the presence of relatively little concrete evidence in its favor, partly because of the elegance and plausibility intrinsic to the clonal selection approach (Burnet, 1957) and partly because of the absence of a persuasive alternative hypothesis. Even if this idea turns out to be correct, many questions concerning the interaction between antigen-reactive cells and antigen remain to be posed. Does antigen enter the cell? If so, how much enters, and where does it go? Must it remain in the cell and/or in its progeny during the course of antibody formation, and if so in what amounts? What factors occasion some encounters between lymphocyte and antigen to be followed by immunity, others by tolerance?

This area of research addressing itself to the interaction between lymphocyte plasma membrane receptors and antigen molecules is one of the most rapidly moving areas of cellular immunology research, and thus difficult to review. It seems certain that it will become of even greater importance in the future, as more effort is put into attempts at enriching cell populations for their content of cells reactive to a particular antigen. For the moment, the experiments we wish to review lead to the following chief conclusions:(1) Most lymphocytes contain surface receptors of immunoglobulin nature. (2) There is a heterogeneity among lymphoid cells in the specificity of these receptors. (3) The specificity of the receptor site probably reflects the capacity of the cell concerned to react to and be stimulated by antigen. (4) During the early stages of an *in vivo,* primary immune response, antibody-forming cells may have substantial amounts of antigen on or in them, but the question of whether this antigen at this stage exerts a functional role remains problematical. (5) During later stages of an immune response, antibody-forming cells contain so little antigen that even very sensitive tests fail to reveal any. It is unlikely that the cells contain more than four molecules of antigen, and they may contain none at all.

The idea that the antibody produced by a cell may be present in readily detectable concentration at the surface of that cell is much more firmly established than the related notion that antibody is present on the surface of certain lymphocytes from unimmunized animals. Thus, though the latter concept is at present of inherently more interest, we thought it wise to consider first the question of antibody-forming cells. We discuss primarily two questions, namely the presence of antibody on the cell surface; and the presence or absence on or in the cell of antigen molecules or antigen fragments.

I. Antibody-Forming Cells from Immunized Animals

A. PRESENCE OF ANTIBODY ON CELL SURFACE

Reiss *et al.* (1950) first noted that lymph node cell suspensions from animals immunized with bacterial vaccines contained a proportion of cells with the capacity to cause intact bacteria to adhere firmly and specifically to their surface. These authors surmised that the cells concerned were the antibody formers. Mäkelä and Nossal (1961, 1962) were able to put this idea to an exact test. They incubated cells from rats immunized against *Salmonella* flagella singly in microdroplets. Antibody-forming cells secreted anti-H antibody into the medium, and thus those test microdroplets containing an antibody-forming cell soon came to possess the capacity to immobilize added motile bacteria having the relevant H antigen. After the identity of a cell as an antibody secretor had been established by the microinjection of a small number of motile (and rapidly immobilized) bacteria into the microdroplet, it was possible to saturate the free antibody by the addition of hundreds of bacteria, thus providing an antigen excess. With very rare exceptions, all the antibody formers possessed the capacity of bacterial immunocytoadherence. In other words, the cell itself became surrounded by a closely adherent corona of bacteria. Conversely, in an animal taken at the height of an immune response, the great majority of cells displaying immunocytoadherence are antibody formers (Nossal *et al.*, 1964c). Interestingly, in the progressive maturation of cells of the plasma cell series, immunocytoadherence becomes evident somewhat earlier than detectable antibody production. Thus, on the second and third day of a secondary response to flagella, or on the fourth day of a primary response, one can find many large, blast cells that are strongly positive for immunocytoadherence. These cells could be shown neither to secrete nor to contain detectable amounts of immobilizing antibody. This suggests both that immunocytoadherence is a sensitive test, and that the rate of antibody synthesis and/or secretion by a cell increases with progressive differentiation. In these early blasts, the antibody coating may not be uniform around the cell. Frequently the site of attachment of bacteria is limited to a small patch, often at one "pole" of an ovoid cell. In contrast, more mature antibody-formers appear to have antibody covering their whole surface. Examples of cells with immunocytoadherence are shown in Fig. 9.1.

More recently, the phenomenon of immunocytoadherence has been adapted in a variety of ways and has been used widely as a test for the detection of antibody-forming cells (Biozzi *et al.*, 1966; Zaalberg, 1964; Diener, 1968). As we shall see directly, it has also been used to deplete cell populations of their content of antibody-forming cells (Wigzell and Andersson, 1969).

The presence of antibody firmly bound to the plasma membrane of antibody-forming cells may turn out to be a useful marker for the analysis of the cellular physiology of antibody secretion. For example, electron microscopic observations of immunocytoadherence of antigens such as ferritin of ^{125}I-labeled proteins might reveal whether the distribution of accessible combining sites were uniform or patchy, and whether there were any morphological features of interest at or near the antibody displaying "pole" of a blast cell. It is of interest to note that receptors for antigen on lymphocytes of unimmunized animals are distributed in a patchy fashion (see p. 184).

In section (II,C) of this chapter we will describe in detail immuno-absorbant columns in relation to fixation and removal of antigen-reactive

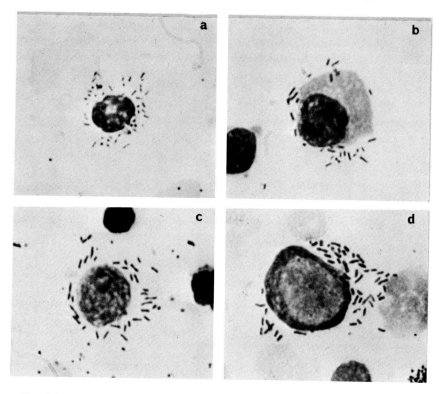

Fig. 9.1. Various types of lymphoid cells forming antibody as judged by immuno-cytoadherence. (a) Small lymphocyte (×1850); (b) plasma cell (×1850); (c) medium lymphocyte (×1850); (d) large blast lymphoid cell (? plasma blast) (×1850).

cells (Wigzell and Andersson, 1969). Here, it suffices to record that one can remove antibody-forming cells (as judged by indirect plaque-forming techniques) by filtering a cell suspension containing these through antigen-coated glass bead columns. The virtually total effective-ness of this procedure suggests that the exposed antibody on the cell surface is a uniform feature of all antibody-forming cells.

B. Presence of the Injected Antigen

We turn now to another main question of this chapter, namely the amount of antigen or antigen fragments which can be found on and in antibody-forming cells. In the early literature on this subject, no one seems to have doubted that antigen or antigen-derived material was present in antibody-forming cells. This was, of course, a *sine qua non* of the direct template hypothesis of antibody formation, and also of those hypotheses which ascribe to antigen an intracellular derepressive role. In the light of the newer theories we have been discussing, the need for the physical presence of antigen within the antibody-forming cell is no longer obvious.

The first two groups that sought to determine the antigen concentration in antibody-forming cells were Roberts and Haurowitz (1962) and Wellensiek and Coons (1964). The former group used tritiated hapten-protein conjugates and looked for antigen spread using radioautographic techniques. They found a wide diffusion of antigen including some in plasmablasts and plasma cells. In later studies (Roberts, 1964) it was also noted that organs such as the spleen, remote from the injection site, contained antibody-forming cells, as judged by immunofluorescent techniques, but most of these did not contain detectable isotopic labeling. In other words, it seemed as if antibody-forming cells might or might not contain detectable antigen. In this system, multiple injections of antigen were needed to induce an active immune response. It was thus not possible to determine whether the labeled antigen inside plasma cells had subserved an inductive role, or whether it had come into association with a previously induced cell by an antigen–antibody reaction, similar to immunocytoadherence, but occurring *in vivo*. Furthermore, these soluble antigens had been injected in milligram amounts into mice, and had spread widely through all lymphoid tissues. Thus any cell with pinocytic activity might have taken up some of the material. There was no indication that antibody-forming cells contained more antigen than other lymphoid cells.

The work of Wellensiek and Coons (1964) was performed using ferritin as antigen, and electron microscope detection of the marker molecules to test their cellular distribution. In the primary response, no antigen could be found in plasma cells. In the secondary response, both plasmablasts and plasma cells were reported to contain ferritin, the former in greater amounts than the latter. It was in fact estimated that mature plasma cells, presumably forming antibody against ferritin, contained up to 12,000 antigen molecules. This is an experiment of relatively simple design, and thus it is not easy to understand why two other groups obtained apparently different results. However, neither Buyukozer *et al.* (1965) nor de Petris and Karlsbad (1965) could find ferritin in immunoblasts or plasma cells appearing after immunization.

Our approach to this problem was to inject into rats a small amount of an ^{125}I-flagellar antigen labeled to high specific activity; to identify antibody-forming cells some days later using micromanipulatory techniques; and to process single antibody-forming cells for quantitative radioautography to determine their content of antigen-derived ^{125}I (Nossal *et al.*, 1965c, 1967). Flagellar antigens are rapidly eliminated from the extracellular fluid, and thus wide spread of isotope with possibly nonspecific uptake was minimized. A single injection of flagellar antigen will induce a vigorous primary response. Thus the need for multiple injections, with consequent difficulties in interpretation, was avoided. These substantial advantages must be counterbalanced against one serious drawback inherent in our experimental design. To achieve the desired labeling intensity, we had to use an external label, ^{125}I, which could become detached, particularly during partial fragmentation of our antigen, and which might or might not have been bound to an immunogenically active portion of the antigen molecule. As discussed in Chapters 2 and 3, there is no evidence to indicate that bound iodide can be detached from an intact protein molecule. Furthermore, five of the six tyrosine residues in flagellin are present in "fragment A" which also contains all detectable antigenic determinants. We believe, in fact, that the distribution of ^{125}I gave a fair indication of the distribution of the flagellar antigen, both because the localization pattern we found was so similar to that noted in several different systems (see Chapter 7) and because most of the isotope stably trapped in lymphatic tissues could be precipitated by specific antisera.

Our study can best be dealt with in two portions. The most clear-cut and readily interpretable results were obtained with the late IgG phase of the primary response (Nossal *et al.*, 1965a). The reasons for this are related to the shape of the antigen dose: antibody response curves for the IgM and IgG phases of the primary response to flagellar antigens (Nossal *et al.*, 1965a). The early primary response, consisting of IgM antibody, can be increased in intensity almost indefinitely with increasing antigen dose, and studies using radiolabeled antigen can thus involve injections of very large amounts of radioactivity. In contrast, near-maximal IgG responses, with high antibody levels persisting for many weeks, can be achieved with submicrogram doses of antigen. Thus, when rats were injected with 0.1 μg or less of labeled flagellin, and killed

1 to 9 weeks later, radioactivity levels in antibody-forming lymph nodes were quite low and single cell suspensions essentially free of noncell-bound radioactivity could readily be prepared. These contained anti-body-forming cells, identifiable by immunocytoadherence. Positive cells were identified, washed by micromanipulation, placed into marked circles on gelatin-coated slides, and processed for quantitative radio-autography. In fifteen experiments involving 216 single antibody-forming cells, only one cell displayed a degree of labeling greater than background. It was calculated that if each cell had included four molecules of iodinated flagellin, the mean grain count over the cells would have been one grain over background. In fact, the total grain count over the 216 cells was found to be slightly *less* than background. Thus if the distribution of label reflected the distribution of immunogenic molecules or fragments, then mature antibody-forming cells during the IgG phase of the primary response in this system contained either no antigen at all, or less than the equivalent of four molecules.

A similar conclusion was reached by studies of Humphrey's group (Humphrey *et al.*, 1967; McDevitt *et al.*, 1966), using a variety of tritiated and iodinated antigens. The most convincing negative experi-ments were performed using the antigen TIGAL (a copolymer of iodo-tyrosine, glutamic acid, alanine, and lysine—see Chapter 2) in which the ^{125}I forms an integral part of antigenically active sites. With this antigen, they were able to achieve an isotope substitution level such that the specific activity of the labeled antigen was higher than in our flagellin studies. Antibody-forming cells were detected by immuno-fluorescent methods and were subsequently processed for radioautog-raphy. These cells were found to be labeled a little *less* heavily than the prevailing background. It was also encouraging to note that ^{3}H- and ^{125}I-labeled synthetic antigens showed no gross differences in label-ing pattern.

A further experiment was that of Hanna *et al.* (1968), who failed to note the presence of ^{125}I-HGG in immunoblasts during immune re-sponses to that antigen, but as they used electron microscopic radio-autography, which needs much more isotope per cell for detectable labeling, these results were not quite so germane to the present argument.

It thus appears that in many established immune responses, antibody-forming cells can function with little or no antigen-derived material in or on them. What is the situation during the earliest, inductive phase of primary or secondary immune responses? We have approached this question in the flagellar system (Nossal *et al.*, 1967) using the same basic approach to study the early IgM response as we had used for the IgG phase. To achieve brisk 19 S responses, 1 to 10 μg of antigen had to be injected. If one were to gain equal sensitivity as had been achieved in the IgG study, this meant the use of 10 to 100 times more radioactivity. It was still possible to detect small numbers of early IgM antibody-forming cells with 0.1 μg or, with great difficulty, after even less antigen. The results of experiments using these small antigen doses can be readily summarized. Of fifty-three antibody-forming cells from animals that had received 0.1 μg or less of antigen, only one was labeled. With the higher antigen doses, however, labeled antibody-forming cells could be seen with increasing frequency, and calculations showed that 25/239 antibody-forming cells in the primary response and 89/345 in the secondary response contained the equivalent of 40–1000 or more antigen molecules. One important result was that antibody-forming cells collected from organs remote from the injection site were less frequently labeled than those derived from the node immediately draining the injection site. It is, of course, fully established that the overall antigen concentration in lymph nodes falls with progressively more remote nodes. Free-floating, antibody-forming cells in the thoracic duct lymph were never labeled. Conversely, nonantibody-forming cells from nodes near the injection site were labeled just as frequently and heavily as antibody-forming cells. In both antibody-forming and nonantibody-forming cells, a substantial minority of the labeled cells showed isotope confined to one or two small foci at the very surface of the cell.

From these experiments involving high antigen doses, it was concluded that the antigen content of many cells might simply have represented an epiphenomenon mirroring the high antigen content of the organ and/or the region from which the cells had been derived. The study showed that antigen *can* be found on and in immature antibody-forming cells, but on the whole did not support the idea that it has to be present for the further correct maturation of the cell. Unfortunately, the technique, of necessity, has to confine itself to cells already forming enough antibody to be detected by the methods used. A more exciting question to ask would have been whether the antibody-forming cell precursor, during the earliest phases of induction, and therefore before it secreted antibody, had to make contact with (and possibly adsorb) antigen. For example, if it had received information, either from a stimulated antigen-reactive cell (see Chapter 6) or an antigen-containing macrophage, this might not have been necessary. Obviously, our experiment cannot answer this question. Perhaps the most important finding of this part of the study was that many cells of blast morphology are synthesizing antibody but contain little or no antigen. It is probable that such cells would have gone on to divide and differentiate further, producing more mature antibody-forming progeny by some antigen-independent mechanism.

II. Lymphocytes from Unimmunized Animals

A. PRESENCE OF GLOBULINS ON CELL SURFACE

1. Demonstration by Immunofluorescence

Much of the evidence that small lymphocytes contain surface immuno-globulins is indirect. In terms of direct evidence, the most exhaustive study of the problem has been reported by van Furth *et al.* (1966a,b), using human material. With immunofluorescent staining techniques specific for the various major immunoglobulin classes, they were able to detect antibody-forming cells of the usual type by their brilliant fluorescence. In addition, however, they noticed a faint fluorescence of many small lymphocytes isolated from thoracic duct lymph, peripheral blood, spleen, and lymph nodes (but rarely from thymus and not from bone marrow). This fluorescence was detected only with reagents that recognized IgM. The authors interpreted this as indicating IgM synthesis by the cells concerned. However, it is not excluded that the very weak reactions might reflect the presence of surface receptors only, rather than concomitant synthesis and secretion of antibody.

2. Effect of Antiglobulin Antibodies

One important line of evidence for the existence of immunoglobulins on the lymphocyte surface comes from the work of Sell and Gell (1965a,b; Sell *et al.*, 1965; Sell, 1967, 1968). They have shown that antisera prepared against allotypic antigenic determinants of the rabbit immunoglobulin molecule can cause small lymphocytes from rabbits possessing the allotypic specificity concerned to transform *in vitro* into blast cells. Extensive washing and preincubation of the lymphocytes failed to remove their reactivity, suggesting that the molecules carrying the allotypic marker were firmly attached to the cells. A surface location was suggested, though not proven, by the fact that contact for only 15 min with anti-allotype sera set the process of stimulation in motion. However, direct tests to demonstrate the presence of bound anti-allotype antibodies after the initiation of stimulation were unsuccessful. In ontogeny, the presence of the allotypic specificity was detectable on or in the cells at an earlier time than it appeared in the serum. Heterologous antisera against rabbit IgG were also effective and could cause blast cell transformation of up to 90% of the small lymphocytes, and anti-light chain, anti-heavy chain, anti-Fab, and anti-Fc sera were all reported to be active. This suggested to Sell (1967, 1968) that all peripheral small lymphocytes carry all the antigenic specificities of the entire IgG molecule. However, the quantitative aspects of this work have been criticized on the basis of the possible release of a blastogen from a minority of initially and specifically stimulated cells. Sell counters such arguments vigorously with a variety of convincing controls. Interestingly, anti-μ chain and anti-γ chain sera also had high rates of activity, and the implication was drawn that all lymphocytes possessed IgG and IgM, and about one-third, IgA as well. The indirect and complex nature of the detection system, however, renders this conclusion somewhat uncertain.

More recently, Gell et al. (1970) have developed an ingenious variant of the rosette technique of Zaalberg (1964) to study the nature of allotypic determinants on lymphoid cells directly, without the necessity of waiting for stimulation of blast transformation. This technique shows great promise and may provide definite answers to the number and variety of such markers on a single cell.

3. Studies Indirectly Relevant to Cell Surface Receptors

The claim that lymphocytes may display on their surface more than one class of immunoglobulin seems at first sight in contrast to the known phenotypic restriction of antibody-forming cells (see Chapter 3). However, nothing is known as to when, in the differentiation of immunocytes, this restriction first becomes manifest. A number of studies have now been performed on immunoglobulin synthesis in vitro by clonal cell lines derived from malignant human lymphoid tumors (Fahey et al., 1966; Takahashi et al., 1969a,b; Fahey and Finegold, 1967). While many of these lines synthesize monoclonal type immunoglobulins akin to myeloma proteins, there are numerous examples of cell lines in which one cell can be shown to simultaneously be synthesizing IgM and IgG, or IgG and IgA. Interestingly, in twenty-seven lines examined, Takahashi et al. (1969a) found no case in which a cell synthesized kappa and lambda light chains simultaneously. Clearly these studies, though interesting, are only marginally relevant to the functioning of normal lymphocytes.

Another indirect line of reasoning that leads us to postulate antibody receptors on nonantibody-forming lymphocytes comes from the work of Mitchison (1967, 1970) on the stimulation of lymphocytes *in vitro* followed by transfer *in vivo* to immunologically neutral hosts. Carefully quantitated experiments have shown that lymphocytes from animals that have been primed, but are not forming detectable amounts of antibody, can be stimulated *in vitro* with antigen, and that this stimulation can be competitively inhibited by hapten. The observations were consistent with the presence of antibody-like sites on or in the primed cells. However, the situation was rendered complex by the demonstration of a major role, in the degree of stimulation, of the carrier portion of the antigenic molecule.

An important but equally indirect observation bearing on the probable characteristics of the surface antigen-binding sites has been reported by Nussenzweig and Benacerraf (1967). They found that the nature and amount of anti-DNP antibodies made by guinea pigs after the injection of DNP conjugated to bovine γ-globulin varied with the dose of antigen. Antibody of highest binding affinity was achieved with 0.05 mg of antigen, considered a low dose in this system. A higher dose, e.g., 1 mg, produced less avidly binding antibody and, furthermore, the "maturation" toward increasingly avid antibody was slower and less marked with the high antigen dose. The postulated explanation for this was that the relative binding affinity of lymphocyte surface receptors for an antigen was the basis for a selective mechanism determining what antibodies would be produced. With antigen present in low concentration, only antigen-reactive cells with high affinity receptors would be stimulated. With high antigen doses, the response would broaden to include also cells with relatively poor affinity receptors. The results fit in easily with clonal selection concepts, but were difficult to understand without postulating the existence of surface receptors which mirrored the synthetic capacities of the cell.

Given that radioautographic techniques are both in principle and in practice much more sensitive than immunofluorescent techniques, it is somewhat surprising that they seem not to have been used in an attempt to demonstrate immunoglobulins on lymphocyte surfaces. Radiolabeled antigens have been used to identify cell-associated antibody or antibody-like factors (Berenbaum, 1959; Pick and Feldman, 1967; Naor and Sulitzeanu, 1967; Byrt and Ada, 1969), but we are not aware of any reports that have attempted to use labeled anti-immunoglobulin antibodies to "stain" lymphocyte surfaces. Perhaps such attempts have been made but have failed because of the substantial background problems which present difficulties in such work.

B. Reaction of Isotopically Labeled Antigens with Lymphocytes

Naor and Sulitzeanu (1967, 1968) were the first to seek a direct confirmation of Burnet's (1957) clonal selection hypothesis by the use of radiolabeled antigens mixed *in vitro* with normal lymphoid cells. If the clonal selection theory is correct, there ought to exist in the spleen of a normal mouse a very small proportion of lymphocytes with the capacity to react with a particular antigen, e.g., bovine serum albumin (BSA). In a primed mouse, not actively forming antibody but ready to react in secondary fashion, this proportion should be specifically increased. Accordingly, Naor and Sulitzeanu took low concentrations of BSA iodinated to high specific activity with ^{125}I, mixed this with suspensions of normal spleen cells for 1 hr at 4°C, washed and performed radioautographs on cell smears. The great majority of spleen cells failed to become labeled. Some 2% became lightly labeled and about one cell per 1000 showed quite heavy labeling. Lymph node cells behaved in similar fashion. Labeled cells included large, medium, and small lymphocytes and macrophages, but the heavily labeled cells were mainly small lymphocytes. Intentional immunization raised the number of "positive" cells if it induced active antibody formation, but not if it simply induced immunological memory. These experiments demonstrated (1) the antigen-binding capacity of some cells; (2) a heterogeneity among lymphocytes in this property; but (3) they did not show that the binding is due to antibody; and (4) they did not distinguish between the positive cells as "natural" antibody formers to BSA or a cross-reacting material as opposed to a true, "virgin" antigen-reactive lymphocyte.

This line of investigation has been taken up in detail by Ada and colleagues (Ada and Byrt, 1969; Byrt and Ada, 1969; Ada *et al.*, 1970; Mandel *et al.*, 1970; Dwyer and Mackay, 1970; Warner *et al.*, 1970) and also by Humphrey and Keller (1970). In the studies of our own group, lymphoid cells from several rat and mouse tissues were tested for their capacity to react in the cold with several antigens, principally hemocyanin (*Jasus lalandii*) and flagellin from *Salmonella* organisms, both being labeled either with ^{131}I or ^{125}I. The reaction was rapid and was not affected by a concentration of sodium azide, which was known to inhibit phagocytosis. As in the studies of Naor and Sulitzeanu, it was found that cells could not be readily placed into two clear categories, negative or positive. Rather, it was noted that the percentage of labeled cells was proportional to the concentration of labeled antigen in the reaction mixture. At a given concentration of labeled protein, however, the number of reactive lymphocytes was relatively constant and characteristic of each tissue. In a typical experiment where labeled flagellin at a concentration of 0.3 μg/ml was mixed with cells (10^8/ml), suspensions of cells from mouse spleen, thoracic duct lymph, and lymph node contained between 0.5 and 2 labeled cells per 10,000. The thymus always contained small numbers of positive cells which were only lightly labeled. In contrast, a high proportion of cells in peritoneal washings reacted with the antigens tested. Particularly when hemocyanin was used, the proportion of cells reacting was found to be very high, being around one cell per thousand for spleen and up to twenty per thousand for peritoneal exudate. The majority of the labeled cells were small to medium lymphocytes.

A limited series of experiments has been performed on germfree animals. These seem to behave no differently from conventional ones.

Bone marrow cells behaved in an anomalous fashion. The proportion of cells reacting with flagellin was over one per thousand but, in contrast to other organ sources, the union of cell and labeled antigen could not be inhibited by anti-immunoglobulin antisera. When bone marrow cells were reacted with labeled hemocyanin, this anomaly appeared less marked.

Interestingly, the reaction of spleen cells was relatively difficult to inhibit by the exposure of the cells to excess unlabeled specific antigen. A 100-fold excess had little effect, but a 10,000-fold excess achieved a reduction of 70–90% in the proportion of labeled cells.

Examination of positive cells in the electron microscope confirmed that most antigen-binding cells in the spleen were small lymphocytes. Bound antigen was present at the surface of the plasma membrane and occurred in discrete patches (see Figs. 9.2 and 9.3).

Evidence was obtained which supported the notion that the mechanism of interaction of antigen with lymphocytes was by means of immunoglobulin at the cell surface. Pretreatment of mouse lymphocytes with a polyvalent rabbit anti-mouse globulin serum inhibited a subsequent reaction of the cells with labeled antigen. Further work established that anti-light chain and anti-μ chain sera were also effective as inhibitors wheras anti-α, anti-γ_1, and anti-γ_2 chain sera were ineffective. Pretreatment of mouse spleen cells with anti-light chain or anti-μ chain sera before adoptive transfer into X-irradiated mice depressed the ability of the cells to respond to a variety of antigens, suggesting that reaction of antigen with IgM receptors at the lymphocyte surface was a necessary step in immune induction.

The reaction may be used as a method for following the proportion of binding cells present in various tissues after injection of antigen.

Work published or in progress is summarized in Table 9.1. The number of comparisons which can be made is limited, as different antigens and different injection schedules were used. In addition, antigen concentrations, extent of isotope substitution, and time of exposure of cell smears to photographic emulsion varied between different laboratories. The major comparison to be made is between control and immunized samples in individual experiments, and here great differences can be seen. For example, 100 days after the injection of ^{125}I-BSA (in Freund's incomplete

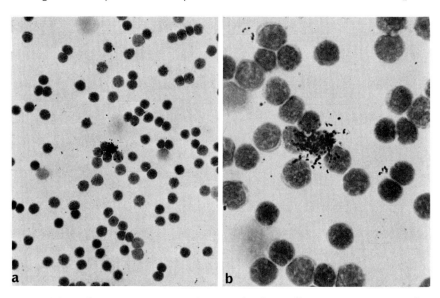

FIG. 9.2. Light microscopic view of antigen-binding cells as seen in a smear after labeling of mouse thoracic duct lymphocytes with ^{125}I-labeled polymerized flagellin. (a) At magnification ×560, used for scanning purposes; (b) at magnification ×1400, used for verification of morphology and for grain counting. The two cells shown are very heavily labeled and would normally be scored as greater than 100 grains.

adjuvant), Naor and Sulitzeanu (1969) found that up to 23% of the lymph node cells bound antigen, though most of these cells bound very little. In spleen the level was 4.5%. Injection of hemocyanin (*M. squinado*) in Freund's complete adjuvant followed by a booster injection also resulted in many more antigen-binding cells in lymph node or spleen compared to controls, but the final proportion was still less than 1%. Dwyer and Mackay (1970) have reported a high proportion of binding cells in blood leukocytes of patients who were injected subcutaneously only 10 days previously with a small dose of flagellin in saline. Several

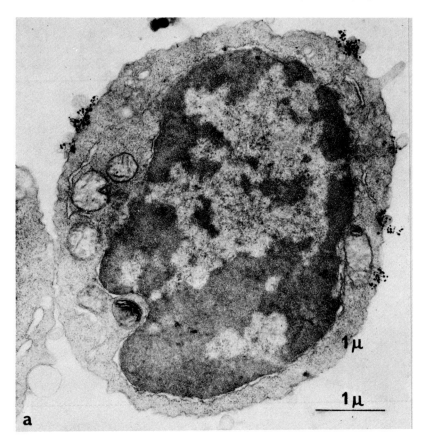

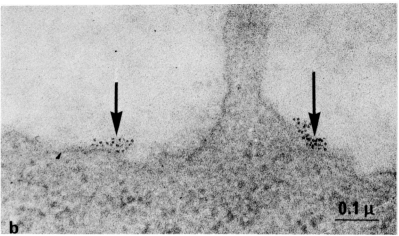

See facing page for legend→

factors may have contributed to this high number, which usually approached around 8% of blood lymphocytes. First, the concentration of antigen used in the binding reaction was high. Second, normal adult humans always have a high level of natural antibody to *Salmonella adelaide* flagellin, which is not the case in mice, and the immune response to the first intentional immunization thus probably starts from a higher plateau. Third, recently stimulated cells may be preferentially released from lymphoid organs and thus present in disproportionately high numbers in the peripheral blood as compared to spleen.

Injection of polymerized flagellin into mice resulted in a very rapid increase in the number of binding cells which was recovered in the spleen. This is known to be an IgM response and it may be that this rapid change was a reflection that most binding cells in nonimmunized mice appear to possess IgM receptors. During the 4-day period after the injection, the positive cells increased in median diameter and this trend was observed as early as 12 hr after antigen injection. Evidence was given which indicated that in this rapid response, some of the binding cells were antibody secretors.

In contrast to the above results, injection of hemocyanin (*J. lalandii*) in Freund's complete adjuvant into rats resulted in a very minor increase in the proportion of binding cells. This may be related to the finding that this was an IgG response. Similarly, injection of the synthetic antigen TIGAL into mice resulted in only a small increase in the number of binding cells recovered from the spleen.

In all *in vivo* experiments of this nature, it should be remembered that a strict comparison of binding cells in organs may not be completely valid because of the possibility of preferential migration of positive cells in stimulated animals.

A tenet of the clonal selection theory, as originally proposed by Burnet, was that cells responding to self-antigens in early life were killed and eliminated. As an extension of this concept, it appeared likely that in acquired tolerance, specific antigen-binding cells might be found to be absent, or at least reduced in numbers. In three results published and from work under way, there is now some evidence in favor and some

---

FIG. 9.3. Demonstration of antigen binding by lymphocytes as seen in the electron microscope. (a) An electron microscope radioautograph of a medium lymphocyte labeled *in vitro* with hemocyanin-^{125}I. The labeled antigen is present in a few discrete patches at the cell surface (glutaralderyde fixation, unstained). ×20,000. (b) Electron micrograph of a portion of lymphocyte which has bound ferritin *in vitro*. Two patches of adherent ferritin are arrowed (glutaraldehyde fixation, unstained, ×115,000).

TABLE 9.I

REACTION OF LABELED ANTIGENS WITH LYMPHOID CELLS FROM IMMUNIZED ANIMALS

Antigen	Experimental subject	Days post-injection	Immunoglobulin class	Source of cells	Proportion of cells labeled (lymphocytes) %	Reference
BSA-^{125}I	Mouse	Control	—	Lymph node	< 0.03	Naor and Sulitzeanu (1969)
		13 days	—	Lymph node	0.6	
		100 Days	—	Lymph node	23	
		100 Days	—	Spleen	4.5	
TIGAL-^{125}I	Mouse	Control	—	Lymph node	0.023	Humphrey and Keller, (1970)
		56 Days	—	Lymph node	0.08	
		Control	—	Spleen	0.019	
		56 Days	—	Spleen	0.031	
Hemocyanin-^{125}I (M. squinado)	Mouse	Control	—	Lymph node	0.005	Humphrey and Keller (1970)
		56 Days	—	Lymph node	0.114	
		Control	—	Spleen	0.006	
		56 Days	—	Spleen	0.45	
Flagellin-^{125}I (S. adelaide)	Man	Control	IgM	Blood leukocytes	0.5	Dwyer and Mackay, (1970)
		10 Days			10	
Polymerized flagellin-^{125}I	Mouse	Control	IgM	Spleen	0.02	Ada et al. (1970)
		4 Days			0.17	
Hemocyanin-^{125}I (J. lalandii)	Rat	Control	IgG	Spleen	0.02	Ada, Byrt, Cooper, and Langman (1970)
		28 Days			0.03	

evidence against this notion. Naor and Sulitzeanu (1969) injected mice during the first week of life with a total of 60 mg BSA. At 6 weeks of age, no antibody could be detected in the sera. In two experiments, cells from the popliteal nodes were found to contain far fewer binding cells than control cell populations (nil compared to 12, and 6 compared to 28 per 10^4 cells). These authors were careful to point out, however, that antigen remaining from the injection schedule may have saturated binding sites on the specific cells.

Humphrey and Keller (1970) induced tolerance in mice to TIGAL (the synthetic antigen TGAL extensively substituted with iodide) and to hemocyanin (*M. squinado*). The first group received intraperitoneal

TABLE 9.II

COMPARISON OF ANTIGEN-BINDING SPLEEN AND LYMPH NODE CELLS
FROM NORMAL MICE AND FROM MICE MADE TOLERANT
TO TIGAL OR HEMOCYANIN (*M. squinado*)[a,b]

	Antigen dose in reaction mixture (ng)	Antigen	Control		Tolerant	
			Spleen	Lymph node	Spleen	Lymph node
Total labeled	64	TIGAL	0.28	0.15	0.11	0.08
cells (>50 grains)	84	Hemocyanin	0.15	0.16	0.26	0.07
Very heavily	64	TIGAL	0.034	0.023	0.015	0.005
labeled cells (hedgehogs)	84	Hemocyanin	<0.006	0.005	0.004	<0.002

[a] Humphrey and Keller, 1970.

[b] Results are expressed as the percent of cells examined which were labeled. For total labeled cells, up to 8000 cells were examined. For heavily labeled cells, up to 90,000 cells were examined.

injections (50 μg TIGAL, each injection) from birth, 3 injections in the first week, 2 in the second and third week and weekly thereafter. No antibody was detected, and littermates on challenge gave no detectable antibody response. The second group received twice weekly intraperitoneal injections of 1.5 mg hemocyanin, and at the time of test no antibody was detected in the blood. Antigen binding cells in spleen and lymph nodes were estimated (Table 9.II). If total labeled cells (cells with >50 grains) were counted, tolerant animals in three out of four cases, appeared to have a reduced number (approximately 50% fewer). If only very heavily labeled cells (hedgehogs) were counted, then in the same three cases, there was an apparent reduction which varied from 50 to 75%. These results could be interpreted as indicating a decrease in the number of high affinity cells in tolerant animals, although a comparison of very small numbers of cells (0 to 5) is perhaps of dubious significance.

Ada *et al.* (1970) induced tolerance in rats to flagellin by two procedures. One group received from birth intraperitoneal injections thrice weekly of 1 μg of the cyanogen bromide digest of flagellin—a total of 21 μg of protein per rat; the other group received at 7 weeks of age and for 4 weeks, 100 μg of this preparation—a total of 2.8 mg of protein per rat. Spleen cells from a few animals per group were tested for their reactivity to labeled flagellin. Most rats in each group were challenged and shown to produce no serum antibody. Similar results were obtained with each group; compared to controls, there was no reduction in the number of spleen lymphocytes from tolerant animals which reacted with flagellin. It is possible in the case of animals made tolerant to flagellin in this way, however, that they may be tolerant to only some determinants of flagellin because they still possess "natural" antibody, as shown by the ability of injected labeled flagellin to lodge in lymphoid follicles.

Separate experiments were therefore carried out (Ada *et al.*, 1970) using hemocyanin (*Jasus lalandii*) as the antigen as there is no evidence that rats contain natural antibody to this antigen. The methods of estimation of antibodies to this antigen used had great sensitivity (hemagglutination, about 10 ng antibody/ml; follicular localization of injected labeled antigen, <1 ng antibody/ml). Rats were injected thrice weekly from birth with 500 μg of hemocyanin. At 8–10 weeks of age, no antibody could be detected. Spleen cells from these rats and from normal rats were reacted with labeled hemocyanin using antigen concentrations varying from 0.5–500 ng/ml. Numbers of cells scanned ranged from 10^4 to $>10^6$. At each level used, spleens from tolerant rats were found to contain as many, and frequently slightly more, labeled cells as did spleens from control rats. This is a particularly significant finding in those experiments where very low amounts of antigen were used in the binding reaction, as presumably only cells with highly avid receptors would react and be detected. Littermates of control and tolerant rats were injected with 100 μg hemocyanin in Freund's complete adjuvant. Control animals produced antibody by 14 days and had high titers by 28 days. Tolerant animals produced no detectable serum antibody, and even more significantly, when they were injected with labeled antigen, follicular localization failed to occur within 24 hr of the injection. Control, challenged animals showed a twofold increase in binding cells in the spleen (Table 9.I); tolerant, challenged animals showed a comparable increase.

Rats that are demonstrably tolerant may therefore contain undiminished numbers of specific antigen binding cells in their spleens. A state of tolerance may not therefore necessarily or always mean an absence of specific binding cells but possibly an inactivation of these cells. If so, it will be of interest to see if such cells can be reactivated. This point will be considered again in Chapter 12.

1. Functional Inactivation

There exist three chief possibilities to explain specific reactions, i.e., those inhibitable by anti-immunoglobulin sera, between certain lymphocytes and antigen. (1) The results could be due to cytophilic antibody. The bulk of the evidence suggests that cytophilic antibody adheres to macrophages rather than to lymphocytes, and in any case strong immunization procedures, involving Freund's complete adjuvant, are necessary to elicit its formation. Moreover, specific functional inactivation experiments (to be described below) practically exclude this possibility. (2) The reactive cells represented antibody-forming cells that had been stimulated *in vivo* by some naturally occurring antigen related to the test antigen. This seems unlikely in view of the high proportion of cells reacting with hemocyanin, an antigen not generally regarded as cross-reacting with food or bacterial floral antigens. Also, the normal proportion of reactive cells in germfree animals speaks against this possibility. (3) The positive cells are really the antigen-reactive cells.

It has long been known (Heineke, 1905) that lymphocytes display marked sensitivity to ionizing radiations. Inactivation of stimulated lymphocytes by pulses of ^{3}H-thymidine of high specific activity have been used to study early events in antibody formation in tissue culture (Dutton and Mishell, 1967b). It thus occurred to Ada and Byrt (1969) to use a similar principle to test the function of cells capable of binding labeled antigen as described above. Thus, suspensions of spleen cells from adult unimmunized mice were reacted for 30 min with polymerized flagellin labeled to high specific activity with ^{125}I. After removal of unbound labeled antigen, the cells were held *in vitro* for 24 hr at 4°C. After this interval, the cells were transferred to lethally irradiated syngeneic hosts. One day later, the host was challenged with unlabeled antigen of the same specificity to test the immunological potential of the transferred cell population, and antibody responses were assessed

8 days later. In every experiment, pretreatment of the cells with radio-labeled antigen either abolished or significantly reduced the subsequent response to the same antigen. Incubation of cells with appropriate concentrations of uniodinated antigen or antigen iodinated with carrier iodide did not affect the immune capacity of the cells. Furthermore, when the immune capacity of the transferred lymphocyte population was tested against a chemically and physically similar, but serologically distinct antigen, a normal antibody response followed. That is, the inactivation of lymphocytes due to adsorption of labeled antigen was shown to be specific. These findings are summarized in Table 9.II.

The simplest explanation of these findings is the following. Antigen-reactive cells specific for the labeled flagellin adsorbed ^{125}I-marked antigen onto their surface. As ^{125}I disintegrates, it gives off, *inter alia*, electrons of relatively weak energy which will be absorbed within a few microns of the isotope source. Thus, specific ARC with antigen on their surface would receive relatively high doses of ionizing radiation and would be inactivated more rapidly and extensively than the other cells.

It is of interest that Humphrey and Keller (1970) also obtained results consistent with the idea that antigen-reactive cells can be killed by irradiation in the manner suggested. They injected very highly labeled but serologically antigenic ^{125}I-TIGAL and noted a specific failure of both primary and secondary antibody responses. The lowered reactivity depended on the degree of isotope substitution and not on the degree of iodination as such. The experiment may have been the *in vivo* counterpart of our experiment. A further factor suggested by Humphrey may be the killing of lymphocytes which come in contact with highly labeled macrophages or dendritic follicle cells.

Both the above sets of experiments suggest that at least some of the cells which reacted with antigen are cells which are vital for the subsequent correct expression of the antibody response. The profound nature of the effect suggests that most, if not all, of the cells which are involved in the initiation of immune induction had been affected, and therefore had presumably taken up at least some isotope. The specificity of the reaction, which left the response to a serologically unrelated but chemically very similar antigen unaffected is difficult to reconcile with any theory other than one requiring restricted range of antigen reactivity per individual cell, such as the clonal selection theory. However, it may be necessary to view the results in terms of collaborative effects between two or more cells as discussed in Chapter 6. It could well be the case that inactivation of one partner in a cell collaboration would be sufficient to prevent antibody formation. There is as yet no evidence to indicate whether the cells capable of binding antigen are thymus-derived, bone marrow-derived or both.

At this stage, the antigen-binding activity of cells from tolerant animals is difficult to interpret. In the flagellin system, we could detect no significant difference in the number of labeled cells from tolerant as compared with unimmunized animals. In the systems investigated by Humphrey and Keller (1970) there was some reduction in the number of very heavily labeled cells in tolerant animals. This reduction was, however, not as profound as that of antibody levels in the tolerant group. Taken at face value, these results might suggest that there exists, in the tolerant animal, specific cells which retain some antigen-binding sites, but which cannot respond under the usual conditions of stimulation. These could represent "tolerant cells," i.e., cells maintained in the tolerant state by nonsaturating quantities of antigen. This possibility becomes more plausible when the difficulty of inhibiting this reaction with excess unlabeled antigen is recalled.

C. Removal of Specific Cells by Immunoabsorbants

Another elegant method approaching the question of the nature of receptors on the surface of ARC has been described by Wigzell and Andersson (1969). It involves the passage of cells through columns of glass or plastic beads coated with antigen. The beads are held with aqueous solutions of antigen, and, without the mediation of any intentional linking procedure, they take up small quantities of protein which they do not release again despite washing. Lymphoid cell suspensions can then be passed through such columns. When these are taken from an animal that had been intentionally immunized with the antigen on the column, the column effluent shows a specific depletion of antibody-forming cells (as measured by indirect plaque techniques) and of "memory" cells (as measured by ability to confer a secondary adoptive immune response). When the cells are taken from an unimmunized animal, the capacity of the column effluent to mount a primary adoptive immune response is specifically diminished. So far, the columns have proved themselves more useful for depletion than for enrichment of ARC. Depletion can be impressive—immune reactivity can fall 10- or 20-fold, though some individual variation between experiments was noted. However, when cells were removed from the column itself, the enrichment factor was, at best, 1.5. This was not unexpected, as it had been noted that passage of cells through such columns involved substantial yield losses, thus showing that many cells became nonspecifically trapped. An encouraging feature of the experiments was that the depletion effect could be diminished by including specific antigen in the medium in which the lymphoid cells were suspended. This suggested a competition between free antigen and bead-bound antigen for cell surface antibody sites. In all, the experiments lead us to the same conclusions as those reported using labeled antigen, namely a dependence of the immune response on cells bearing antibodylike receptors on their surface.

Abdou and Richter (1969) have used antigen-coated glass bead columns to fractionate antigen-reactive cells from the rabbit bone marrow. They achieve specific depletion as noted above, but also claim considerable enrichment in eluate fractions obtained by disruption of the column and vigorous shaking. Some experiments seemed to indicate enrichment factors of 25 or greater. It is not easy to see why these authors obtained enrichment so readily where previous work had failed, and confirmation of the findings is eagerly awaited.

D. Hapten Inhibition Studies

An extensive series of indirect studies have addressed themselves to the nature of the supposed receptor site on antigen-reactive cells. This literature is too extensive and too far from our central theme for us to review. However, we wish to draw attention to one important series of investigations by Mitchison (1967; 1969) which raises some complications to the simple ideas of clonal selection apparently supported by the experiments of Ada and Byrt and of Wigzell just summarized.

Mitchison has used lymphoid cells from preimmunized animals and has investigated conditions of restimulation *in vitro*, prior to adoptive transfer of the cells to X-irradiated hosts. If hapten–protein conjugates are used, free hapten is an effective inhibitor to restimulation. A cross-reacting hapten inhibits to the degree expected from its serological properties. These results are in agreement with the idea that antigen stimulates cells by uniting with an antibodylike site. However, in these stimulations, the nature of the carrier has a profound effect. If an unrelated carrier is substituted, the hapten–carrier complex stimulates much less effectively. This is so even when carrier (both immunizing and unrelated) is separated from the hapten by an immunologically inert "spacer." However, if a population of cells preimmunized against the unrelated carrier is added to the reaction mixture, there is a restoration of the capacity for anti-hapten antibody formation. Mitchison believes that there is a collaboration between cells reacting against the carrier and those reacting against the hapten. He conceives of this as possibly due to better antigen "focusing," the cell with anti-carrier specificity trapping the antigen and bringing it to the cell preadapted to react against the hapten. Experiments of rather complex design suggest that the anti-carrier cells may be thymus-derived and the anti-hapten cells bone marrow-derived. Thus Mitchison seeks to explain the bone marrow: thymus cell-to-cell interactions discussed in Chapter 6 as a special example of collaboration between anti-carrier and anti-hapten cells. The reader is referred to Chapters 6 and 12 for further discussion of this field.

E. Specific Inhibition of Antibody Response by Affinity Labeling of Lymphocyte Surface Receptors

Two independent studies (Plotz, 1969; Segal et al., 1969) have approached the question of the specificity of receptors for antigen on lymphoid cells by using the principle of affinity labeling. This method was first developed to study the binding sites of antibody molecules (Wofsy et al., 1962). The principle is that a hapten with a chemically reactive side group is mixed with antibody, and the reactive side group causes the formation of a covalent bond between hapten and susceptible groups at or near the antibody-combining site. Thus, essentially, the reversible interaction between hapten and antibody is rendered irreversible. The present adaptation of the method involved an interaction of antigen-reactive lymphocytes with the affinity-labeling reagents, and thus putatively an irreversible binding of hapten to the antibody receptors on lymphocytes. It was shown that such a reaction specifically inhibited the immune response to hapten–protein conjugates, without causing nonspecific damage to the lymphocyte population. This type of experiment strengthens the notion of antibody-receptors on lymphocytes, but is not relevant to the unipotency or multipotency of antigen-reactive cells. It may find its greatest usefulness in an analysis of the chemical nature of the antibody receptor on lymphocytes.

III. Summary

In this chapter, we have concerned ourselves with two chief questions, namely the evidence for antibodylike receptors on antigen-reactive lymphocytes, and the antigen content of antibody-forming cells. Evidence that immunoglobulins exist on the surface of lymphocytes is still largely indirect. One line of relevant work is that relating to the blastogenic effects of antiimmunoglobulin and antiallotype sera. Most other lines relate to the antibody specificity of such surface receptors. We have reviewed work dealing with the surface adsorption of radiolabeled antigens onto lymphocytes, the removal of immunocompetence from cell populations by passing cells through antigen-coated columns, and the stimulation of lymphocytes to form antibody by various hapten–protein conjugates. All this experimentation suggests that lymphocytes do possess antibody on their surface, and that there is great heterogeneity in a lymphocyte population. It further suggests that the removal of cells with receptors for a given antigen from a population eliminates the immunocompetence of that population for that antigen. This is in favor of the clonal selection hypothesis of antibody formation, but there are one or two disturbing features. First, the proportion of lymphocytes capable of specifically adsorbing certain antigens can be very high—as much as one cell in fifty in the case of peritoneal cells and hemocyanin. Second, the importance of the carrier effect in stimulation of lymphocytes needs to be explained. These matters will be taken up in Chapter 12.

Experiments on the antigen content of antibody-forming cells have shown that whereas antigen can enter antibody-forming cells and their precursors under some circumstances, this is neither a necessary nor a sufficient condition for antibody formation. Both immature and mature plasma cells and lymphocytes can form antibody while their content of antigen is below the limits of detection of even the most sensitive tracer techniques. It remains possible that each antibody-forming cell contains up to several hundred antigen-derived amino acids, conceivably linked to some critical intracellular control site, but it is no longer reasonable to argue that each polysome synthesizing antibody chains has an antigenic determinant associated with it. Thus the direct template hypothesis of antibody formation appears to be incorrect.

An incomplete and certainly still speculative interpretation of the experiments dealing with the interaction of antigen and lymphoid cells would then be as follows. Lymphoid cells possess receptors of immunoglobulin nature on their surface which are capable of uniting with antigen molecules. Indirect but persuasive evidence argues for the view that different cells bear different receptors, and that cells with receptors specific for a given antigen are necessary for a correct immune response to that antigen. In vivo interactions between these cells (hopefully the ARC) and injected, labeled antigen can at present only be guessed at. It is quite possible that some of these cells adsorb antigen *in vivo*, transform into blasts, begin to secrete antibody, and are recognized, as in our *in vivo* studies (Nossal *et al.*, 1967), as antibody secretors with one or more surface foci of antigen. It is equally possible that sooner or later this antigen becomes detached, diluted out or catabolized, leaving us with an antibody-forming cell *not* containing antigen, and in fact not needing it for its continued healthy functioning. There is nothing in our data to contradict this view, but there are too many missing experimental links for us to press it too firmly.

The line of work dealing with the identification of antigen-binding lymphocytes using radiolabeled antigens, and especially that dealing with their specific inactivation through exposure to high radiation doses, appears to be the most direct approach yet devised to test the clonal selection hypothesis. It is likely to yield many important results over the next few years.

CHAPTER 10

THE ROLE OF ANTIGEN IN IMMUNOLOGICAL TOLERANCE

I. General Features of Immunological Tolerance

A. BACKGROUND

It is by now well established that antigen can cause not only immunization, but, under suitable circumstances, an opposite event, namely immunological tolerance. Immunological tolerance represents a condition in which the capacity of an animal to react to a normally effective antigenic stimulus has been specifically diminished or abolished by prior administration of that particular, or a related, antigen. This subject has such great theoretical and practical implications that a considerable literature has accumulated on it, and the most important findings have been summarized in recent reviews and symposium monographs (Landy and Braun, 1969; Dresser and Mitchison, 1968; Bussard, 1963; Smith, 1961; Hasek et al., 1962). In this chapter, those aspects dealing with antigen dose, antigen presentation, and antigen distribution will receive special emphasis.

Early work of an initially nonimmunological character (Owen, 1945; Traub, 1938) established that living foreign viruses or cells, present in an animal's tissues from early embryonic life onward, enjoy a privileged existence even after the animal has matured. Reflection on these findings caused Burnet and Fenner (1949) to predict the experimental demonstration of tolerance. They reasoned that if an antigen were introduced into an embryo before the immune apparatus had developed, the animal would be "tricked" into later regarding that antigen as a "self" component. Thus, the animal would fail to form antibody to that particular antigen, even if it were reintroduced at a later time in a form and dose adequate for immunization of normal controls. The experiments of Billingham, Brent, and Medawar (1953) showed that tolerance, at least with respect to transplantation immune responses, could indeed be induced by injection of living allogeneic lymphoid cells into mouse embryos. Soon thereafter, it became clear that similar principles could be used to induce tolerance toward defined protein antigens (Hanan and Oyama, 1954; Smith and Bridges, 1958).

A major step forward was the realization that tolerance could also be induced in adult animals. Important early work was that of Glenny and Hopkins (1923) and Felton (1949), but the matter first came in sharp focus with studies of adult animals that had been subjected to X-irradiation (reviewed by Schwartz, 1966) or cytotoxic drugs (Schwartz and Damashek, 1963). Such animals, temporarily rendered incapable of an active immune response, could be made tolerant with doses and forms of antigen comparable to those effective in embryonic or newborn animals. The next important contribution was the finding of Dresser (1961b) that certain antigens, when prepared in soluble form and given by the intravenous route, could induce tolerance in adult animals even in the absence of prior immunosuppression.

Current research on immunological tolerance is moving from the phase of phenomenological description to that of detailed analysis of mechanisms. Accordingly, a greater proportion of studies are now concerned with defined, purified antigens and quantitative analysis of immune capacity. Some of these are considered below. Description of in vitro models of tolerance induction will follow in Chapter 11.

Most tolerance studies can be considered in two phases: tolerance induction, and testing of the degree of tolerance. In the first phase, the investigator administers antigen, frequently giving repeated injections over intervals of some weeks. Parameters varied or examined over this interval include antigen dose, size, presentation, persistence, fate, and specificity; or recipient animal's species, age or immunological integrity.

In the second phase, the investigator seeks to test to what extent the antigen he has given has altered a subsequent immune response to the same, or a related antigen from the expected norm. Usually this involves giving a challenge of antigen in highly immunogenic form, for example in Freund's complete adjuvant. After an appropriate interval, the level of serum antibodies in treated animals is compared to that of normal controls. It is important to realize that tolerance can be partial as well as complete. A partially tolerant animal is one which forms significantly less antibody after challenge than do controls, and a completely tolerant animal one which makes no detectable antibody after challenge. The division is arbitrary and depends on the sensitivity of the detection technique. The point is that, at the level of the whole animal, tolerance and antibody formation are not mutually exclusive states, though they might be at the level of a single lymphocyte. A fairly complete list of the antigens and species used for current tolerance models is given in Table 1 of Dresser and Mitchison's (1968) review. Suffice it to say here that the models successfully used include numerous species such as mouse, rat, guinea pig, rabbit, and chicken, and all manner of antigens, such as soluble or particulate protein, carbohydrate or haptenic antigens. It is probably fair to say that the current models on which most work is being done all involve mice or rats, and one of three groups of antigens, namely heterologous serum proteins, pneumococcal polysaccharides, or bacterial flagellar antigens.

B. Some Key Results Summarized

In view of the complexity of much of the material to be reviewed, a brief summary of some of the key findings relating to antigen trapping and tolerance induction *in vivo* may be helpful at this point.

(1) The newborn animal traps and retains antigens poorly. This is probably due both to anatomical immaturity of the reticuloendothelial system and low levels of natural antibodies.

(2) This poor antigen trapping facilitates diffuse penetration of antigens throughout all organs and tissues, including the thymus and peripheral lymphoid organs.

(3) A phase of diffuse penetration of antigen right throughout the extravascular fluid compartment is a feature of most experimental protocols leading to tolerance induction, be this in newborn or adult animals. However, this phase can be quite short with some antigens and its importance is not yet clear.

(4) Some antigens are removed rapidly from the extracellular fluid

compartment, even though not captured by the RES. An example is monomeric flagellin in the newborn rat. This is due to catabolism and excretion, presumably chiefly by serum enzymes. To induce tolerance with such antigens, it is usually necessary either to give frequently repeated antigen injections over a period of some weeks, or to use relatively large amounts given as a single dose.

(5) If labeled antigen is injected into an animal in which the tolerant state is already established, its distribution and fate will depend on the level of natural or immune antibody present in the animal concerned at the time of injection. No inherent deficiency in antigen capture exists in the RES of such animals.

(6) The lymphoid follicles may represent an important mechanism for concentrating antigen, keeping it in an extracellular location, and maintaining it in its native state. In some situations, the follicles may perhaps help tolerance induction.

(7) The phenomenon delineated by Mitchison (1964) of two zones of antigen dosage capable of inducing tolerance appears to be a general one. However, with one type of antigen, the flagellar proteins, the doses required to achieve tolerance in both zones may be much lower than in the case of serum protein antigens, or synthetic polypeptide antigens.

(8) In newborn and adult rats, tolerance to antigens derived from *Salmonella* flagella can be achieved with doses that are surprisingly small. Daily injections of 10^{-15} gm/gm of body weight/day, injected for 4 weeks, can be effective.

(9) Molecular size has an important bearing on *in vivo* effects of antigen. It may be too early to lay down rigid rules describing the relationship, but specific examples will be cited to support the view that lower molecular weight forms tend to be more tolerogenic, at least in adult animals, than similar material injected in higher molecular weight or particulate form.

II. Antigen Dose and Tolerance Induction

A. HIGH AND LOW ZONE TOLERANCE

We owe to Mitchison (1964) and Dresser (1962a,b) the concept that antigen can cause tolerance in two distinct zones of antigen dosage. High zone tolerance is achieved with very high doses of antigen and can reach a profound degree quite quickly, e.g., within 24 hr. Low zone tolerance is induced with "subimmunogenic" antigen doses, which normally must be injected repeatedly over several weeks to exert an optimal effect. High zone tolerance tends also to be more complete and longer lasting than low zone tolerance, which is usually partial and more transient.

It is much easier to describe these tolerance effects in operational terms than to explain their mechanism. However, the following considerations (many of them borrowed from Mitchison's original article) may provide helpful orientation.

(1) The immunological status of an animal toward a given antigen must be viewed in statistical terms. If antigen injections have caused an overall increase in the number of lymphocytes able to react to that antigen, the animal is said to be immune. If the number of reactive cells is significantly decreased, the animal is said to be partially tolerant; and if the number has been reduced to zero, it is fully tolerant.

(2) At the level of a single reactive lymphocyte, immunity and tolerance are mutually exclusive states. A single injection of antigen into an animal usually causes a change toward immunity in some cells, and of tolerance in others. The net effect of the injection will depend on the relative frequency of the two types of events.

(3) The processes of immunization can hide and even impede concurrent processes of tolerance induction. For example, antibody-forming cells divide and thus immunization is amplified, whereas, at least on classic views, the property of tolerance cannot be passed from cell to cell. An animal in which half the competent cells have been rendered tolerant and half the cells immune will, on challenge, simply behave a little less hyperreactive than a second animal in which half the cells were rendered immune and half were unaffected. There is thus no way of detecting the many "tolerance events" in the former animal. Also, antibody may have important effects on antigen distribution and thus on an antigen's *in vivo* effects. For example, it has been claimed that IgM antibody may enhance antibody production (Henry and Jerne, 1967) possibly by promoting more efficient antigen handling by the RES.

(4) There is no fundamental difference between adult and neonatally-induced tolerance. It is probable that the main reason why tolerance appears to be so much easier to induce in neonatal animals is because the competing process of antibody formation takes place to a lesser extent. If circumstances are chosen in the adult where immunization is rendered impossible (cytotoxic drugs, whole body X-irradiation or certain molecular forms of antigen), tolerance induction is the normal outcome of an antigen course, and the tissue antigen concentrations

required are of the same order as in newborn animals. In several experimental systems, it is clear that the antigen dose needed to cause tolerance is in no way reduced by drugs or irradiation (Dresser and Mitchison, 1968).

(5) The initial event in the induction of immunity or tolerance is probably an encounter between antigenic determinant and antibody receptor on the surface of the reactive lymphocyte. It is known that, for induction of antibody formation to occur, we are not dealing with just one single event of derepression. Apparently, antigen plays a continuing role throughout the whole of the differentiation of the antibody-forming clone. Similarly, the tolerance change, whatever, it may be, might not occur instantly but over a period. Furthermore, the occupancy of a surface site by antigen must be regarded as a reversible event, not only by virtue of the reversibility of antigen–antibody interactions but also because of the possibility of active site regeneration. Finally, the membrane perturbation or other changes resulting from occupancy of a surface site of antigen will be influenced by the size and shape of the antigen and by the avidity of binding. All of these variables and complexities make it hazardous to propose simple models. Nevertheless, the general facts of high and low zone tolerance can be examined by postulating that a cell will be rendered immune if, over a time t, it encounters between a and b "hits" with antigen (where $b > a$), but will be rendered tolerant if it is subjected to 1 to $a - 1$ hits, or to $> b$ hits, over the equivalent time, t (Nossal, 1969). Perhaps the cell possesses some integrating device which senses the number of sites on its surface occupied by antigen over the time t.

B. The Influence of the Mode of Presentation of Antigen at Various Dosage Levels

Following this somewhat speculative preamble, we can now consider details of low and high zone tolerance induction in the flagellin system (Shellam and Nossal, 1968; Shellam, 1969a,b; Ada and Parish, 1968; Parish and Ada, 1969b, Diener and Armstrong, 1969; Feldmann and Diener, 1970). This can be taken in four portions, pertaining, respectively, to newborn rats, normal adult rats, lymphocyte-depleted adult rats, and tissue culture systems. It will become clear that, apart from antigen dose, two factors which significantly affect the process of tolerance induction are the molecular weight of the injected material and the presence of antibody. Both of these may influence the mode of presentation of the antigenic determinant at the lymphocyte surface.

In newborn rats, the doses needed to induce tolerance vary considerably with the frequency at which antigen is given. If only a single injection is used, 100 μg to 1 mg of monomeric flagellin must be given to induce significant tolerance in adult life. If twice-weekly injections are given from birth up to age 8–10 weeks, a complete and long-lasting tolerance will ensue. The most interesting results, however, are obtained when antigen is injected every day during the neonatal period.

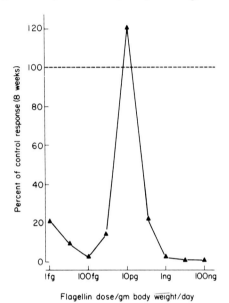

FIG. 10.1. Induction of immunological tolerance to monomeric flagellin by multiple injection in the newborn rat. Note two zones of antigen dosage causing tolerance (see text).

When animals are given various daily doses of monomeric flagellin for 2 weeks and are then placed on a uniform tolerance-maintaining schedule of twice-weekly monomer injections, it can be seen that the neonatal injection course induces tolerance in two distinct zones of antigen dosage. Very minute antigen doses, namely 10^{-14} to 10^{-12} gm/gm body weight/day, cause significant "low zone tolerance." All doses above 10^{-9} gm/gm body weight/day cause profound "high zone tolerance." Doses in between these two levels cause no detectable alteration of the subsequent immune response; nor do doses of 10^{-15} gm/gm body weight/day or below. A typical experiment is shown in Fig. 10.1.

If, instead of a tolerance-maintaining regimen commencing at 2 weeks, a course of daily, weight-graded doses is continued, the basic profile of two zones of tolerance is maintained, but the dosage requirement for each zone shifts somewhat upward. With 6-week injection courses, low zone tolerance is achieved with 10^{-11} gm/gm body weight/day and high zone tolerance with 10^{-8} gm/gm body weight/day. Doses in between cause neither immunization nor tolerance.

Even more remarkable results were obtained when the antigen polymerized flagellin was used in the newborn period (Shellam 1969a). Here, the experimental protocol chosen was quite simple. Daily, weight-graded doses of antigen were given over the first 2 weeks of life, and at 2 weeks a uniform challenge dose of 100 μg of polymerized flagellin was given to all groups. Serum antibody levels were determined just before challenge and 1 and 6 weeks later. Again, low and high zones of tolerance were found. Low zone tolerance was induced by doses of 10^{-17} to 10^{-15} gm/gm body weight of antigen, the optimal daily dose being 10^{-16} gm/gm/day. Impressive high dose tolerance required very much more antigen, i.e., 10^{-8} gm/gm/day or more. However, polymerized flagellin is clearly an extraordinarily effective antigen in low zone tolerance induction in newborn rats, being even more potent than monomeric flagellin.

An antigenically active fragment of flagellin (fragment A), prepared by cyanogen bromide cleavage and of molecular weight 18,000, has been extensively investigated for its tolerogenic properties in adult rats (Parish, 1969), but less extensively in newborn animals. We do know it will cause effective high zone tolerance in the neonatal period.

In the normal adult rat, the only flagellar antigen to cause impressive tolerance is fragment A. Here, low zone tolerance can be induced with 10^{-15} gm/gm/day injection daily for 4 weeks, and high zone tolerance with 10^{-7} gm/gm/day. Intermediate doses result in very high antibody titers rather than in tolerance. A typical experiment is shown in Fig. 10.2. Whereas normal rats are rendered only partially tolerant by even very high daily doses of monomeric flagellin, this situation can be altered by lymphocyte depletion (Shellam, 1969b). In a rat given antigen subsequent to 5 days chronic thoracic duct drainage, excellent high zone tolerance to monomer can be obtained. Though the low zone has not been fully investigated, a hint of some tolerance has been obtained in preliminary experiments. Similarly, pretreatment of adult mice and rats with anti-lymphocyte serum facilitates tolerance induction. The exact way in which lymphocyte depletion favors tolerance induction is not known.

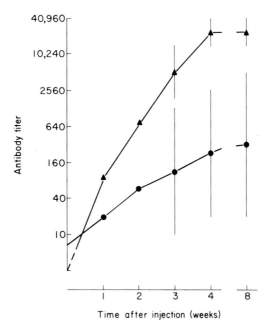

FIG. 10.2. Tolerance in rats to flagellin. The production of antibodies to flagellin by rats injected daily for 28 days with fragment A isolated from a CNBr digest of flagellin, and then challenged with an injection of flagellin in Freund's complete adjuvant. Vertical bars are standard deviations. (After Parish and Ada, 1969b.) ▲, Control rats; ●, rats preinjected with fragment A.

Tolerance induction *in vitro* will be considered in Chapter 11, and further speculations on the possible mechanisms of high and low zone tolerance will be given in Chapter 12.

III. Antigen Distribution and Tolerance Induction

A. THE FATE OF TOLEROGENIC ANTIGEN

While the mechanism by which antigen induces tolerance is still unclear, it may be useful to contrast the distribution of injected antigen molecules under circumstances where the effect of such injections is tolerance induction with the distribution, already discussed in Chapter 7, of immunogenic antigen. Unfortunately, and contrary to our earlier expectations, the localization patterns do not readily fit into two clearly distinguishable categories.

1. In Adult Animals

The fate of tolerogenic antigen in adult animals can assume any one of three basic patterns depending on the nature of the antigen used. The first group of studies to be considered relates to heterologous serum protein antigens, such as bovine serum albumin (BSA) which readily causes tolerance in adult mice, rats or rabbits. When such antigens are injected, particularly after removal of molecular aggregates, they are poorly phagocytosed. Indeed, Frei et al., (1965) were able to show that denatured and aggregated material, palatable to the RES, was immunogenic, whereas those molecules that continued to circulate for long periods were tolerogenic. This conclusion was reached as a result of a "biological filtration" experiment in which radioiodinated BSA was injected intravenously into rabbits. The portion that was *not* removed from the circulation was recovered from the serum of the first recipient (the radioactive marker serving as a dosage calibrator) and was injected into a second recipient. This recipient failed to become immunized; it appeared that the biologically filtered material acted like a "pure" tolerogen. Interesting though this experiment is, one would like to see it extended to cover a wide spectrum of antigen doses and animal species (Dresser and Mitchison, 1968).

Largely as a result of these experiments, the notion has become widely accepted that antigen meeting a lymphoid cell directly and without mediation of the reticuloendothelial system will cause tolerance; whereas antigen which has been associated with cells of the RES will cause immunity. This idea may well be correct in certain restricted situations, but unfortunately cannot be regarded as a general truth. As we shall see in Chapter 11, an *in vitro* system exists in which lymphoid cells deprived of macrophages can be rendered either immune or tolerant depending on the type of antigen and on antigen dose. Also, it has been shown that small quantities of antigen can stimulate macrophage-free lymphocyte suspensions *in vitro*, allowing the subsequent evolution of antibody formation in an irradiated animal. Naturally, with such an experimental design, it cannot be entirely eliminated that, despite extensive washing of the injected lymphocytes, antigen is carried over to the host animal. Macrophages of the host could then become involved. However this formulation is much clumsier than the simpler view that nonprocessed antigen had stimulated the lymphocytes directly. Thus, in some systems (as discussed more fully in Chapter 8) macrophage-processed "superantigens" may play an important, and perhaps obligatorily immunogenic, role; whereas, in others, nonprocessed antigen reacts with lymphocytes, and the decision between tolerance and immunity depends chiefly on dose effects.

We have performed extensive studies on adult rats injected with BSA-^{125}I in putatively tolerogenic doses (Ada et al., 1964c, Mitchell, Abbot, and Nossal, unpublished). The key finding is one of extremely diffuse permeation of label. Blood and lymphatic vessels and sinuses are heavily labeled, and all areas of all lymphoid tissues show diffuse spread of antigen. Clark (1966) has shown that even the thymus is not spared; intranuclear label can readily be found in thymic cortical lymphocytes by electron microscopic radioautography. Such a distribution is certainly consistent with the hypothesis of Frei et al. (1965).

The second group of studies is relevant to the fate of tolerogenic antigens which share the characteristic of poor digestibility and long persistence inside macrophages. Examples are pneumococcal polysaccharide and the linear D-amino acid copolymer of tyrosine, glutamic acid, and alanine (D-TGA) recently studied by Janeway and Humphrey (1969). Here the pattern of localization is the reverse of that described for BSA. After a brief, initial phase, antigen becomes localized inside phagolysosomes of reticuloendothelial cells. It is widely believed that these may act as a reservoir for the slow, constant release of antigenic fragments, thus maintaining tolerogenic concentrations available for lymphoid cells.

The third, and in some respects most extraordinary, localization pattern for tolerogenic antigen in adult animals is that shown in the *Salmonella* flagellar system. The only antigen of the flagellar group that induces convincing and complete tolerance in healthy adult rats is fragment A, the largest polypeptide resulting from cyanogen bromide cleavage of the intact flagellin molecule (Parish and Ada, 1969a), possessing a molecular weight of about 18,000 and all of the demonstrable antigenic determinants on the whole flagellin molecule. Study of the fate of this antigen (Ada and Parish, 1968) injected after labeling with ^{125}I and in microgram amounts, showed that only a small proportion ($<0.1\%$) of the injected pulse found its way to the lymphoid organs. Fragment A and flagellin drained from subcutaneous injection sites at similar rates, but the degree of retention of fragment A in lymph nodes was lower than that noted with flagellin. Radioautographs showed that fragment A was taken up very strongly by lymphoid follicles, but poorly by lymph node medullary macrophages. From comparison of radioautographs, it appeared that fragment A and flagellin were trapped equally well in folliscles, and that the lower overall retention of fragment A was due to poor retention by macrophages. We have suggested that, in this system, the follicles may represent the sole site in the body where antigen can be kept extracellular, native, and in reasonably concentrated form (Ada and Parish, 1968). It is difficult to escape the conclusion that follicle-retained antigen can, under some circumstances, be tolerogenic. Some of these features are illustrated in Fig. 10.3.

2. In Newborn Animals

Detailed examination of the fate of the antigen molecules that may be involved in inducing tolerance in newborn animals is rendered diffi-

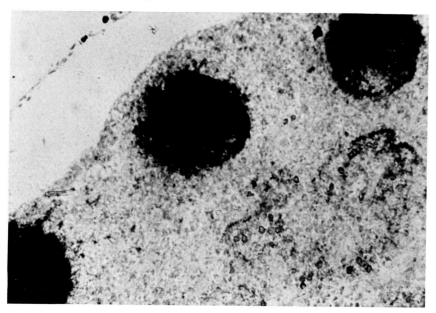

FIG. 10.3. Localization of ^{125}I-labeled fragment A monomeric flagellin in the lymphoid follicles of adult rat popliteal lymph node.

cult by virtue of the very small antigen doses which suffice to set tolerance induction in motion in some systems. Using *Salmonella* flagellar antigens as model substances, we shall describe the fate of radioiodinated material injected in doses sufficient to achieve high zone tolerance. The first point to be noted is that even here, we are dealing with very small amounts of protein, particularly if repeated injections are given. Fate of antigen experiments are much easier to interpret when only one pulse of labeled material is injected, and so our initial tracer experiments (Mitchell and Nossal, 1966) used 100 μg of ^{125}I-monomeric flagellin given to rats once on the day of birth. Previous work (Nossal *et al.*,

1965d) had shown that this was the lowest dose that would be sufficient for tolerance induction using the (admittedly inefficient) single injection protocol.

Rapid elimination of antigen was certainly one reason why single doses were inefficient relative to repeated doses. Radioactivity counting of whole newborn animals after a ^{125}I-flagellin injection showed that 90% of the original counts were eliminated from the animal within 1 week and 99% within 2 weeks. Despite the administration of excess inorganic iodide in the drinking water of the mothers of the rats, the strong possibility exists that a proportion of this residual 1% was iodine that had been liberated from the antigen and reutilized, as the thyroid gland of the neonatally injected rats always showed heavy labeling. Counts of specific tissues and of blood also showed rapid elimination of label. The spleen, for example, within several hours of intraperitoneal injection, contained about 0.1% of the injected amount of antigen, but 1 week later this proportion had fallen by a factor of about 100. None of the lymphoid organs showed impressive antigen-concentrating or antigen-trapping powers. However, the radioactivity-elimination rates were slower between 2 and 5 weeks of life than they had been over the initial 2 weeks. Interestingly, size of injected antigen had little influence in determining overall antigen retention. Both whole organ counts and specific tissue radioactivity showed very similar patterns of behavior with each of the four iodinated antigens: whole flagella, polymerized flagellin, monomeric flagellin, or BSA.

Radioautographic analysis of antigen distribution confirmed the widespread penetration and poor retention of the antigens. In the spleen, for example, sections taken over the first 2 days showed heavy and very diffuse label covering all the lymphoid and other cells present. (Fig. 10.4). Peak levels of labeling, equivalent to many thousands of antigen molecules per area of a single cell, were reached 2 hr after antigen injection. Diffuse labeling 10 days later was down by a factor of 100. Three weeks after antigen injection, some diffuse label could still be seen.

We calculated that (at this time point), the amount of antigen remaining in lymphoid tissues after an initial injection of 100 μg of antigen was between 1 and 20 molecules of antigen per cell area, depending on the tissue and the antigen used. By 4 to 5 weeks after antigen injection, scattered label had fallen to background levels. As mentioned in Chapter 7, no "blood–thymus barrier" for antigens could be found in newborn animals.

Some specific antigen retention did occur in certain cells. In the spleen, for example, occasional moderately heavy collections of grains could be seen in the marginal zone surrounding white pulp islands. Similarly, lymph nodes showed scattered labeled macrophages after the single injection. It seems that the activities of these developing antigen-trapping

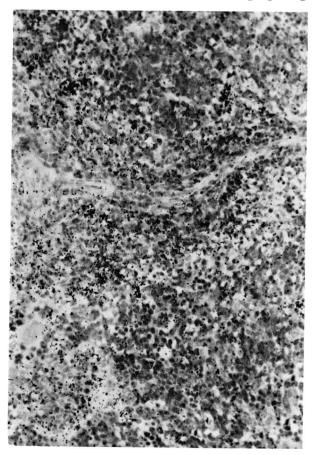

FIG. 10.4. Radioautograph of spleen of newborn rat 2 days after injection of ^{125}I-labeled monomeric flagellin. Note heavy label scattered diffusely over all the lymphoid cells.

cells were not sufficiently strong to account for most of the antigen elimination. Even with particulate flagella, phagocytosis after an initial neonatal injection was not impressive and diffuse scattering of label was the outstanding feature.

There is a puzzling difference between the findings just described for flagellar antigens and BSA, all good tolerogens in newborn animals, and that noted in newborn mice by Janeway and Humphrey (1969) using D-TGA. This material appears to be efficiently phagocytosed by young animals, yet it is clearly tolerogenic. It is well known that newborn and even fetal animals possess the capacity to phagocytose whole bacteria. The reason why flagellar particles, even in the presence of passive antibody, are so poorly retained in newborn rats is not clear.

In the induction of high zone tolerance to flagellar antigens in newborn rats, the rapid elimination of antigen just described means that multiple injection protocols are much more effective than single doses. Thus, high zone tolerance to monomeric flagellin in newborn mice requires 100 μg given as a single dose at birth, 1μg per dose on a twice-weekly regimen (Nossal et al., 1965b) and doses ten to a hundredfold less again on a daily injection schedule (Shellam and Nossal, 1968). We do not know the level of cell differentiation which is necessary before tolerance can be induced, but it seems probable that antigen must modify the rapidly enlarging population of lymphocytes in a continuing fashion over the first weeks of life. This suggests a need for well-maintained antigen levels, clearly more readily attained with a multiple injection protocol. Radioautographic study was performed on rats killed at various intervals during a twice-weekly tolerance-inducing course (Mitchell and Nossal, 1966). The recipients had received 1 μg of ^{125}I-flagellin at each injection. The radioautographs of animals killed over the first 3 weeks reflected fluctuating levels of essentially diffuse labelling. As the animals matured, however, specific antigen trapping became more apparent. About the fourth week of life, follicular and medullary antigen retention could be noted, as could exclusion of antigen from the thymus. However, at this time, the two antigen-capturing mechanisms had not yet reached maturity, and their comparative inefficiency allowed considerable diffuse permeation of antigen. By about 6 weeks of age, an essentially adult antigen-processing system had appeared, and antigen pulses injected after these times were found very largely in the RES.

It would have been of interest to examine the fate of antigen responsible for low zone tolerance in the flagellin system. However, the doses involved here are so minute that, even with heavily radioiodinated material, radioautography is not practicable because of the low tissue antigen concentrations reached. It is quite possible that subnanogram doses would be handled differently from microgram doses. For example, newborn animals may possess minute concentrations of opsonins, which may have been "swamped" by microgram doses, but may have encouraged subnanogram doses to be concentrated in follicle *anlagen* or in the spleen marginal zone.

Our work on antigen distribution during tolerance induction has revealed a number of important differences in behavior between young and mature rats with regard to their handling of an antigen such as monomeric flagellin. In adult animals, after a short phase of diffuse permeation, practically all material is captured by the RES; either through the phagocytosis-lysosome activation mechanism of macrophages or through the surface-capture mechanism of lymphoid follicles. The main bulk of the lymphocytes is, in fact, protected from exposure to antigen by this efficient antigen trapping, as levels of antigen free in the extracellular fluid compartment fall very rapidly. In the newborn and suckling rat, active antigen capture is not efficient, and diffuse permeation of injected antigens is the rule. All lymphocytes, including those in the thymus, are exposed to antigen after a single pulse. Naturally, the intensity of this exposure depends on the dose. Bearing in mind the limitations of quantitative radioautography and also the problems of possible deiodination of antigen or antigen fragments, the following first approximations may nevertheless be of some interest.

When tolerance is induced in newborn rats with a single injection of monomeric flagellin, the minimal dose effective (for a challenge injection in early adult life) is 100 μg. Following such a dose, the lymphocytes of the animal concerned are initially exposed to a concentration of about 10,000 molecules of antigen/cell. The level of freely circulating antigen falls by 80% or more over the first day (as judged by quantitative radioautography) and to around 100 molecules or so per lymphocyte at the end of a week. It remains above 1 molecule per cell for 3 weeks. We must bear in mind that about 10,000-fold less antigen, if given daily, is enough to cause high zone tolerance in this system. On the hypothesis, by no means a proved one, that this antigen would be handled similarly to the bigger dose by the recipient animal, one could still claim that all lymphocytes would be exposed to a concentration of about 1 molecule antigen/cell over the first few hours after a pulse, and that the expected antigen concentrations over the duration of the experiment would fluctuate between 1 and 0 molecules/cell.

The dilemma in understanding the basis of tolerance comes not with this high zone phenomenon, but with ultralow zone tolerance. Here, the diffusely penetrating antigen concentration could be 10,000-fold less again, and we encounter problems in understanding how each reactive lymphocyte could meet antigen at all during the period of tolerance induction. The possibility has been raised that this ultralow zone tolerance to flagellin is not tolerance, but a form of enhancement (Simonsen, 1969). On this postulate, the injection antigen causes the production of antibody, undetectable by routine techniques, which exerts a powerful negative feedback action when the challenge injection of antigen is given. Evidence for this is lacking, and it seems unlikely that the negative feedback induced could be powerful enough to block large doses of antigen, even in adjuvants. Another possibility that has been raised is that tolerant cells could pass on the property of tolerance to other cells, but evidence for this is also not available. Finally, it is conceivable that over a long period, an antigen molecule, held in a follicle or elsewhere, could cause tolerance sequentially in several or even many cells. None of these explanations is entirely satisfactory, and the phenomenon clearly needs much further study.

B. THE LOCALIZATION OF LABELED ANTIGEN IN ALREADY TOLERANT ANIMALS

It is largely owing to the work of Dr. J. H. Humphrey that we now have a clear and reasonably complete picture of how an *already tolerant* animal handles antigen. This will depend to a large extent on whether the tolerance course has incidentally caused a little antibody formation. It is by now well established that during tolerance induction in the majority of an animal's lymphoid cells, a minority may be immunized and thus a little antibody in the serum is not imcompatible with a substantial degree of tolerance. We have found (Ada *et al.*, 1965) that a proportion of tolerant rats exhibit *increased* follicular localization of flagellin, a finding which seemed hard to interpret until it became clear that a tendency for follicular localization was probably the most sensitive test available for the presence of antibody in an animal (Humphrey, 1969). Though, in the majority of these tolerant rats, we could detect no trace of antibody by conventional serological methods, we presume they must have made a little antibody, which was enough to give them excess follicular-localizing capacity. It is also possible that rats were fully tolerant of those antigenic determinants important for bacterial immobilization, but had made antibody to other determinants of flagella. In the rest of the adult, tolerant rats, antigen localization was normal. The RES capture of flagellin was never detectably reduced. We interpret this to mean that the opsonins normally present in untreated rats and responsible for follicular localization are the result of stimulation by cross-reacting, naturally occurring antigens. This seems not to be affected by the tolerance course. Thus, in our system, the RES of the tolerant animal exhibits no overt defect in antigen handling.

Interpretation of the sequence of events is easier when an antigen capable of evoking antibody production but *not* initially rapidly jetted into follicles is used. Such is the case with hemocyanin (Humphrey and Frank, 1967). When this is labeled and injected into previously untreated rabbits, diffuse permeation and some macrophage entry is observed. Only after several days, and thus presumably following the initial formation of antibody by the recipient animal, does follicular localization occur. When, however, the labeled antigen is given to an animal previously rendered fully tolerant by unlabeled antigen, follicular localization never eventuates. Diffuse antigen distribution and gradual disappearance by catabolism is all that the radioautographs of lymph node and spleen show. However, the RES of these animals still appears to be perfectly normal *vis-a-vis* this antigen, because if passive antibody is given, then follicular localization is rapidly observed. This study stresses the great importance of antibody in determining follicular localization.

There is thus ample evidence that antigen uptake and retention by the RES is not deficient with respect to an antigen to which the animal is tolerant. However, there could still exist some deficiency in antigen handling too subtle to be detected by radioautographic methods. For example, macrophages of tolerant animals could exhibit some biochemical abnormality preventing manufacture of immunogenic factors. One important study (Mitchison, 1967) speaks against this view. With some model systems, it appears that a "superantigen," extracted from antigen-containing macrophages, is a more powerful stimulant to reactive lymphocytes, molecule for molecule, than the native antigen. In such systems, it appears that the macrophages of tolerant animals yield quite normal "superantigen" on appropriate extraction. In all, there seems little reason to doubt that tolerance is a defect in the reactivity of a lymphocyte, rather than the macrophage population of an animal.

C. Is There Antigen in "Tolerant Cells?"

Whether tolerance represents the specific elimination of certain preadapted cells (Burnet, 1959), or an altered reactivity in an existing cell, is not yet decided, though the former view seems to be gaining ground. If the latter view is correct, we should have to pose the question: Is a cell held tolerant by antigen?

In the newborn rat–flagellin model system, one conclusion seems certain. In a fully tolerant animal killed 2 or more weeks after the end of the tolerance course, no trace of antigen can be detected in the lymphoid cells, at least by the available methods. It seems clear that in rats made tolerant in adult life, particularly with low zone protocols, the same holds true. In other words, antigen does not have to remain in or on the lymphoid cell concerned to maintain the tolerant state, except, perhaps, in minute and undetectable concentration at some critical control site. Clearly, just as antibody formation does not depend on a direct template of antigen, so tolerance does not depend on a high inhibitory concentration of antigen in antigen-reactive cells.

Though many authors have studied the relative organ concentrations of labeled antigens in adult vs. newborn animals, the literature fails to reveal studies directly relevant to the quantitative radioautographic approach which could answer the questions of antigen content of "tolerant cells." Robbins *et al.* (1963) reported a slower catabolism of some antigens in newborn as opposed to adult animals, consistent with previous work of Smith's school in stressing the importance of antigen persistence for tolerance induction, Several studies have suggested that antigens reach the thymus more readily in newborn than in adult life (Staples *et al.*, 1966; Nossal and Mitchell, 1966), though this may in some cases simply be a result of slower blood clearance. While our claim that antibody-forming cells need not contain antigen has been disputed, we are not aware of any study that disagrees with our contention that "tolerant cells" (if such exist) do not contain appreciable antigen.

IV. Antigen and the Specificity of Tolerance

In much of the recent literature on immunological tolerance, there has been some question as to whether the specificity of tolerance induced by an antigen is exactly equivalent to the specificity of immunity induced by that antigen. In most experiments, there is no problem about the immunological capacity of the tolerant animal with respect to unrelated antigens. Nevertheless, there are a number of studies, which superficially at least, suggest that the "recognition unit" in tolerance involves a "wider area" of antigen surface than the area able to bind to an antibody combining site. Perhaps the best-studied of these phenomena is the apparent termination of tolerance by a cross-reacting antigen (Weigle, 1961, 1965; Linscott and Weigle, 1965; see also Cinader and Dubert, 1955, and Schechter *et al.*, 1964a,b). For example, rabbits rendered fully tolerant of BSA by neonatal injections, when injected with sulfanyl-arsenyl BSA, commence to make antibodies which at first are directed mainly at the haptens, but as immunization proceeds, react more and more strongly with the native BSA. The induction of autoantibody formation by injections of antigens in Freund's adjuvant, with consequent probable partial denaturation, may rest on a similar mechanism. The original implication to Weigle was that the formation of antibody involves two steps: an initial recognition of the molecule as a whole, and subsequent formation of antibody to its individual determinants—tolerance affecting only the first step. A second complex phenomenon has been described by Rajewsky *et al.* (1967). Working with the enzyme lactic dehydrogenase as antigen, he was able to show that of the two subunits of this molecule, one behaved as a carrier and one as a hapten. In other words, the first subunit was immunogenic but the second could cause antibody formation only when linked to the first and not by itself. In animals rendered tolerant to the "carrier" moiety, it was found that even the "hapten–carrier" whole molecule could not cause antibody production. Normal immune reactivity thus depended on the animal's capacity to recognize *each* of *two* antigenic sites on the whole antigen molecule. Mitchison (1969) has argued that this type of dependence of the total immune response on two (or more) sites on the antigen mosaic is merely a specialized example of thymus–bone marrow interactions (as already discussed in Chapter 6). We have ourselves (Austin and Nossal, 1966) described a somewhat similar situation. Rats rendered tolerant to the *Salmonella* flagellin serotype *fg* respond suboptimally to two other *Salmonella* flagellar antigen serotypes, *i* and *d*, even though the three appear to be serologically unrelated. The probable explanation of this is that in all three flagellins there are common determinant groups, acting as a type of "silent carrier." Such silent carrier determinants would evoke an immune response not detectable by tests such as bacterial agglutination (or immobilization) or by passive hemagglutination. Tolerance to them might have much the same effect as tolerance to the "carrier" type subunit of lactic dehydrogenase. In fact, antisera to *Salmonella* flagellins do contain precipitating antibodies to all other *Salmonella* flagellins, even though the Kaufmann-White scheme shows no cross-reactivity whatsoever (Pye and Ada, unpublished).

Clearly then, a state of tolerance toward one part of a complex antigenic mosaic can influence a subsequent immune response to other determinants on such a mosaic. In the broadest sense, therefore, the immune system recognizes and reacts to whole molecules, though it still seems highly likely that individual lymphoid cells recognize and react to individual antigenic determinants. Does this viewpoint help in the interpretation of the Weigle phenomenon? In some respects it may, because it is now clear that an animal may behave as tolerant toward an antigen as a whole without necessarily being tolerant to every single determinant on it. The extra "helper function" set in motion by attaching strongly antigenic groups to a tolerated protein molecule may, particularly after prolonged immunization, allow antibody formation against one or more determinants on the original molecule against which tolerance has perhaps never been complete. The threat to the clonal selection theory from this type of experiment becomes less as one realizes (1) the complexity of the immune response to a whole macromolecule and (2) that tolerance is more often a quantitative reduction in immune capacity rather than a complete and permanent lesion.

V. Summary

In this chapter, we have regarded immunological tolerance from the viewpoint of the insights into the phenomenon that can be gained by studying the effects of antigen dose, antigen molecular weight, and antigen fate *in vivo*.

Several examples are discussed in which tolerance can be obtained with either high or low dosages of antigen. We describe in particular detail the extraordinary and poorly understood phenomenon of ultralow zone tolerance to flagellar antigens in which amounts of antigen as low as 10^{-16} gm/gm body weight/day can induce significant partial tolerance.

The distribution of labeled antigen molecules during the *in vivo* induction of tolerance fails to reveal a single common pattern which covers all experimental circumstances. In many models, wide diffusion and prolonged extracellular persistence of tolerogenic antigen is seen, making it likely that lymphoid cells are rendered tolerant by contacting free, nonprocessed antigen. In other circumstances, the chief concentration of antigen during tolerance induction is in the lymphoid follicles, raising the possibility that antigen, firmly attached to and concentrated at the surface of dendritic follicle cells, is responsible for tolerance induction. Finally, in some tolerance models using essentially poorly digestible substances, the bulk of the antigen ends up in macrophages. In such cases it is probable that the slow leakage of antigenic material is responsible for tolerance induction and maintenance.

Animals already tolerant to an antigen appear to process new doses of that antigen in a fashion which depends critically on the level of natural or acquired antibody to it. If the animal shows full tolerance with no trace of antibody to any determinant of the labeled molecule, the injected antigen will circulate widely and be distributed as if it were an autologous constituent. If, during tolerance induction, some antibody were formed (as is often the case), traces of persisting antibody will cause rapid follicular localization of antigen. When the macrophages of tolerant animals are given further antigen, the immunogenic properties of material extracted from such macrophages are no different from those of material derived from normal macrophages fed the same antigen.

Studies with radiolabeled antigens suggest that if "tolerant cells" exist, they are not held tolerant by large quantities of antigen in or on them. In fact, in many situations of complete tolerance, no antigen at all is detectable in any lymphoid cell.

Studies on the specificity of tolerance show that tolerance to some determinants of an antigenic mosaic can affect the immune response to other nontolerated determinants linked to the same molecule. Analysis of this and related phenomena highlights once more the importance of cell collaboration in some immune responses.

CHAPTER 11

ANTIBODY PRODUCTION AND TOLERANCE IN DISSOCIATED CELL SYSTEMS

Despite the great interest in the mechanisms involved in the immune response in animals which has been evident for the last 20 years, there are still very large gaps in our knowledge. Surprisingly rapid advances have been made in some aspects, notably in the elucidation of the structure of antibody molecules and the nature of antigenic determinants. Such investigations are largely carried out *in vitro;* the area of ignorance is in the details of antigen–cell and cell–cell interaction. As has been shown with so many other systems, the ability to carry out a complex reaction *in vitro* offers the hope of isolating and examining separately many of the variables involved in the reaction. This has been the aim of numerous immunologists who have used a variety of approaches, varying from tissue fragments or slices to cell suspensions.

It is only in the last half decade that techniques have been described which are repeatedly successful in the hands of numerous workers. Both Dutton (1967) and Fishman (1969) have recently reviewed *in vitro* systems and discussed many aspects which are not of immediate concern to our main interest. In this chapter, we will pay particular attention to those reports which indicate the nature and properties of the cells involved, the way in which antigen is handled, and especially to those systems which offer most hope in determining the molecular events involved in the inductive stages of antibody production and secretion.

There has been general agreement for some time about two findings. (1) Antibody production could be shown to occur in lymphoid tissues or cell suspensions removed from stimulated animals and incubated *in vitro*. (2) Lymphoid tissue removed from an animal previously injected with a particular antigen could be stimulated *in vitro* by exposure to the same antigen to give a secondary immune response (e.g., O'Brien *et al.*, 1963). Claims that a primary response could be elicited *in vitro* have been more recent. Stevens and McKenna (1958) found that if rabbits were injected intravenously with endotoxin, the spleens removed 24 hr later, diced, and the fragments incubated briefly *in vitro* with bovine γ-globulin as antigen, small amounts of antibody rapidly appeared. This work on the rapid formation of antibody by cells in culture was not confirmed. Globerson and Auerbach (1965) later developed a reproducible system with some similar features. Spleen explants from adult mice previously injected either with phytohemagglutinin or with adjuvant, upon subsequent exposure to sheep red blood cells, produced hemagglutinins or hemolysins. This system was later simplified (Globerson and Auerbach, 1966) when it was shown that use of larger organ fragments eliminated the need for nonspecific stimulation without a decrease in the antibody titers achieved. Probably the most convincing of the early demonstrations that a primary response could occur *in vitro* was the work of Fishman and colleagues (Fishman, 1959, 1961; Fishman and Adler, 1963; Fishman *et al.*, 1965), already referred to in Chapter 8. In essence, a phenol extract of a bacterial virus–macrophage mixture was shown to stimulate the production of specific antibody when added either to cell suspensions or to cultures of lymph node fragments in an appropriate environment. Tao and Uhr (1966b) found that incubation of bacteriophage $\phi\times174$ with cultures of lymph nodes obtained from nonimmunized rabbits resulted in the production of specific antibody. It would have been of further interest if lymph nodes from young or germfree animals had also been used. In fact, Saunders and King (1966), at the same time, reported that primary *in vitro* synthesis of antibody had been achieved in a mouse spleen–thymus organ culture explant after exposure to a coliphage, R17. The tissues were obtained from mice less than 1-week-old and the presence of both spleen and thymus was necessary.

I. Systems for Studying the Immune Response in Cultures of Dissociated Cells

The finding which ushered in the "modern era" of cell culture work in immunology was the report of Mishell and Dutton (1966) describing for the first time suitable conditions for the cultivation of dissociated cells which allowed antigenic stimulation to take place and cell multiplication and differentiation to occur. These authors (Mishell and Dutton, 1967; Dutton and Mishell, 1967a,b) used spleen cells from unimmunized mice and red blood cells from a variety of sources as antigen. The main features of their system were (1) the use of Eagle's medium, supplemented with certain amino acids and 10% fetal calf serum; (2) particular atmospheric requirements (7% O_2; 10% CO_2; 83% N_2); (3) a suitable and rigidly defined cell concentration; (4) mild agitation of the cultures held in petri dishes; and (5) daily addition of certain nutrients. With this system, the number of plaque-forming cells to sheep red blood cells (Jerne and Nordin, 1963) rose to >1000 per 10^6 mouse spleen cells within 4 days, and this is of the same order seen in spleens from mice injected with this antigen. The effect was specific and proliferation of cells was a demonstrable feature. Different populations of cells were stimulated in response to two noncross-reacting groups of red cell antigens.

The system devised by Mishell and Dutton has proved to be reproducible and is now used in many laboratories. There are two other systems, one a variant, which we shall describe because work involving their use has contributed information of particular interest.

Instead of a culture dish, Marbrook (1967) used a glass tube sealed at the bottom with a dialysis membrane and this dipped into excess medium present in a larger vessel. The cells settled on to the membrane and this allowed adequate cell contact without agitation; it proved unnecessary to have supplementary feeding. Using sheep red blood cells as antigen, Marbrook achieved plaque numbers almost as high as those reported by Mishell and Dutton. Marbrook's technique has been used extensively by Diener, Armstrong, Shortman, and their colleagues as will be described later in this chapter.

The other system is one developed by Bussard and colleagues (Hannoun and Bussard, 1966; Bussard and Hannoun, 1966; Bussard, 1967; Nossal et al., 1970; Bussard et al., 1970). It involves short-term (1 to 3 days) culture of lymphoid cells in a viscous medium that has the property of simultaneously nourishing the cells and revealing antibody formation as it occurs. Essentially, lymphoid cells are mixed with sheep erythrocytes, guinea pig complement, and a tris-buffered Eagle's medium containing carboxymethyl cellulose (CMC) at a final concentration of 1.5 mg/ml. This extremely viscous sol is either (1) squashed between slide and coverslip, sealed, and incubated at 37°C (closed CMC method) or (2) spread thinly and evenly on a cover slip which is then immediately placed under liquid paraffin (open CMC method), where the preparation is accessible to a micromanipulation pipette. Incubation of such preparations for $\frac{1}{2}$ to 3 hr is an efficient method of revealing the presence of cells which had been forming hemolytic antibody against sheep cells *in vivo*. Incubation for longer periods of 1 to 3 days is followed, in some circumstances, by the appearance of plaques of hemolysis which can be shown to be due to the *de novo* commencement of antibody formation by cells at some time after initial explantation into culture. As will be seen below, the most intriguing result obtained by this technique is the demonstration of plaque formation by many peritoneal cells of unimmunized mice.

II. Important Features and Limitations of Dissociated Cell Systems

It is now possible to note some of the factors, other than conditions of culture maintenance and cell growth described in the preceding section, which have contributed to the success of *in vitro* investigations in recent years.

A. ASSAY FOR ANTIBODY AND ANTIBODY-SECRETING CELLS

Although there are now numerous methods for assaying antibodies which have a sensitivity considerably less than 1 μg antibody/ml, a major technical advance was the ability to detect and enumerate antibody forming/secreting cells. In red blood cells, the system "par excellence" is the plaque-forming technique originally developed by Jerne and Nordin (1963) and by Ingraham and Bussard (1964). The development of this technique immediately made the red blood cell, despite its complexity, the antigen of choice in many laboratories. The ability to obtain complement-dependent lysis of red cells coated with endotoxin extended the usefulness of this technique. A long sought for goal was to obtain complement-dependent lysis of red cells coated with any antigen by the appropriate antibody. There are now numerous publications which have described methods for obtaining plaques, using cells sensitized with haptens (Merchant and Hraba, 1966) or a variety of protein antigens (e.g., Golub *et al.*, 1968). The methods so far described for proteins still seem to suffer from some limitations, chiefly because very high concentrations of protein are needed to achieve adequate antigen coating of red cells.

There are other techniques which in all probability would detect antibody-forming cells to a wide variety of antigens. One such technique is to use isotopically labeled antigen which would be expected to adhere to cells forming specific antibody against it. Cells reacting in this way are detected by radioautography of cell smears (Berenbaum, 1959; Pick and Feldman, 1967; Naor and Sulitzeanu, 1967; Byrt and Ada, 1969; Humphrey and Keller, 1970; Dwyer and Mackay, 1970). Similarly, Baker et al. (1966) detected antibody-forming cells by virtue of their ability to adsorb antigen-coated bentonite particles. However, these techniques suffer from the great disadvantage that detection and enumeration of positive cells can only be made at high magnification so that the scanning of more than 10^5 cells is very tedious.

At the time of writing, the only other technique for detection of antibody-forming cells which is comparable to the hemolytic plaque procedure in ease of performance and the detection of positive cells is the method of Diener (1968) for the detection and enumeration of antibody-forming cells to *Salmonella* bacteria H antigens. The conditions of cell culture are similar to those described by Marbrook (1967) for sheep red blood cells but the antigen used and the procedure for the detection of positive cells differ. As described, the antigen used is polymerized flagellin, prepared from the flagella of different strains of *Salmonella* organisms (Chapter 2). Antibody-forming cells are detected by the technique of bacterial adherence (Mäkelä and Nossal, 1961). In brief, a suspension of spleen cells (from either spleens of injected animals or from *in vitro* cell cultures exposed to polymerized flagellin) are washed and mixed with a suspension of motile bacteria of the appropriate specificity. Coronae of bacteria form around the antibody-secreting cells and upon incubation in an agar medium in petri dishes, these give rise to discrete colonies of bacteria which are detected at low magnification (Diener, 1968; Diener and Armstrong, 1967). Few reactive cells ($<1/10^6$ cells) are found in the spleens of unimmunized mice but the numbers rise to between 10^2–10^3 cells/10^6 recovered cells after 4 days incubation with antigen at 37°C.

B. Rapidity of the Antibody Response

Because of the difficulty of maintaining optimum conditions for cell culture over long periods, antigens have been used which result in the rapid formation and secretion of antibody. In most cases the antibody is IgM and cell culture is rarely continued beyond 6 days. This is of course a limitation of the procedure. In cases where a delayed antibody response is expected, this may be detected by subsequent transfer of the cells into X-irradiated, syngeneic hosts.

C. NATURE OF THE ANTIGEN

The requirements of very sensitive assays for antibody (or for enumeration of antibody-secreting cells) and for a rapid antibody response have in most cases greatly restricted the choice of antigen which can be used *in vitro* studies. For these reasons, foreign red blood cells (or sensitized syngeneic red cells) or particulate viral or bacterial preparations possess special advantages.

III. Major Findings Using Dissociated Cell Systems

Most investigations which have contributed substantially to our knowledge of the role of antigen and of the cell-cell interaction in cell cultures have used spleen cell suspensions. These have been obtained from unimmunized or from immunologically deficient animals. In some experiments, spleen cell populations were fractionated and/or other cell types added to them. Lymph node cell suspensions are less satisfactory than spleen. So far, bone marrow and thymus cell suspensions, either separately or mixed, have proved inadequate. Cells in peritoneal washings contain a variety of cells, some of which may have special properties. Investigations involving their use will be discussed separately.

Mainly two types of antigens have been used—red blood cells (frequently sheep) or bacterial flagellar antigens–and most work to be discussed utilized either or both of these.

Work with dissociated cell systems is still, in many respects, in preliminary stages, but important results have already been achieved.

A. ANTIGEN CONCENTRATION

In both the Mishell-Dutton and Diener-Armstrong systems, the standard spleen cell concentration used was 1–2 × 10⁷ cells/ml. Under these conditions, the response was antigen dependent.

Using sheep red blood cells as antigen (Dutton and Mishell, 1967a) the first measurable response was obtained with 10^4 red cells and in-creasing responses occurred with doses up to 10^6 cells. Higher doses did not cause increased numbers of plaque-forming cells. Under these conditions, maximum plaque numbers occurred by day 4 and did not increase on further culture. This is remarkably similar to the *in vivo* pattern. In both cases, 0.1–0.5% of the cells were plaque formers. If spleens were removed from mice 2–3 days after *in vivo* stimulation, cell suspensions made, and then exposed *in vitro* to another aliquot of sheep red blood cells, up to 20% of the spleen cells could be shown to be plaque formers by day 4. This is a much higher proportion than could be obtained *in vivo* by any schedule of antigen injection tried.

In the Diener-Armstrong system, the effect of varying antigen con-centration (polymerized flagellin) was quite dramatic. At a level of 2–20 ng antigen/ml, the peak level of 500 antibody-forming cells per 10^6 harvested cells by day 4 was achieved. If 1 μg antigen/ml was used, very few antibody-forming cells were detected at 4 days (Diener and Armstrong, 1969). This suppression by high antigen concentration was specific as the same culture responded to two other antigens, sheep red blood cells and polymerized flagellin from another strain of *Sal-monella* (*S. waycross*). The results are reproduced in Fig. 11.1. This depressing effect of large doses of the antigen seemed to be indistin-guishable from tolerance, as defined in *in vivo* work and a second test was consistent with this interpretation. Armstrong and Diener (1968) had earlier elaborated a method for the detection of antigen reactive cells to polymerized flagellin. This test was based on those earlier de-scribed (Playfair *et al.*, 1965; Kennedy *et al.*, 1965, 1966) for the de-tection of hemolytic foci in the spleens of lethally irradiated syngeneic mice given spleen and sheep red blood cells. Using this technique, Arm-strong and Diener (1969) showed that the number of antigen-reactive cells responding to polymerized flagellin (*S. adelaide*) in mice which had received spleen cells previously incubated with 3 μg of this antigen was significantly depressed, compared to that of animals which had received cells exposed to the immunogenic dose of 20 ng.

The *in vitro* system allows an approach to the kinetics of tolerance induction. Diener and Armstrong (1969) have held spleen cells at either 37° or 4°C for various intervals with "tolerogenic" concentrations of antigen. Control cultures without antigen were held for equivalent in-tervals and temperature. Then, the spleen cells were washed and placed in Marbrook-type (1967) cultures for 3 to 4 days with the normal, im-munogenic dose of 20 ng of polymerized flagellin/ml. The experiments thus measured the extent to which an early, brief exposure to a tolerance regime had influenced subsequent immune performance in tissue culture. At 37°C, some reduction in response capacity was already evident by 15 min, and near maximal suppression had occurred by 3 hr. At 4°C, the initiation of tolerance took somewhat longer, but near maximal effects were evident by 6 hr. The simplest explanation for these rapid effects is that the first stage in tolerance induction is the union of polymer

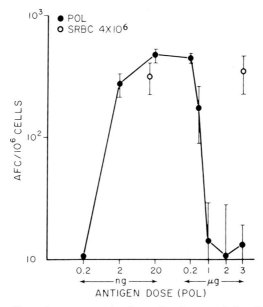

FIG. 11.1 The effect of increasing the dose of polymerized flagellin (POL) of S. *adelaide* on the *in vitro* antibody response. Cell suspensions were tested for the number of antibody-forming cells present after 4 days of culture. The arithmetic mean number of antibody forming cells per 10^6 harvested cells to POL is plotted ●————●, and to 4×10^6 sheep R.B.C., ○. Vertical bars indicate 95% confidence limits. (Diener and Armstrong, 1969).

particles in supraoptimal amounts with antibody receptors on the surface of reactive lymphocytes.

Britton (1968) has described a similar, rapidly induced tolerance to bacterial lipopolysaccharide antigens. In these experiments, normal lymphoid cells were exposed to various doses of detoxified antigen *in vitro*, and were then adoptively transferred to X-irradiated syngeneic recipients. It was found that 100 μg of antigen/10^6 lymphoid cells was an optimal paralyzing dose. A period of 12 min was found to be insufficient for tolerance induction. After 2 hr *in vitro* at 37°C with antigen, 96% suppression of reactivity was obtained, but when cells and antigen were

held for an equivalent period at 4°C, only 75% suppression ensued. Pretreatment of lymphocytes with trypsin destroyed the ability of antigen
to cause *in vitro* paralysis. These results seem in broad agreement with
the findings in the flagellin system.

B. Properties of the Antigen

The different result obtained with sheep red blood cells and polymerized flagellin is due to a number of factors as will be shown later
but one of these is the question of size of the antigen. An advantage
associated with using flagellar antigens is that there are a number of
derived fragments which are of known chemical composition and physical properties and whose *in vivo* biological properties have been characterized (Chapter 2). Polymerized flagellin, flagellin, and fragment A
(derived from flagellin) have been tested for their ability to induce
antibody formation or tolerance in mouse spleen cultures. As reported
above, polymerized flagellin may cause both immunity and tolerance,
the dose being the deciding factor. Flagellin is moderately active at
inducing antibody formation and fragment A is inactive. Fragment A
fails to cause tolerance (Diener and Feldmann, 1970) *in vitro,* and
flagellin is less tolerogenic than polymerized flagellin. These results are
in direct contrast to those obtained *in vivo* and the reason for this may
become clear when the results of tolerance induction in the presence
of antibody are described (p. 236). The results of Scott and Waksman
(1968), though preliminary, should be mentioned here. These authors
incubated spleen cells with very large amounts (100 mg) of bovine
γ-globulin for 2 hr at 37°C. This did not cause tolerance as shown
by transfer of the treated cells into X-irradiated, syngeneic hosts. If,
however, the antigen was injected *directly* into isolated whole spleens
and cells from these spleens transferred to X-irradiated syngeneic hosts,
no antibody response occurred upon challenge with the antigen. The
specificity of this effect was not reported.

IV. Cellular Reactions

A. Types of Cells Present and Their Ability to React with Antigen

There are at least four types of cells present in lymphoid tissues
which, from *in vivo* antigen localization studies (Chapter 7) and from
cell transfer studies (Chapter 6) are known or are inferred to react

with injected antigen. These are (1) macrophages as present in the lymph node medulla and the red pulp of the spleen; (2) dendritic cells as present in the follicles of lymph nodes and the white pulp of spleens; and lymphocytes (or lymphocytelike cells) which are present in both spleen and lymph nodes and may be either (3) thymus or (4) bone marrow derived. When preparing a cell suspension from spleen or lymph nodes, not all cell types which are present in the intact organ are recovered in the suspension. Those that are present in suspension and can be shown to be able to react with or bind labeled antigen (4°C, 30–60 min exposure) are mainly small lymphocytes with a small proportion of medium lymphocytes, and macrophages and polymorphonuclear leukocytes (Naor and Sulitzeanu, 1967; Byrt and Ada, 1969). The dendritic follicle cells are not recovered in spleen cell suspensions in detectable numbers so that reaction of antigen with these cells, which is such a visually dramatic event in *in vivo* studies, does not play a role in these *in vitro* antibody responses which use suspended cells.

To our knowledge, there is as yet no detailed report on the distribution of antigen among spleen cells in suspension under conditions (described above) which result either in antibody formation or in tolerance (see however, p. 181). It is well known however that macrophages will actively phagocytose red blood cells or particulate antigens under these conditions. Extrapolation of published data (Byrt and Ada, 1969) would suggest that under conditions of antibody formation to polymerized flagellin, some lymphocytes ($<1/1000$) would bind 1000–5000 "molecules" of the antigen. Under conditions leading to tolerance, the same cells would bind 10 or more times this number of "molecules." (Molecules are estimated here as units of flagellin in the polymer preparation; polymerized flagellin is polydisperse but an average size particle might contain about 300 residues of flagellin.)

B. Cell–Cell Interaction in Dissociated Cell Systems

The data reported in previous chapters leave little doubt that for certain immune responses to occur there must be some cooperation between cells. There is now substantial evidence from tissue culture work that this is the case; in fact, a major contribution of such studies has been to elucidate the roles that macrophages play in immune induction.

It is a general finding that to achieve antibody formation in tissue culture the concentration of cells must be sufficient to allow cell-cell contact. There is a dramatic cut-off point in cell numbers below which antibody formation will not be demonstrated. For example, using 25×10^6 lymphoid cells and an immunogenic dose of polymerized flagellin, 380 antibody-forming cells/10^6 cells were detected at 4 days of incubation; with less than 5×10^6 lymphoid cells, no antibody-forming cells were detected (Diener and Armstrong, 1967).

Cell separation procedures have lent weight to the concept of cell-cell interaction. Haskill (1969), using equilibrium centrifugation in continuous gradients of bovine serum albumin (Shortman, 1968), was able to show that spleen cell suspensions contained antigen-sensitive cells which differed in their buoyant density. If measured by their ability to initiate responses in animal transfer experiments, antigen-sensitive cells to sheep red blood cells showed six distinguishable populations. If tested in tissue culture, however, not all these populations were active. One density fraction was active by itself. With other fractions, definite synergistic effects could be shown on mixing different cell fractions (Haskill et al., 1970). However, interpretation of results was rendered difficult because it was not clear whether one was observing macrophage–lymphocyte interactions, or lymphocyte–lymphocyte interactions (e.g., of thymus or bone marrow type). Shortman and his group are currently engaged in a study which combines macrophage–lymphocyte separation techniques and density separation and it appears likely that a "thymuslike" collaborating cell fraction will be able to be defined.

Raidt et al. (1968) used a discontinuous albumin gradient for the separation of spleen cells from unimmunized animals or from animals earlier injected with sheep red blood cells. Both antibody-forming cells and antigen-sensitive cells from unimmunized animals banded in the denser region of the gradients. Both cell types present in the spleens of immunized animals banded in the light region of the gradient. This change in density occurred within 12 hours after the immunization of the donor animals and was antigen specific. Haskill (1969) also observed this change in density during immunization but presented evidence to indicate that the density change, with some cells, might not be antigen specific. The reason for the different findings has not been resolved.

In their most recent work, Mishell et al. (1970) have obtained cooperative effects using cells separated by flotation in discontinuous albumin gradients. Addition of small numbers of cells from the light density band to cells in the densest band greatly increased the numbers of plaque-forming cells obtained. The precursor cells were shown to come from the most dense band. Allowing for differences in the gradient system used, the results are in close agreement with those of Haskill et al. (1970).

Other methods for cell separation—attachment to glass or plastic surfaces, filtration through glass bead columns—have also been used and these have given a clearer picture of the role which macrophages may play in the inductive aspect of antibody formation.

1. The Role of Macrophages in Immune Induction and Tolerance

The requirement demonstrated earlier in adoptive transfer experiments for macrophages to be present in a cell population for antibody to be produced to red blood cells, has been elegantly demonstrated in an *in vitro* system by Mosier (1967). Mouse spleen cells were separated into two portions by allowing the cells to stick to a plastic or glass surface. Two fractions, adhering and nonadhering, were obtained. The adhering population was especially rich in macrophages while the nonadhering contained mainly lymphocytelike cells. Alone, neither fraction would give rise to antibody-forming cells after addition of sheep red blood cells. When mixed, the yield of antibody-forming cells was of the same order as that given by the unfractionated population. That the macrophages play a functional role of immunological importance was shown by the following experiment. To the macrophage-enriched population was added sheep red blood cells, the mixture incubated until many macrophages could be shown to have engulfed red blood cells. Nonmacrophage-associated red cells were removed. The residual population of macrophages containing ingested red cells, was added to the lymphocyte-rich cell fraction. On incubation, antibody-forming cells appeared. Close examination of this system showed that during the incubation period cell clusters occurred (Mosier, 1969). About 10% of these clusters contained most of the antibody-forming cells in the cell population and many clusters contained one or more large monocytic cells together with several lymphocytes. The prevention of clustering by mechanical means or by excess antibody to the antigen blocked the immune response. Pierce (1969a) reported results of a similar nature, using adherent and nonadherent cells from mouse spleen. In addition, the interesting observation was made that, in contrast to cell cultures from unimmunized mice, cultures of nonadhering cells from primed mice exhibited increasing antibody responses, and these were more pronounced as the interval after priming cells increased. Pierce and Benacerraf (1969) showed that the formation of cell clusters was necessary only for the first 24–48 hr during which time lymphoid cells became "activated" and thereafter developed into antibody-forming cells independent of antigen and macrophages.

Hartman et al. (1970) separated adhering and nonadhering cells from mouse spleen using glass beads or plastic surfaces. Marked cooperative effects were obtained on adding small numbers of adhering cells to nonadhering cells. Precursor cells, as expected, were present predominantly in the nonadhering cell population.

Sulitzeanu *et al.* (1969) have shown that clusters of lymphocytes around macrophages may occur during a secondary response *in vitro*. In this experiment, the lymphocytes were derived from the blood of rabbits previously injected with bovine serum albumin.

These results inevitably raise the question—what does the macrophage do? Is it really necessary? Shortman, Diener, and colleagues (Shortman *et al.*, 1970; Diener *et al.*, 1970) examined the requirement for macrophages in cell culture systems using two different antigens, red blood cells and polymerized flagellin. Three procedures for obtaining subpopulations of mouse spleen cells were used—equilibrium centrifugation in gradients of bovine serum albumin and filtration through glass beads under conditions which effected separation either according to cell size ("size" columns) or on the basis of active adherence to the glass bead surface ("adherence column"). In the latter case, the adhering cells could subsequently be recovered from the column. Marked differences were found between the behavior patterns of the two antigens.

A study was first made of the nature and distribution of cells which phagocytosed the antigens under the conditions of tissue culture. Nearly all cells phagocytosing sheep red blood cells were classified as macrophages or monocytes and these banded in the less dense regions of the gradient. In contrast, more than 90% of the cells which phagocytosed polymerized flagellin were polymorphs and were recovered in the denser regions of the gradient. The ability of the different fractions to initiate an antibody response, either in tissue culture (*in vivo*) or in adoptive transfer experiments (*in vivo*) was tested. Despite the complex patterns obtained, there were clear differences between the two antigens. For polymerized flagellin, there was little difference between the patterns of cells reacting *in vivo* and *in vitro* and this approximately followed the distribution pattern for lymphocytes. The response for sheep red blood cells *in vitro* was restricted to cells in the upper region of the gradient whereas cells active in the *in vivo* response were more evenly distributed through the gradient. This latter finding was similar to that observed in rats by Haskill *et al.* (1970). This pattern suggested different cell requirements for these two antigens and this was confirmed and extended using cell populations separated by glass columns.

Under specific conditions, it was found that passage of mouse spleen cells through an "adherence" column would reduce, on a morphological basis, the level of macrophages fourteenfold and of polymorphs, fortysevenfold in the effluent. No cells capable of phagocytosing sheep red blood cells were found in the effluent, but the fraction did contain a very low number of polymorphs which would phagocytose polymerized flagellin. When the original cell population, cells in the effluent and cells recovered from the column (adherent cells) were tested, it was found that the two antigens had very different cell requirements. (1) Effluent cells could produce antibody to both antigens when tested by adoptive transfer. (2) When tested in tissue culture, the effluent fraction *adequately* supported antibody production to polymerized flagellin but *did not* support antibody production to sheep red blood cells. Adding adherent cells to nonadherent cells restored the activity for sheep red blood cells. (3) The antibody-forming cells for sheep red blood cells were in the effluent fraction, showing that the adherent cells were an accessory type of cell. (4) Spleens from irradiated mice could act as a source of these accessory cells. It had been earlier observed by Roseman (1969) that active adhering cells could be obtained from heavily irradiated mice.

Glass bead "size" columns were used to separate small lymphocytes from larger cells (including larger lymphocytes and phagocytic cells). Small lymphocytes so obtained were able, though to a reduced extent, to support antibody production to polymerized flagellin, both *in vivo* and *in vitro*. The response of these cells in tissue culture to sheep red blood cells was very low but was restored by addition of accessory cells (macrophages) from an "adherence" column. Finally, in agreement with the notion that the accessory cell recovered from "adherent" columns was a macrophage, it was shown that these cells banded in density gradients in the region where macrophages had previously been shown to band in greatest numbers.

The results suggest strongly that phagocytic cells are needed as well as lymphocytes for a response to sheep red blood cells. This was most clearly shown *in vitro* in reconstitution experiments but the evidence also showed clearly that this cell could be provided by the irradiated host in adoptive transfer experiments. In contrast, such an accessory cell does not appear to be necessary for a response to polymerized flagellin.

Of a number of possible explanations for these different requirements, an attractive one is simply the question of size—that the appropriate antigen of the sheep red blood cell membrane needs to be reduced to an appropriate size before effective presentation to the lymphocyte can occur. If this were so, then processing red blood cell membranes in the test tube to yield a range of products of different sizes might yield a preparation which could induce antibody formation in the nonadherent cell population in the *absence* of accessory cells. There are numerous ways of isolating antigenic fractions from cell membrane (e.g.,

Fetherstonhaugh, 1970) and Palmer (1970) has recently described two procedures which yield two preparations which will specifically stimulate the nonadherent cell population, thus obviating the requirement for macrophages. The first is a microparticulate preparation, comparable in particle size to polymerized flagellin, is almost as immunogenic as intact erythrocytes, and yields plaque numbers with pure lymphocyte suspensions only marginally lower than those with unfractionated spleen cells. The second, a soluble fraction not sedimentable in the ultracentrifuge, is somewhat less immunogenic *in vitro* and totally macrophage independent. Work is currently in progress to see if a larger aggregate of the flagellar antigen can be prepared and shown to have macrophage-dependent immunogenicity.

In addition to the findings reported above, Diener *et al.* (1970) also demonstrated that effluent cells from an "adherence" glass bead column could be made tolerant using doses of antigen similar to those used with unfractionated cell populations. That is, it seems most unlikely that macrophages are necessary for the induction of either antibody formation or of tolerance to polymerized flagellin.

2. The Role and Origin of Lymphocytes

The results of Claman, of Miller and Mitchell and of others reported in Chapter 6 demonstrated the requirement of two cell types in transfer experiments, using red blood cells as antigen. It is clear that a deeper insight into this aspect will be achieved using tissue culture systems.

As reported above, Mosier (1967) was able to separate mouse spleen cells into adhering and nonadhering populations and to show that both types of cells were necessary to achieve an antibody response to sheep red blood cells. Mosier and Coppleson (1968) went onto demonstrate the complexity of the nonadhering cell population. They made serial dilutions of one population and cultured these dilutions in the presence of excess numbers of the other population. The slope of the regression lines obtained by plotting the logarithm of the limiting cell dose against the logarithm of the antibody-forming cell response was used to predict the order of cell interaction required to produce the response. For adhering cells, the value of 1.07 was obtained, for nonadhering cells, 1.89, and for the unseparated population, 2.59. This was consistent with a requirement of 1 adhering cell and 2 types of nonadhering cells. Dutton *et al.* (1970) however, obtained rather variable results in similar experiments.

To define further the nature of the nonadhering cells, Mosier *et al.* (1970) have studied the response of separated cell populations from normal and from thymus-deprived mice. The latter were prepared by thymectomy of adult CBA mice, followed after 2 weeks by 800 r total body X-irradiation and then 5×10^6 syngeneic bone marrow cells injected intravenously. These mice could be reconstituted by a thymus graft. As expected, spleen cells from thymus-deprived mice (Tx) responded poorly to sheep red blood cells whereas the same mice, reconstituted with a thymus graft, responded well. Adherent cells from Tx mice subsequently reconstituted, when added to nonadherent cells from Tx mice, responded poorly to this antigen; similar results were also found by Munro and Hunter (1970). In contrast, adherent cells from Tx mice when added to nonadherent cells from Tx mice reconstituted with a thymus graft, responded well. These results demonstrated that the cellular deficit in thymus-deprived mice resided only in the nonadherent cell population.

Munro and Hunter (1970) also found that spleen cells from thymus-deprived CBA mice responded poorly to sheep red blood cells. Addition of syngeneic thymus cells sometimes restored competence to such spleen cells whereas allogeneic thymus cells never did. However, allogeneic spleen cells added to spleen cells from Tx mice, had a synergistic effect and the interesting, preliminary observation was made that the function of the allogeneic spleen cells in this system was not abolished by 1000 r of whole body X-irradiation, although this dose completely abolished any *in vitro* response of these spleen cells when these were incubated alone. In these systems it is known that the antibody-secreting cell is bone marrow derived and divides rapidly. The irradiation results suggest that in the *in vitro* system, it is not necessary for the thymus-derived cell to proliferate—a different finding to that obtained earlier by Mitchell and Miller in transfer experiments (Chapter 6).

Hirst and Dutton (1970) have also recently found that a deficiency of cultures of spleen cells from adult mice thymectomized at birth to produce plaque-forming cells to sheep red blood cells could be restored by the addition of irradiated nonadhering cells obtained from the spleens of normal mice.

There is little doubt that tissue culture systems will allow further elucidation of the nature of cell–cell interaction in the immune response.

C. INHIBITION OF THE IMMUNE RESPONSE BY ANTIBODY TO THE ANTIGEN

It is well established that an *in vivo* primary antibody response can be inhibited if antibody to the antigen is injected at an early stage

(Chapter 3). The effect of antibody in the *in vitro* system has also been studied, using sheep red blood cells and polymerized flagellin as antigens.

Mishell and Dutton (1967) initially reported that anti-sheep red blood cell antibody, if mixed for 1 hr at room temperature with an immunogenic dose of sheep red blood cells, suppressed the subsequent appearance of antibody-forming cells to this antigen. Pierce (1969b), Lang *et al.* (1969), and Feldmann and Diener (1970) have examined this effect in more detail, with rather different results. Using mouse anti-sheep red blood cell sera, Pierce established the following points: (1) addition of antibody prevented the appearance of antibody-forming cells; (2) the effect was specific; (3) increasing the antigen dose overcame the suppressive effect of a given amount of antibody; (4) Exposure of cells to antibody for 4–6 hr was needed before substantial suppression occurred; and (5) antibody added 12 hr after addition of red cell to the culture was completely effective, but if added 48 hr after addition of the antigen, no suppression occurred. These results suggested that the antibody acted at an early stage in the immune process, possibly at the stage of interaction of antigen with macrophages. Lang *et al.* (1969) published very similar results which point to a similar interpretation. Pierce (1969b) in addition used cell fractions separated by the technique described earlier by Mosier (1967), i.e., ability of some cells to adhere to a plastic surface. He was able to distinguish clearly between the lymphocyte-rich (nonadherent) and macrophage-rich (adherent) cell populations with respect to their ability to react with antibody. For example, adherent cells were incubated with antigen for 30 min, washed, new medium added, and incubation continued for 24 hr. To these were added nonadherent cells, which had previously been incubated with antibody for 24 hr and washed thoroughly. No suppression of antibody formation occurred in such cultures. Suppression did occur, however, if adherent cells were first incubated with antibody for 24 hr, washed, new medium with antigen added for 30 min, the cells washed, and nonadherent cells then added. Furthermore, if adherent cells which had been exposed to antibody were heated at 56°C for 1 hr, suppressive activity was released from the cells.

These data suggest strongly that antibody suppresses the *in vitro* immune response by neutralizing the antigenic stimulus at the macrophage-dependent phase of the response. The mechanism is not clear. Lang *et al.* (1969) point out that suppression occurs when only a minor fraction of the antigen is covered by antibody.

It seems however that antibody can also act at a different level—by a process akin to immunological tolerance, as first suggested by Rowley and Fitch (1964). Feldmann and Diener (1970) have studied in considerable detail the suppressive effect of antiserum prepared in mice on the response of mouse spleen cells *in vitro* to both polymerized flagellin, and sheep red blood cells. They established the following points: (1) Antibody inhibits both responses specifically—that is, antibody to one antigen left unchanged the response to the other by the same spleen cell preparation. (2) Very small amounts of antiserum were effective. (3) With both antigens, under conditions where antibody, added with antigen, inhibited the normal response by 90%, the doubling time of the remaining cells was unchanged compared with uninhibited cell populations. (4) If specific antibody was added to the culture after the addition of either antigen, an inhibitory effect was noted throughout the *whole* incubation period, although it decreased in magnitude as the time interval between addition of antigen and antibody increased. (5) Using polymerized flagellin, the addition of excess antigen in the presence of a standard amount of antibody did *not* overcome the suppressive effect. That excess antigen levels were achieved was shown by the fact that adding fresh spleen cells to the inhibited culture resulted in antibody production. (6) The addition of an antigen (polymerized flagellin)–antibody complex, prepared in antibody excess, resulted in an "antibody response tolerance" curve, similar to that shown by this antigen alone but displaced with respect to antigen concentration. However, if polymerized flagellin was incubated with specific antibody in the presence of spleen cells for varying lengths of time, suppression occurred because the same cells, if subsequently washed and exposed to an immunogenic dose of this antigen, did not respond. Suppression was detected as early as 15 min and increased with longer periods of incubation. It was shown that the lack of response to the immunogenic dose of antigen was not due to the carryover of antibody from the initial treatment—adding more spleen cells resulted in a normal response. The same result was obtained using sheep red blood cells as antigen, although similar control experiments to those with polymerized flagellin could not be carried out with this antigen.

These results were most simply explained by antigen and antibody acting on the lymphocyte. To provide further evidence for this, cells were incubated with antigen and specific antibody for 12 hr, washed, and injected into syngeneic, irradiated mice. The mice were challenged with the appropriate antigen and both serum antibody titers and the number of antigen reactive cells in spleens determined. As judged by both criteria, depressed responses were obtained when either antigen was used. As a further check, and to relate *in vitro* to *in vivo* studies, antibody was injected into mice followed at 3 hr by an injection of the appropriate antigen. Twelve hours later, the spleens from these mice were removed, single cell suspensions made, and injected into syngeneic irradiated mice. Again depressed responses were obtained using either antigen.

Interesting results were obtained when spleen cells were briefly treated with specific antiflagellar antibody and fragment A of flagellin. While fragment A by itself was quite neutral in the *in vitro* system, causing neither immunity nor tolerance, fragment A plus specific antibody was tolerogenic in quite low dosage (Diener and Feldmann, 1970). This was true only for sharply defined antigen and antibody doses. We are thus now in a position to compare and contrast the *in vivo* with the *in vitro* effects of the flagellar antigens. As regards immunogenicity, these parallel each other; polymerized flagellin is more immunogenic than monomeric flagellin, which in turn is more immunogenic than fragment A. As regards tolerogenicity, there is at first sight a discrepancy, with fragment A being the best tolerogen *in vivo* (see Chapter 10), but polymerized flagellin the most effective *in vitro*. This dilemma disappears when one considers that *in vivo,* natural antibody to flagellar antigens is always present in adult animals. *In vitro*, in the presence of antibody, fragment A is an excellent tolerogen and at least as effective as polymerized flagellin.

It is difficult to escape the conclusion from these results that antibody may act by directly reducing the number of immunocompetent cells for the antigen concerned. Feldmann and Diener suggest that antigen is required to focus the relevant antibody onto the target cell. This applies to both antigens used—polymerized flagellin, the response to which *in vitro* is independent of macrophages, and sheep red blood cells which, to be immunogenic *in vitro*, require macrophages. It is at present confusing that the protocols of Feldmann and Diener using sheep red blood cells appear to be at variance with those of Pierce and/or Lang *et al.* or at least three major points (Nos. 4, 5, and 6 above). Otherwise the evidence of the three groups seem substantial enough to conclude that antibody can suppress the *in vitro* response to sheep red blood cells at two different stages—one a peripheral effect (macrophages) and the other central (lymphocytes). It should be pointed out that neither Pierce nor Lang *et al.* report any attempt to demonstrate whether, in addition to the peripheral effect, there was *also* a central effect.

The idea that antibody in correct concentration can serve to increase the number of molecules of antigen bound to a lymphocyte with antibody receptors is plausible, so long as the antigenic molecule concerned has more than a single antigenic determinant on it. So far, it is by no means clear how excess antigen on the lymphocyte surface leads to tolerance. This point will be considered again in Chapter 12.

V. Work with Peritoneal Cells

Bussard and Lurie (1967), using the CMC monolayer culture system described on p. 220, noted that cells harvested from the peritoneal cavity of normal, unimmunized mice, apparently began to form IgM antibody to sheep erythrocytes some 8 hr after initial incubation. The number of active plaque-forming cells (PFC) rose to peak figures of about 1000 per million peritoneal cells cultured 2–3 days later. This system has since been investigated in considerable detail (Bussard, 1967; Nossal et al., 1970; Bussard et al., 1970). Micromanipulation transfer experiments have proved beyond reasonable doubt that the PFC are synthesizing IgM antibodies active against sheep cells, and that the phenomenon does not simply reflect a high natural background activity among peritoneal cells. However, the discovery that in the open CMC system, peak plaque numbers can be seen already at 20 hr and in the absence of all division sets the phenomenon apart both from the other models of primary in vitro immune responses, and from the in vivo primary response as we understand it today. It has been found that the number of peritoneal PFC revealed in such cultures varies greatly from mouse to mouse. Some mice yield fewer than 200 plaques/10^6 cells. The "standard" figure for young adult CBA mice from the Pasteur Institute is 3000/10^6 and retired breeder mice of the same strain consistently yield 50,000/10^6 or more PFC. It is not yet established what events in pregnancy or lactation cause this grossly elevated performance. The rapid rise to peak plaque numbers, and the existence of a proportion of PFC that form antibody even in the presence of high concentrations of actinomycin D argue for a condition of preimmunization among the mice, and the considerable variability of the phenomenon, particularly from laboratory to laboratory, raises the possibility of some cross-reacting food antigen.

The following further points regarding this phenomenon can be made:

(1) Cells from other lymphoid sources, such as spleen, lymph nodes, thymus, bone marrow or Peyer's patches, taken alone or in a variety of combinations, are consistently negative. The only other cells that

work are cells harvested from the pleural cavity (Bendinelli and Wedderburn, 1967).

(2) Successful appearance of peak plaque numbers is dependent on an optimal cell concentration, though not on the presence of glass-adhering (macrophage) cells.

(3) Germfree mice can be successfully used.

(4) The phenomenon can be induced only against sheep erythrocytes, and not toward erythrocytes of other species.

It is tempting to make comparisons between this strange capacity of peritoneal cells with the finding noted in Chapter 9 that antigen binding of some antigens is very frequent among peritoneal cells. Unfortunately, however, the true basis of both phenomena is still poorly understood.

VI. Summary

The latter half of the 1960's saw the steady improvement of *in vitro* culturing techniques for organ pieces and this was partially responsible for the subsequent appreciation of the functional complexity of lymphoid cell populations. Mishell and Dutton were the first to describe a reproductible system using dissociated cells, one which gave results in terms of number of antibody-forming cells which were comparable to *in vivo* values. A modification by Marbrook has also been widely used. Spleen has been the most satisfactory source of cells for these systems. Partly because of the ease of detection and enumeration of the cells forming specific antibody, two antigens have been mainly used. These are red blood cells and polymerized flagellin. Both antigens cause a rapid IgM response.

Table 11.I summarizes some of the main findings presented in this chapter and compares these, when appropriate, with *in vivo* findings. There are some striking differences when flagellar antigens are used. In adult animals, polymerized flagellin is an excellent immunogen and is not tolerogenic. *In vitro*, this antigen may cause either antibody production or tolerance, depending *solely* on the dose used. Flagellin, *in vivo*, is a good immunogen and poor tolerogen; *in vitro* it may induce either response though rather poorly. Fragment A is inactive *in vitro*, though a good tolerogen *in vivo*.

The suppression of antibody on a primary antibody response observed *in vivo* is also seen *in vitro*. Two groups, working solely with red blood cells as antigen, found very suggestive evidence that the suppressive

TABLE 11.I

A COMPARISON OF THE *In Vivo* AND *In Vitro* RESPONSES TO TWO TYPES OF ANTIGEN

Antigen	In vivo			In vitro					
						Cell types required			
							Lymphocytes		
	Immunogenicity 1°c	Immunogenicity 2°d	Tolerogenicity (Adult)	Immunogenicity 1°c	Tolerogenicity (Adult)	Macrophages	Spleen	Thymus derived	Bone marrow derived
SRBC[a]	+++	+++	−	+++	−	+		+	+
SRBC + antibody	−			−					
SRBC fragment (Palmer)	+++	+++	−						
POL[b]	+++	+++		+++	+++	−	++		
POL + antibody	−			+++	+++	−	++		
Flagellin	++	+++	−	+	−	−	++		
Fragment A	±	++	++	−		−	++		
Fragment A + antibody					++				

[a] SRBC, sheep red blood cells.
[b] POL, Polymerized flagellin.
[c] 1°, primary antibody response.
[d] 2°, secondary antibody response.

effect occurred at the initial stages of interaction of antigen with cells, i.e., with macrophages. Another group using both red blood cells and flagellar antigens have convincing evidence that antigen reacted with the antibody at the lymphocyte surface to cause inactivation, i.e., tolerance. Using a population of lymphocytes freed from macrophages, an immunogenic dose of polymerized flagellin could, in the presence of antibody, cause tolerance; furthermore, fragment A which by itself is inactive *in vitro*, was able to cause tolerance if added with a given amount of antibody.

It is well established that the immune response involves cell cooperation. Though antibody production and tolerance to flagellar antigens could be obtained using a lymphocyte-rich macrophage deficient population, an antibody response to red blood cells required the presence of macrophages. In fact, antibody production occurred only if clustering of macrophages and lymphocytes was allowed. A most important advance was the demonstration that preparation of sonicated red blood cell membranes would induce antibody formation in a suspension of lymphocytes freed from macrophages. These findings relegate the role of the macrophage to that of an accessory cell.

Spleen cells from thymus-deprived mice responded poorly in *in vitro* cultures to sheep red blood cells, whereas spleen cells from mice restored with a thymus graft responded normally. The results of all work so far is consistent with a two-cell (lymphocyte) model of interaction—a thymus derived cell and a precursor cell.

There are numerous gaps in Table 11.I. It is confidentially expected that they will shortly be filled and the table expanded as this is perhaps the most rapidly moving front of this aspect of immunology.

CHAPTER 12

ANTIGEN AND LYMPHOID CELLS—A SYNTHESIS AND PROSPECTS

I. Antigen Pumps and Cell Responses—Chief Requisites of Systems Design

One of the chief points that this book has tried to make is that when antigen enters the body, it does not simply behave like a gas entering a vacuum. In fact there are elaborate mechanisms which affect distribution, storage, catabolism, and disposal of antigen and which must therefore obviously influence the immune response. It is interesting to speculate on what the chief requisites for a "perfect" antigen-handling system might be, and to see how the observed antigen-handling systems described in Chapter 7 and elsewhere meet these requirements.

A. Physiological Requirements

We will start with the assumption that evolution designed the humoral antibody system to help vertebrate species cope better with bacterial and viral pathogens. Two considerations will influence our arguments:

(1) that efficient scavenger cell systems antedated adoptive immunity in phylogeny; (2) that humoral immunity may be an elaboration on a prior evolutionary development, namely cell-mediated immunity, which may have the different prime function of immunological surveillance against neoplasia. A perfect system for antigen handling would, on teleological grounds, be geared primarily toward small particulate microbes, present in relatively low total dose in the tissues, and toward the endo- and exotoxins produced by such microbes. This suggests that the investigator seeking a model which might approximate a natural immune response situation should use a "strong" immunogen, such as a bacterial or viral protein. On the other hand, the system can also cope with both artificial and synthetic antigens. Frequently, however, high doses and/or the use of adjuvants are required. Nevertheless, an analysis of the fate and action of such weak antigens has provided important clues to the mechanisms involved in the immune response.

The antigen distribution system must ensure not only antibody formation, but must also be flexible enough to provide for tolerance to self components, immunological memory, and some form of feedback control to prevent excess antibody synthesis. The self-tolerance requirement applies not only to molecules like albumin which are present in large amounts but also to potential immunogens such as insulin present in low concentration in blood and extracellular fluid. If it were not for the need for self-tolerance, the requirements of the system could be much simpler. For example, one of the key functions of the macrophage and other antigen-trapping mechanisms may simply be to prevent a flooding of the lymphoid system with antigen in potentially tolerogenic amounts. At the same time, there may be occasions when it is necessary to conserve antigen and to use the limited amounts available to best purpose. These various systems requirements can be dealt with in somewhat more detail under the headings of activation and inactivation, amplification, and damping.

B. Activation and Inactivation

To discuss the mechanism of action of antigen in initiating antibody formation, we put forward three simple postulates, none of them proved, to provide a framework for discussion. (1) A necessary but not a sufficient condition for activation of an immune response is for an antigenic determinant to meet an antibody-receptor on the surface of a lymphocyte. (2) Such a lymphocyte must then make a choice between three courses of action —(i) no response, (ii) tolerance, and (iii) increased antibody production and secretion. (3) If activated (i.e., 2, iii), the variable portion of the light and heavy chains of the antibody subsequently produced and secreted are identical to the equivalent portions of the lymphocyte surface receptor initially hit by that antigen. Viewed in this light, antigen is seen essentially as a genetic regulator of lymphocyte metabolism.

1. Postulated Mechanisms for Signal Discrimination

It is clear that not all encounters between antigenic determinants and reactive lymphocytes lead to immunity, otherwise haptens would be excellent immunogens. Similarly, not all encounters lead to tolerance. What properties, then, confer on an antigen the power of activating a lymphocyte, or alternatively of repressing it? Several ideas have been proposed. Bretscher and Cohn (1968) have suggested that the immunity signal is when two (or more) combining sites of one receptor antibody molecules on a lymphocyte react with two (or more) antigenic determinants, thus "stretching" the receptor molecule and causing an allosteric change. The stretched conformation would result when the receptor combined with a polymer of antigen, formed by its prior reaction with anti-carrier antibody. Natural polymers, on this model, would be immunogenic without carrier antibody. When a receptor molecule has only one of its combining sites occupied by antigen, this is deemed to be a tolerance signal, resulting in a different allosteric change in the receptor. Thus monomeric antigens in the absence of carrier antibody would be obligatory tolerogens. The most powerful arguments against this proposal come from the work of Diener, Armstrong, and Feldmann outlined in Chapter 11. They have used as immunogen a polymeric particle, polymerized flagellin, which is a powerful immunogen *in vivo*. When lymphocytes, in the absence of macrophages, are exposed to this antigen they make a decision between immunity and tolerance depending purely on the concentration of antigen present. The polymeric entity is a powerful tolerogen in concentrations above 1 μg/ml, but an immunogen in concentrations of 1 to 100 ng/ml. Anti-carrier antibody is not present in such cultures; the brief period required for a decision between immunity and tolerance, and the fact that this decision can be made at 4°C, argue strongly against the idea that the lymphocyte population actually synthesizes anti-carrier antibody in amounts sufficient to influence the decision. In other words, anti-carrier antibody does not seem to be playing a role. Moreover, in this system the polymer is clearly not an obligatory immunogen, nor the monomer an obligatory tolerogen. Finally, added specific antibody (which certainly would contain an anti-carrier component), far from aiding immune induction, in fact swings the balance in favor of tolerance. Thus, on every count the experimental results contradict the predictions of the Bretscher-Cohn model. Nevertheless, this model does serve a useful purpose in enunciating the concept that the mode of presentation of antigen at the cell surface could cause contingent allosteric changes in receptors or possibly other plasma membrane constituents.

A second model for discrimination between immunogenic and tolerogenic signals has been presented by Roelants and Goodman (1970). This preserves the notion of an important role for carrier determinants in immunogenicity, and is based partly on work on cell-to-cell collaboration discussed in Chapter 6. On this model, an antigen will act as a tolerogen unless presented to the antibody-forming cell precursor by an antigen-reactive cell. This antigen-reactive cell has picked up the antigen by virtue of possessing receptors for some carrier determinant on the antigen. The model has much in common with the ideas of Mitchison (Chapter 6); the authors believe they have discovered an artificial antigen, poly-D-glutamic acid, and that rabbits do not possess an antigen-reactive cell which can recognize this substance. Poly-D-glutamic acid, they claim, behaves as a "pure" tolerogen, although one would like to see an investigation of the *in vivo* effects of a much larger series of dose and time schedules. This model also does not seem to explain the *in vitro* flagellin data. Moreover, it suggests that cell-to-cell collaboration of thymus–bone marrow type is essential for every immune response, whereas this is clearly not the case. This last objection can be dealt with by supposing that the two collaborating cells may sometimes both be of thymus–independent type. The chief objection to the model is that it does not give enough weight to the profound importance of antigen concentration in tolerance.

The third model, which has been put forward in various ways (Mitchison, 1964, 1967; Burnet, 1967, 1969; Nossal, 1969; Marchalonis and Gledhill, 1968; Diener and Feldmann, 1970) gives primary emphasis to the dose of antigen at the surface of the reactive cell. It is postulated that the cell has some sensing device by which it knows how many surface receptors are occupied by antigen. The correct evolution of clonal expansion in an immune response requires that the number of receptor sites effectively hit by antigen remains between a and b. Any dose of antigen resulting in a-1 or less hits might cause a "sterile activation" of the cell, which embarks on the events of immunity, but, in the absence of further hits, becomes inactivated or dies. This would represent low zone tolerance. Similarly, $>b$ hits would cause high zone tolerance.

The nature of the "weight-sensing integrator" that counts the number of hits is left vague. In an elaboration of this view, Diener and Feldmann suggest that the way in which passive antibody aids tolerance induction is by "focusing" antigen on the surface of the cell, and by allowing a lattice to build up which might cause interlinkage of different receptor units at the lymphocyte surface, with consequent inactivation of the cell. Low zone tolerance to monomeric molecules is believed to be possible *only* with the help of passive antibody, namely natural antibody in most *in vivo* situations. We feel that the key to progress in this area will be further study of antigen presentation.

The normal number of specific antigen-binding lymphocytes found in fully tolerant animals, a surprising finding, has raised anew the question of whether tolerance is a reversible inactivation of a cell, or a

TABLE 12.I

THRESHOLDS OF ANTIGEN DOSE FOR ANTIBODY FORMATION[a]

Antigen	Minimum immunizing dose (gm)
Salmonella O antigen	10^{-15}
Salmonella polymerized flagellin	10^{-10}
Pneumococcal polysaccharide ⎫ Diphtheria toxoid ⎭	10^{-8}
Bovine γ-globulin	10^{-5}
Bovine serum albumin	10^{-4}

[a] Single injection.

complete destruction. The latter idea has been favored because of its simplicity, and because low zone tolerance is difficult to explain without it. The antigen-binding data suggest inactivation with maintenance of surface receptors. Receptor preservation is teleologically sensible only if reversibility is postulated. The reversibly paralyzed cell has long been proposed by Sercarz (Byers and Sercarz, 1970) and others. Further progress in cell separation methodology should allow a direct experimental answer to emerge.

2. Differences between Different Antigens

Dresser and Mitchison (1968) have reviewed the minimal doses of various antigens required to cause immunization of an animal when given once and without Freund's adjuvant. Table 12.I is taken from their review and from our own experience. In its extremely simplified form it makes a profound point, namely that eleven orders of magnitude separate the "strongest" immunogens from the "weakest." It is a constant surprise to us that this variety in the inherent immunogenicity of antigens has received so little emphasis in the literature, and that it remains to this day entirely unexplained. A challenging theory has recently been put forward by Jerne (1970) which postulates that the germline genes for immunoglobulins code for antibodies with activity against the major histocompatibility antigens of the species concerned. This would account for a high immunogenicity in any antigen which cross-reacted with the test animal's species spectrum of histocompatibility antigens. Such cross-reactivities ought now to be systematically looked for.

3. Antigen-Concentrating Devices

Clearly, some of the stronger immunogens are extraordinarily efficient, molecule for molecule, in stimulating antibody formation. This may be aided by antigen-concentrating and retaining devices in lymphoid tissues. Among these we can list dendritic follicle cells, the spleen marginal zone, and the macrophages. Factors influencing antigens to reach one or more of these concentrating devices include particulate nature, denaturation, and the presence of natural or immune antibody. On the other hand, many antigens fail to be concentrated by these devices, but become rather generally distributed throughout the body. Factors favoring this type of distribution in the adult animal are low molecular weight (nonparticulate), native conformation, absence of natural antibody, and structural similarity to a "self" macromolecule.

Though important exceptions are encountered, it is usually easy to obtain adult tolerance using antigens that become generally distributed, whereas those attractive to the reticuloendothelial system are more often highly immunogenic. Antigen held on the surface of one cell, say a macrophage, may affect a lymphocyte in a special way when the two cells meet. However, the newer tissue culture findings have shown that it is no longer feasible to equate immunogenicity directly with "RES-processing," or tolerogenicity with absence of such processing.

C. AMPLIFICATION

The ideal activating system in antibody formation would be one in which a vigorous response could be induced early in an infection. There are several mechanisms which can be regarded as positive feedbacks for early immune responses. First, there is the suggestion (Henry and Jerne, 1967) that the rapidly synthesized, IgM antibody can have a stimulatory role, presumably by promoting more efficient antigen trapping and utilization in lymphatic tissues. Second, the carrier effect, where the presence of an active immune response to one portion of antigen molecule aids the response to another portion, represents a type of amplification or cascade effect. Third, the immunological memory mechanism, whereby antigen causes the production not only of antibody-forming cells but also of an increased number and/or reactivity of antigen-reactive cells, is an obvious amplification mechanism. There is a substantial body of indirect evidence linking germinal centers with memory cell genesis, and most likely follicle-trapped antigen acts efficiently in triggering these cells. A somewhat worrying finding is that the number of antigen-binding cells in animals displaying memory is clearly elevated and until the functional tests for enumeration of antigen-reactive cells improve considerably, detailed analysis of the cellular basis of memory will remain difficult.

D. DAMPING

It would clearly be wasteful and indeed dangerous if antibody formation during an infection continued to increase exponentially without check. Two negative feedback systems in fact exist, and both depend on antibody itself. On the one hand, antibody free in the serum and extracellular fluid can complete with antibody receptors on the surface of lymphocytes for available antigenic determinants. Thus the end product of antigen's action on lymphocytes, namely antibody, exerts a form of end-product inhibition, not in a biochemical or enzymic sense within the actual antibody-forming cell, but at the level of the whole responding system. Moreover, this competition may have a strong geographic component. It is eminently possible that antibody be in excess over antigen in the extracellular fluid compartment, but that antigen be in excess in some localized microenvironment of lymphatic tissue.

The second negative feedback role of circulating antibody is more subtle, and involves antibody-aided induction of immunological tolerance. This mechanism has been best worked out *in vitro* but may play a role in certain *in vivo* situations also. Here antibody is seen as a mechanism serving to focus or concentrate antigen on the surface of a reactive lymphocyte. The lymphocyte surface receptor binds antigen, which in its turn attracts free antibody, and so a lattice is built up at the lymphocyte surface. With multivalent antigenic molecules, this could result in a greater total number of binding sites on the lymphocyte surface being occupied by antigen.

II. The Reaction of Antigen with Cells

There are three cell types which have been implicated in the processes of induction of antibody formation or of tolerance and which have been shown to react with antigen—the macrophage, the dendritic follicular cell, and the lymphocyte. It seems now very likely that the critically important reaction between antigen and these cells is a cell surface phenomenon. This is certainly the case with the dendritic cell, is most likely to be correct in the case of the lymphocytes (especially as antigen has not been detected in antibody-secreting cells), and the case for macrophages is now persuasive in some *in vitro* models. Apart from the special case of cytophilic antibody, there is no known special receptors for antigen on the surface of macrophages, dendritic cells appear to have a recognition site for the Fc portion of immunoglobulin molecules, and lymphocytes possess an immunoglobulin receptor which is self-produced.

One finding now stands out clearly and may be regarded as a landmark in immunology. The principal inductive step for both antibody production and for tolerance involves the lymphocyte(s) and can take place in the absence of both macrophage and dendritic cell. Thus, the macrophage and dendritic cell must be regarded primarily as helper and/or controller cells.

A. The Macrophage—The Immunologist's Dilemma

Macrophages have been implicated in the immune response. One extreme view is that they are simply scavenger cells; perhaps the opposite extreme is that these cells form an informational RNA for transmission to lymphocytes. This has been a confusing situation which now seems to be largely resolved. It now seems simplest to regard the macrophage primarily as a nonspecific helper cell.

A major function of the macrophage is to act as a scavenger cell, to destroy foreign or damaged material. A result of this activity would be to remove some of the "load" from the antibody-producing machinery and prevent tolerance. In so doing, the cell does in effect act as a competitor to lymphocytes, as has been demonstrated on several occasions. Some degraded fractions of the injected antigen may act as immunogen. This is clearly so in the case of red blood cells—a rather unnatural immunogen—but possibly, a similar situation would exist with invading bacteria. It has been pointed out on numerous occasions, particularly by Sela, that fragments of an antigen, degraded to the stage where their original conformation was substantially altered, would be less likely to act as inducers compared to the original antigen. Presumably they could induce the formation of low-affinity antibody.

The recent work of Askonas, Unanue, and colleagues is sufficiently persuasive for us to support, with some reservation, their proposal that intact "soluble" antigen held at or near the cell surface serves as the inducer in an antibody response. Reasons for caution are that this type of localization has not been clearly observed during examinations of many sections of lymph node or spleen after injection of labeled antigen; and that some peritoneal cells which are the source of the immunogen may not be macrophages but the lymphocytytelike cells described by Mandell and colleagues. The former reason may not be a valid objection—it could readily be proposed that in lymphoid organs, the proportion of antigen associated with the macrophage cell surface may be small and/or may be rapidly "handed on" to a susceptible lymphocyte. Although these experiments suggest mainly a role for macrophage-associated antigen which leads to antibody production, this may not always be the case. Some substances such as poly-D-amino acid polypeptides are actively phagocytosed by these cells and yet preferentially cause tolerance.

Are mocraphages functionally heterogeneous? In discussing peritoneal exudate cells, Fishman has proposed that there are scavenger macrophages, processing macrophages, and antibody-forming "macrophages," and that antigen associated with these may have different fates and/or functions. This may be a misuse of the word macrophage. It is more realistic to assume that peritoneal washings and exudate contain a wide spectrum of cells and that very little is known about the functional behavior of some of these cells. For example, a very high proportion of cells (2%) in mouse peritoneal washings react with hemocyanin. Yet, most of these, when examined in the electron microscope, are morphologically similar to medium lymphocytes. Similarly, a very high proportion of peritoneal cells, when cultured in the presence of foreign (sheep) red blood cells, may secrete specific antibody.

What about informational-RNA and antigen-RNA from macrophages? As antibody formation can be obtained *in vitro* to polymerized flagellin and to a fraction of sheep red blood cells using preparations of mouse spleen cells containing very few macrophages, we support strongly an opinion earlier put forward by Humphrey (1969). He regarded the demonstration that an informational-type RNA could be extracted from macrophages which had been incubated with antigen, though fascinating, to be irrelevant to the question of how antigen normally interacts with immunocompetent cells so as to stimulate an antibody response. Furthermore, the *in vitro* findings cast doubt on the physiological and immunological relevance of antigen-RNA complexes, despite the findings that such complexes have an increased immunogenicity.

There is finally the additional aspect that macrophages may provide nonspecific stimulatory factors and these may be of considerable importance in a microenvironment.

In summary, we propose that the role of the macrophage in immune induction is that of a helper cell—a means of antigen presentation and of nonspecific stimulation.

B. The Dendritic, Follicular Cell—The Immunologist's Cinderella

If it could be said that in recent times the period 1964–1968 were the "years of the macrophage" and 1968 – ? the "years of the lymphocyte," it is significant that at no time has a consideration of the dendritic follicular cell occupied much time in the thoughts of most immunologists. And yet it is perhaps the most striking phenomenon seen by those who have studied the distribution of injected labeled antigens. Although a variety of preparations has been shown to localize in lymphoid follicles, the mechanism most likely to be of physiological importance is that antibody acts as the glue which holds antigen externally to the cell membrane. It is considered likely that antigen so held would be able to interact with cells, presumably lymphocytes, which might pass through this region. What is the function of antigen so localized? (1) It is not a *necessary* condition for a primary response. Antibody responses to a number of antigens, e.g., hemocyanin, denatured serum albumins, occur *prior* to the antigen becoming localized in the follicle. (2) It is not a *sufficient* condition for a primary response. This was elegantly shown by Askonas and Auzins (reported by Humphrey, 1969). Mice were primed with a hapten–protein conjugate NIP-bovine γ-globulin, and 3 weeks later when anti-NIP antibody was present, the mice were given ^{125}I-labeled NIP-bovine γ-globulin in one footpad and in the other, NIP-human serum albumin. The mice made no antibody to the albumin but gave a large response to the globulin, though both antigens became extensively localized in the follicles because of the anti-NIP antibody present. Furthermore, injection of antigen either with antibody or into passively immunized animals, causes marked follicular localization of the antigen, but the production of antibody is inhibited. (3) Another possibility is that antigen in the follicle may be particularly well placed to stimulate cells already primed elsewhere to go on to produce antibody. A study of cell migration in chick spleen (White et al., 1967) suggests that antibody-producing cells in the medulla may eventually appear adjacent to antigen-retaining dendritic cells. In addition to this finding, it is well known that a secondary antibody response may be induced when specific antibody is present. Injection of antigen at this time leads to extensive follicular localization and this is consistent with the notion that antigen in this region could stimulate primed cells. (4) A further possibility, not necessarily at variance with (3) above is that antigen in follicles may induce tolerance by reacting with unprimed but competent lymphocytes. This suggestion was first raised (Ada and Parish, 1968) in an attempt to explain ultralow zone tolerance to flagellin in adult rats induced by the injection of so few as 10^8 molecules of fragment A (from flagellin). To explain this finding, it seemed necessary to postulate some molecules of antigen being able to contact many lymphocytes; and to achieve this, some extracellular site for antigen concentration would be necessary and the ability of fragment A to localize in lymphoid follicles was pertinent. This possibility warrants more discussion. It is known that antibody may act to limit an immune response by "feedback inhibition." It seemed appropriate that this might happen, not by affecting cells already stimulated by antigen but by inactivation of unprimed, competent lymphocytes, i.e., tolerance (Ada and Parish, 1968). This notion has received a very considerable boost from the in vitro work of Diener and Feldmann, discussed in Chapter 11, to the effect that an immunogenic dose of antigen, in the presence of antibody, causes tolerance. It was particularly impressive that fragment A which per se was inactive was able to cause tolerance when antibody was present. It is tempting to extrapolate from this to the in vivo situation. A sequence of fragment A molecules held on the dendritic cell membrane by antibody might in effect be not very different to a polymerized flagellin–antibody complex. The structural rigidity of the cell wall–antibody–antigen complex could be a deciding factor in determining whether a reacting lymphocyte was inactivated rather than stimulated.

It may not be possible to come to a decision about the role of antigen localized in lymphoid follicles until more is known about the traffic of cells in and out of follicles and perhaps until that traffic can be manipulated. In this connection, it is important to note that the dendritic-cell rich "cap" of germinal centers is a place which at least some injected, labeled lymphocytes can reach, and where a proportion go on to blast transformation.

C. The Lymphocyte—The Immunologist's Hope

Excluding the macrophage and the dendritic cell, there is still the cooperativity of thymus- and bone marrow-derived cells to be considered. The reaction of these cells with antigen will, immunologists fondly hope, answer the question—what is the nature of the critical union between cell and antigen which leads to the proliferation and differentiation of a cell so that antibody is formed in large amounts and secreted?

What in summary do we know now? (1) There are two cells which may cooperate in this way. (2) One type, or both, can be shown to react directly with labeled antigen. The results of many other experiments are most easily explicable on the basis that both do. (3) With one exception (Schlossman *et al.*, 1969), the work presented so far is explicable in terms of the receptor on these cells (or at least on the antibody-secreting precursor cell) being a sample of the immunoglobulin which the cell, if stimulated, will produce and secrete in larger amounts (4) The possibility exists that the receptor on the surface of the thymus-derived cell may differ. Cells mediating delayed hypersensitivity or graft rejection could be inhibited if they were first pretreated with anti-light chain sera. This is in contrast to the inhibition of cells mediating an antibody response by pretreatment with either anti-light chain or anti-μ chain sera.

These results have been interpreted to mean that the thymus-derived cell acts as a device for focusing antigen onto the antibody-secreting cell precursor. Thus to be effective, antigen must be at least bivalent and act as a bridge between these two cells. This being so, one would expect to see evidence of coupling between lymphocytes in sections of lymphoid tissues from animals after injection of labeled antigen. To date, this has not been reported. Possibly such occurrences may be transient, alternatively, they may occur in areas where there is extensive localization of antigen in macrophages (and hence labeled lymphocytes might be masked and not easily detected). Finally, the focusing idea may be wrong. This is again an area in which the *in vitro* approach will be more likely to yield direct evidence. Overall, little would be conceptually changed if one thinks of the thymus-derived "helper" cell *not* as physically carrying the antigen around the body but as secreting a special (? IgX) anti-carrier antibody which aids in the correct focusing of the antigen, e.g., on dendritic follicle cells. This view gets over the considerable dilemma that with *in vivo* studies of antigen localization, antigen is never seen in the "traffic areas" of lymphoid organs, i.e., in those areas where thymus-derived cells are known to go. It must however be admitted that direct evidence for "IgX" secretion is totally lacking.

III. Lymphocyte Heterogeneity—The Clonal Selection Question Rephrased

Immunobiology is a branch of science in which the expression "final proof" must be used with even greater caution than usual. Final proof of the basic tenets of the clonal selection theory (Burnet, 1957) may not be forthcomming for some time. Nevertheless, the evidence in favor of the idea that antigen stimulates a subset of lymphocytes with pre-formed antibody receptors on them is now so compelling that it is difficult to think of any plausible alternative mechanism. Interestingly, both those workers who favor somatic mutational and/or somatic crossing-over mechanisms to account for amino acid sequence variation in immuno-globulins, and those groups who favor the existence of a great multi-plicity of germline immunoglobulin genes, now seem to agree that the role of antigen can best be understood if a given, single antigen-reactive cell exhibits only one or at most a few types of antibody on its surface. Perhaps the time has come to ask not whether clonal section theory is correct but rather how does it work? That question revolves around the number of antibody-combining sites which must be present in an animal to give it full immune competence; around the phylogeny and ontogeny of cells with reactivity to antigen; around the different func-tional categories of lymphocytes; and around the mechanism of acti-vation and inactivation of a cell by antigen. The last issue has already been dealt with (Section I of this Chapter).

A. Cross-Reactivity among Lymphocyte Receptors

Perhaps the greatest difficulty that opponents of clonal selection have had with the theory revolves around the issue of how many different sorts of combining sites are needed to provide a library of reactivities sufficient for antibody production to any antigenic determinant. Two recent discoveries seem to us to have reduced this difficulty considerably. The first is the unsuspected degree of low avidity antibody activity of randomly chosen myeloma proteins against haptens such as dinitrophenol (DNP). Admittedly this finding may be complicated by the possibility that myeloma proteins may not represent a true cross section of normal immunoglobulins, but the finding that 10–15% of mouse myelomas may have some anti-DNP activity is nevertheless remarkable. The second is that the more one looks for cross-reactivities, the more one finds them. Thus, recent studies have stressed cross-reactivites between histocompatibility antigens and bacterial wall antigens; bacterial antigens and erythrocyte antigens; dinitrophenol and nucleoproteins and many others. When the problem is viewed from the point of view of the lymphocyte surface, it may simply come down to a question of whether, with a given antibody receptor and the presence in its vicinity of a given concentration of antigen, the frequency of binding events is sufficient to exceed a certain threshold. If so, the cell will be activated, and its product, by definition, is an antibody to the antigen concerned. Once clonal expansion has commenced, the possibilities for further mutation and selection are excellent, particularly if one bears in mind that most high avidity antisera are produced through intensive and prolonged immunization schedules involving adjuvants. The findings of idiotype support the myeloma findings that for any one antigenic determinant, there exists many antibodies, and though formal proof is less easily obtained, it stands to reason that for any one immunoglobulin there exist many antigens which will fit. On this view, it is *impossible* to assign a particular *number* to the proportion of lymphocytes which react with a given antigen, as this will depend critically on the concentration of antigen. We interpret our findings of an increasing number of *in vitro* antigen-binding cells with increasing antigen concentration in exactly this light.

B. PHYLOGENY OF CELL DIVERSITY

Much has been written on the phylogenetic origins of the immunoglobulins but relatively little on that of reactive cells. The two are clearly related, and the problem is rendered difficult to study because of the apparent quantum jump between the highest prevertebrate and the lowest vertebrate available at the present time. We suggest there may be considerable value in approaching the phylogenetic origin of lymphocyte diversity by a quantitative study of antigen binding by prevertebrate mononuclear cells under conditions similar to those we have used (Chapter 9). As the possibility exists that adaptive immunity evolved essentially as a bodily surveillance mechanism, reactivity of such cells against various cell membrane fractions would be of interest.

C. ONTOGENY OF CELL DIVERSITY

We do not propose to discuss the controversy as to the detailed genetic mechanism leading to antibody diversity. In fact, the points for and against the Dreyer-Hood programmed activation of one of a large multiplicity of germline genes, the Edelman-Gally somatic crossing-over between a limited number of tandemly duplicated genes, and the Burnet-Cohn model of somatic mutation together with Jerne's variant on that theme, have been well summarized in a recent review by Mäkelä and Cross (1970), which is a good source of detailed references. The main contribution that the cell biologist can make to this area is to provide accurate data as to the life history of immunocyte precursors during ontogeny. Here we should draw attention to the work of Moore (Chapter 6) who has shown the origin of hematogenous stem cells from the blood islets of the yolk sac and the seeding of specific organs with yolk-sac derived cells during defined time gateways in ontogeny. Any calculation of numbers of divisions among lymphocyte precursors, possible mutation frequencies, selective influences, etc., must now reckon with the fact that in the mouse, only 9 days or so elapse between initial seeding of the thymus *anlage* with the first few yolk-sac derived stem cells and birth. Even admitting that immune competence is not achieved until some days after birth, this observation sets severe limits to the number of divisions, and thus mutation and selection, that can occur among cells committed to lymphocyte differentiation. On a somatic mutation model, it slants one's view toward abnormally high mutation rates, possibly commencing already in multipotent stem cells. Moreover, the observation that there is little morphologic evidence of cell death in early embryonic thymuses must be regarded as at least a minor embarrassment for Jerne's theory, which proposes a high rate of cell death (negative selection or paralysis selection) among the first-born immunocompetent cells, many of which would have reactivity against the animal's own histocompatibility antigens.

It seems likely that phenotypic expression of surface receptors is limited to cells which have differentiated through the influence of thymic or bursaltype inducers, and in both antigen-reactive cells and antibody-secreting cells, phenotypic restriction in immunoglobulin gene expression seems to be extreme. Questions about the number and kind of immunoglobulin genes (i.e., the genotype) of cells can be asked not only of these two classes of differentiated cells, but equally logically about all their precursors, beginning from the fertilized egg. The present problem is that no techniques exist which can directly test theories about the genes of a single normal mammalian cell. Techniques, such as *in vivo* colony formation, exist in which a hemotogenous stem cell forms a large cell clone which can eventually reconstitute a crippled immune system. However, the number of sequential divisions involved is large, and the possibility of extensive somatic mutation or crossing-over exists. As our knowledge of the embryonic stem cells of the yolk sac, and of *in vitro* methods increases, it should be possible to construct experiments in which the emergence of immune competence in cell clones can be monitored more precisely. This should allow a more reasoned judgement as to the feasibility of somatic mutation as the generator of diversity among lympyhocytes.

D. HETEROGENEITY AMONG THYMUS-INDEPENDENT CELLS

Immunological specificity in populations of thymus-derived, recirculating long-lived lymphocytes has been demonstrated beyond doubt. It has not been as easy to establish the same point for bone marrow-derived, thymus-independent (bursaltype) lymphocytes. For example, one study (Weigle, 1970) has established the property of tolerance among bone marrow cells, but others have failed to demonstrate either memory or tolerance in bone marrow-derived populations under experimental circumstances where these properties could readily be shown in the thymus-derived cell line. Despite the uncertain picture, it seems likely that both cell lines will eventually be shown to exhibit clonal individuation of surface receptors. The only other plausible alternative is transfer of an episome from antigen-reactive cell to antibody-forming cell precursor.

E. THE IMPORTANCE OF MEMORY CELLS

Germfree mice, which are still far from antigen-free, exhibit a gross diminution in the size of the pool of recirculating lymphocytes. Though it is hard to quantitate the point, it is likely that the number of thymus-independent cells in the peripheral compartment is also much lower than in conventional mice. Despite this, the immune competence of such mice is normal. Therefore, it is clear that the majority (perhaps the great majority) of lymphoid cells in the peripheral compartment are there only beause of antigenic stimulation. They are either memory cells, antibody-forming cells, or executive cells of cellular immunity, and "virgin" antigen-reactive cells must represent a small minority of the total. Cross-reactions among antigens are common, and it seems likely that many (perhaps most) allegedly primary immune stimuli act at least in part on cells that are, in fact, memory cells. Fazekas de St. Groth's (1967) work on original antigenic sin is best interpreted in this way. Tests which ask questions about the proportion of total lymphocytes in a normal adult animal which react with a given antigen will be profoundly influenced by this consideration, and the development of antigen-free animals (if it proves to be technically feasible) is eagerly awaited.

IV. A Plan for Progress

There are now two distinct approaches to studying the antibody response, and particularly the role of antigen in this process. One is the *in vitro* approach which in the short period of 3–4 years has already made very substantial contributions. The other is the *in vivo* approach, which is now made more easy to interpret because of the *in vitro* results. The adoptive transfer technique acts as a bridge between these two approaches, on the one hand, enabling donor cells to be manipulated *in vitro* but requiring the animal to act as a suitable nursery for the full expression of those cells' potential.

A. TISSUE CULTURE SYSTEMS

Many of the questions posed by immunologists over the last decade or so will be answered in the future using *in vitro* techniques. It has been possible to isolate and recover macrophages and to add them to depleted cell preparations. As, for the first time, antibody responses have been obtained without macrophages, it should now be possible to analyze in some detail biochemical events in or on this cell which are relevant to immunological processes.

The unavailability of dendritic follicular cells in suspension is at present a deficiency in the tissue culture approach. This may in part be remedied by a tissue slice approach but perhaps a more satisfactory way would be the preparation of artificial dendritic cells. As antigen-cell interaction in follicles is most probably a surface phenomenon, it should not be beyond the wit of immunologists to devise a substitute.

It is now possible to obtain from lymphoid organs suspensions of cells in which the proportion of cells morphologically described as lymphocytes approaches 100%. Such preparations are functionally heterogeneous. (1) In secondary lymphoid organs (spleen, lymph nodes), there are thymus- and bone marrow-derived cells. These can be distinguished from each other by means of a thymus-specific antigen. Techniques will need to be developed for their physical separation before we can answer the question—how does cooperation occur. Similarly, differences in cell receptors on these cells will be resolved in detail only when separate populations are available. Perhaps the greatest challenge in this area is to define the receptor on susceptible cells, not simply in terms of an immunoglobulin molecule but rather as a receptor complex. How is the receptor held at the cell surface? Is it in close or loose association with the cell membrane? Is the initial inductive event simply a change in conformation of the Ig molecule? If so, there must be some mechanism for transmission of such a disturbance. Can we devise models to determine its molecular–biological nature? (2) The second area of functional heterogeneity is the specificity of the immunoglobulin receptor. In a spleen from an unstimulated mouse, how many bone marrow-derived cells possess identical receptors? The number is small, but how small? To provide answers for questions such as these, it will be necessary to develop cell enrichment procedures—antigen-coated glass bead colums, etc.—to high degrees of efficiency, particularly for cell recovery and thus enrichment.

B. The *in Vivo* Approach

Although many of the most fundamental questions will be answered by *in vitro* techniques, there are many aspects, particularly those of a practical nature, which must still be investigated *in vivo*. We wish to know especially what are the properties of an antigen which make it a good or poor immunogen *in vivo*? How can a poor immunogen be improved and a good immunogen be converted to a tolerogen? These questions are important in any consideration of the preparation of good vaccines or of tissue transplantation. The role that macrophages and dendritic cells play in antigen handling may be decisive in these circumstances.

In view of the complexity of whole animal experiments, a more ideal situation is the technique developed by Morris and colleagues for the "isolation" of an individual lymph node by cannulating afferent and efferent lymph ducts. In this situation, antigen or cells can be introduced as a pulse of known duration and effluent cells and antigen monitored. The node can be removed for sectioning and radioautography. In this system, most of mormal lymphoid physiology is retained. This approach should be particularly valuable in studying cell migration paths and the influence with antigen and/or antibody localized in defined areas may have on cell migration and subsequent behavior.

C. Clinical Implications—Immunoregulation

So far, the main clinical implications of immunology have been in three areas: immunization (active and passive, including continuous passive immunization in agammaglobulinemia); immunosuppression; and what might be termed "immunodamping" with antiinflammatory and antihistaminic drugs. The last decade's work in cellular immunology has so far had relatively little impact on clinical practice, in the sense that most agents in present clinical usage had either been discovered empirically or been borrowed from the cancer field. Two noteworthy exceptions are anti-D serum in the prevention of Rh disease and antilymphocyte serum. However, it is to be hoped that further practical results will flow from the present immunology research explosion.

Here it may help to introduce the term *immunoregulation*. One of the main purposes of this book has been to show that antibody formation at the level of the whole animal is exquisitely regulated through complex physiological mechanisms. The two great regulators are antigen and antibody. The more we understand antigen handling and presentation, on the one hand, and antibody formation and feedback, on the other, the more our power to manipulate immune responses at the whole animal level should grow. The stakes involved in clinical immunoregulation are high—specific tolerance in transplantation, allergy and autoimmunity, specific or nonspecifically heightened immunity in cancer, and partial immune deficiency states. The molecular biologist may well give us "the complete solution of immunology" (Jerne, 1969) in the sense of a satisfactory and final explanation of the origin of antibody diversity, but it will remain for the cell physiologist aware of the design of the whole animal's lymphoid system to harness this knowledge for workable clinical immunoregulation.

PREPARATION OF FLAGELLAR PROTEINS FROM *Salmonella* ORGANISMS

This appendix is designed for those who may wish to prepare the different flagellar antigens described in this monograph. It details the technique currently in practice in our laboratories as this differs in some respects from the procedure published previously (Ada *et al.*, 1964a).

I. Bacterial Culture

Bacterial cultures from our laboratories are prepared for freeze drying by growing the organisms first in nutrient broth, then transferring 0.5 ml of this culture into blood agar plates, and incubating overnight at 37°C. A thick suspension of the organisms is prepared in fetal calf serum containing 7.5% glucose and 0.1-ml samples of this suspension are freeze-dried.

When an ampoule is opened, the culture is suspended in about 5 ml of nutrient broth and incubated for 1–2 hours at 37°C. A small sample is then inoculated onto the edge of a motility plate (diameter = 8 cm).

Upon incubation of this plate at 37°C, the growing edge of bacteria should have moved most of the way across the plate within 4 hr. This depends upon the "sloppiness" of the supporting medium. The following composition is given only as a guide as the desired result depends upon the brand of reagents used. (Composition of medium for motility plates, 200 ml of Difco heart infusion broth containing 12.5 gm of gelatin and 0.7 gm Difco Bacto agar, the pH adjusted to 7.2.) After this incubation period, the motility plate is left overnight at room temperature to allow firming of the medium. Thereafter it is stored at 4°C and may be used for 7–10 days.

For production of flagella, the complete growing edge of bacteria from a motility plate is cut out, added to 300 ml of serum broth (10% bovine serum in heart infusion broth), and incubated for 7–8 hr at 37°C. This suspension is then added to culture medium in stainless steel trays at the rate of 20 ml per tray. Each tray (about $35 \times 25 \times 4$ cm) contains 1 liter of a medium consisting of 1.5% agar (Difco Bacto) in heart infusion broth (Difco) and has a close-fitting lid. The trays are incubated at 37°C until the bacterial growth is fairly confluent. For *Salmonella adelaide*, this is frequently 40 hr but may be longer or shorter for other strains. If substantial bacterial autolysis takes place, the subsequent isolation of the flagella is more difficult. On some occasions, it has been found advantageous to inlude gentian violet (1 ml of 0.1% per liter of medium) in the medium. This may reduce bacterial contamination and in some experiments has resulted in a higher yield of flagella.

II. Harvesting of Bacteria and Isolation of Flagella

After removal from the incubator, the trays are allowed to stand for about $2\frac{1}{2}$ hr to allow the medium to firm. Saline containing 1/10,000 merthiolate is added to each tray and the bacteria scraped off the surface of the medium with a bent glass rod so that the yield per tray is about 100 ml. The combined suspensions are blended for about 2 min in a container fitted with blades rotating at about 7000 rpm. The conditions for shearing off the flagella do not appear to be critical except that unduly long periods may disrupt some bacteria. The suspension is filtered through a pad of fine glass wool to remove small pieces of agar and the bacterial bodies then removed by three centrifugations for 7×10^4 g min at 0°–4°C. (All values are calculated to the midpoint of the contrifuge tube.) The final supernatant should be translucent.

Flagella are deposited from the supernatant by centrifugation in a Beckman ultracentrifuge, rotor No. 30 (2.4×10^6 g min). The pellet is resuspended in merthiolate-saline and this solution clarified (1×10^5 g min). The flagella are again deposited, resuspended, and the solution clarified and the flagella again deposited. The final pellet is slightly opaque with usually a dark central area. It is resuspended in 0.01 M phosphate buffer, pH 7.5, containing 1/100,000 merthiolate, deposited once more as above, and resuspended in this last solvent. From 12 trays, the yield may be 30 ml of a suspension containing 10 mg protein/ml. To estimate the protein concentration, the flagella preparation is diluted, 1 N HCl added to give a final concentration of 0.05 N, the solution centrifuged (5×10^6 g min), neutralized and the extinction at 215 mμ read (ϵ_{215} mμ, 1 cm = 94).

III. Preparation of Polymerized Flagellin and Flagellin

The flagella suspension is acidified by adding one-twentieth the volume of 1 N HCl, centrifuging for 5×10^6 g min, and neutralizing the supernatant with 1 N NaOH. Polymerization of the protein is achieved by adding saturated ammonium sulfate solution to a final concentration of 15% (v/v) and standing at room temperature for 1 or more days. The protein solution rapidly becomes translucent. The polymer is sedimented using the same conditions as for flagella (2.4×10^6 g min), the pellet resuspended in and dialyzed exhaustively against distilled water. The protein concentration is estimated (215 mμ) and the preparation frozen. The monomer, flagellin, is prepared immediately before use by acidification and neutralization as described above. If stored, the flagellin will slowly polymerize, the rate depending on the concentration of both protein and salt. Repeated freezing and thawing of samples also causes polymerization.

The purity of the flagellin preparation is determined by polyacrylamide gel electrophoresis at pH 2.7 in 8 M urea (Neville, 1967) using a 13% running gel. A single band only should be present (Parish and Ada, 1969a).

IV. Preparation of Fragment A from Polymerized Flagellin

Details have been established for one strain only (*S. adelaide*), and are described in full elsewhere (Parish and Ada, 1969a). If it is desired to obtain only pure fragment A, it is convenient to use a column containing only Sephadex G100. In the following experiment 1.5 ml of a CNBr digest of polymerized flagellin (35 mg) in 70% formic acid was applied to a column (80 × 3.2 cm) of Sephadex and the column eluted with 50% formic acid. The rate of passage of solvent was 14 ml/hr. It has been found advisable to keep the column at an even temperature and in a darkened room. All solutions containing high concentrations

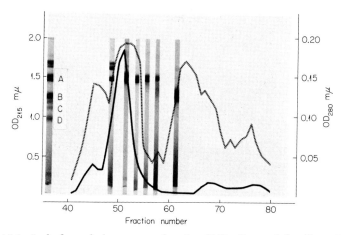

FIG. A1.1. Sephadex gel chromatography of a CNBr digest of flagellin. The curves show the O.D.$_{280\ m\mu}$(————) of the column effluent (in 50% formic acid) and O.D.$_{215\ m\mu}$ (----------) of the same samples after dialysis. Superimposed on these curves are polyacrylamide gel electrophoresis patterns of different fractions. At the left hand side is the pattern of whole CNBr digest, and the major fragments are marked. Fractions 51–57 from the column contain only fragment A.

of formic acid should be deaerated before use. Fig. A.1.1 shows the absorption of the effluent at 280 mμ, and, after dialysis of each sample against water and centrifugation to remove dextran solubilized by the formic acid, of the dialyzed samples at 215 mμ. It has been generally found that the second half of the major peak absorbing at 280 mμ is pure fragment A, as judged by polyacrylamide gel electrophoresis (see above) and a yield of about 9 mg should be obtained. The preparation of fragment A may be stored frozen.

THE TECHNIQUE OF ELECTRON MICROSCOPIC RADIOAUTOGRAPHY

The technique used is basically that of Salpeter and Bachmann (1964) with a few modifications. Pieces of radioactive tissue are cut and processed for electron microscopy using standard methods; viz., fixation in either OsO_4 or glutaraldehyde, dehydration in alcohols, and embedding in epoxy resin. Ultrathin sections are cut, stained, and mounted on collodion-coated glass slides, covered with a thin layer of evaporated carbon and then with a thin layer of Kodak NTE–nuclear track emulsion. Slides are kept in a light-tight box at 4°C for the required exposure time, after which they are developed, sections are stripped from the glass, and mounted for viewing in the electron microscope.

I. Preparation of Glass Slides

Standard glass microscope slides are first cleaned using a mild abrasive such as that marketed under the brand name Bon Ami. The slide is worked for about 1 min between finger and thumb with a little added abrasive, and then thoroughly rinsed, and allowed to dry. The end of the slide first held for support becomes the holding end for all future occasions of handling and no other part of the slide should be touched by hand thereafter. The slide is then held by tongs and introduced into a hot flame and firepolished for about two-thirds of its length with frequent reversals to prevent bending. This process takes about 2 min.

II. Collodion Coating

After cooling, the slide is dipped to about two-thirds its length in a solution of 0.2% collodion in ethyl acetate and is then slowly withdrawn. The slide is held vertically in air to complete the evaporation of the solvent and then placed in a covered box until required for use.

III. Mounting of Sections

This is conveniently done under a dissecting microscope. Ultrathin sections of silver to pale gold coloration are cut, using standard ultra-microtomy techniques and then stained floating freely in 5% aqueous uranyl acetate for from 2 to 12 hr as convenient. They are then washed by passing through two beakers of distilled water and mounted on the prepared slide about 1 to 2 cm. from the end. Manipulations are carried out with a platinum wire loop of 5 mm. diameter. Finely drawn glass probes assist in maneuvering the sections. The water droplet with the ribbon of sections is retained within the loop by surface tension. The loop is brought near the surface of the slide, contact is made with the underhanging surface of the water droplet, and the sections settle on the slide as excess water is withdrawn by means of a fine-bore, freshly pulled capillary tube. The wire should not be allowed to touch the collodion as this is easily torn when wet. The position of the sections is marked by lightly scoring an encompassing circle on the underside of the slide. Reference data may be scored at the holding end of the slide, again on the underside.

IV. Carbon Coating

Slides are then placed in a high-vacuum coating unit and covered with a 50 Å layer of evaporated carbon.

V. Emulsion Coating

The slide is dipped into the diluted emulsion (at 60°C) for half its length, withdrawn slowly and steadily, and held vertically to dry. After drying, the slides are stored in light-tight boxes with a desiccant, "Drierite."

VI. Development

The slides are developed to the following regimen.

Kodak Dektol diluted $1 + 2$ at 20°C	$1\frac{1}{2}$ min
3% CH_3COOH	10 sec
Water	5 sec
Amfix	30 sec
Water	2 min

VII. Mounting for Viewing

If the slide is retained in a humid atmosphere for about 30 min, this assists in the stripping process which may be carried out under a dissecting microscope. Using a needle, a circle slightly larger than the diameter of the support disc is scored round the ribbon of sections, and a drop of water placed on the score line gradually infiltrates under the collodion. The complex sandwich of collodion, section, carbon, and emulsion strips from the glass and can then be mounted on the support disc of choice. The use of a support disc of 1 mm central aperture allows complete, uninterrupted viewing of the section and is very useful for light microscope correlation studies. If the section complex is reluctant to strip from the glass a drop of 1% hydrofluoric acid placed on the scored line greatly assists the stripping procedure.

VIII. Preparation of the Emulsion

The Kodak NTE emulsion (Eastman Kodak Co., Rochester, New York) as supplied requires diluting for use. The procedure is as follows. A bench centrifuge is preheated to 60°C; this can conveniently be done in one-half hour using a hairdrier and cowl. A water bath at 60°C contains a flask of distilled water, 12 centrifuge tubes each containing

9 ml distilled water, and the pot of emulsion concentrate. After preheating the centrifuge, working under a Wratten No. 1 safelight, the emulsion pot is opened and 1 ml added to each tube. After the pot of concentrate has been secured, work may proceed under a Wratten OA safelight. The 12 tubes are spun for 45 min at about 4000 rpm. The supernatants are then discarded and 1 ml distilled water is added to each tube in turn and the pellets are resuspended. This water is also at 60°C and the sedimented buttons are maintained at this temperature while awaiting resuspension. The total volume is then poured into a suitable glass container and a further 2 ml distilled water is used to rinse all the tubes and this is added to the pool. The diluted emulsion is now checked to determine if further dilution is required. A test slide is dipped and the resultant dried emulsion film is viewed in white light. The coloration of the reflected surface indicates the thickness of the emulsion layer. Water is added until the test slide shows a silver color and part of this film is then viewed in the electron microscope to ascertain that it is, in effect, a monolayer of undeveloped silver halide crystals. The diluted emulsion is stored in a light-tight container at 4° and heated to 60°C for use.

IX. Modifications of the Method to Allow Study of Cells Previously Held in Cell Suspensions

Frequently only minute numbers of cells are available for examination as, for example, when the peritoneal cells from a single mouse may have to be split to provide a number of samples. The technique to be described allows such small cell numbers to be processed for electron microscopy without loss of tissue.

After the appropriate exposure to a radioiodinated antigen or some other marker, the cells are carefully washed and resuspended in 50% serum. Small aliquots of the cell suspension (approximately 1 ml), containing $0.5-2 \times 10^6$ cells are then placed in Spinco cellulose nitrate tubes ($\frac{3}{16}$ in. $\times$ $1\frac{5}{8}$ in.) and gently centrifuged for 1–2 min. A loose pellet of cells remains at the bottom of the tube. Gentle centrifugation is essential to prevent the cells from packing too tightly. The supernatant is then removed and is replaced with fixative (e.g., glutaraldehyde). The fixative is changed twice and the pellet is allowed to fix for 1–2 hours. The bottom of the tube containing the fixed cells is cut off and washed in buffer following which the cells are post-fixed in osmium. The pellet, still in its cap of cellulose nitrate is then dehydrated in increasing concentrations of acetone. The cellulose nitrate tube dissolves in absolute acetone and the pellet can then be embedded in araldite. This procedure allows small samples of cells to be handled, since it does not involve manipulation of the pellet itself. The pellet remains intact and losses of tissue due to fragmentation of the sample are avoided. Further processing is carried out as described above.

SOME PROPERTIES OF RADIOISOTOPES USED COMMONLY FOR RADIOAUTOGRAPHY, WITH SPECIAL REFERENCE TO TRITIUM AND ^{125}IODINE

Radioisotopes emitting electrons are convenient to use as markers for proteins or other substances which may be present in tissues or cells, and for the detection and localization of which radioautography is to be used. Table A3.I (Cairns, 1962) lists some properties of six electron emitters. There is a considerable difference in the half-lives of these isotopes. This is of importance as the extent of substitution of a radioisotope in a given substance necessary to achieve a particular specific activity is proportional to the half-life of the isotope. Another property of importance is the energy of emission of each isotope as this will determine the resolution which will be obtained in radioautographs. The use of three of these isotopes has been described in this monograph, namely ^{3}H, ^{125}I, and ^{131}I. Further information about the two of these isotopes which give best resolution, namely ^{3}H and ^{125}I,

TABLE A 3.I

Isotope	Half-life day^{-1}	Proportion disintegrating per day	Ci/gm atom	Maximum energy keV
^{3}H	4.5×10^{3}	1.5×10^{-4}	2.9×10^{4}	18
^{125}I	60	1.1×10^{-2}	2.2×10^{6}	34
^{14}C	2.0×10^{6}	3.4×10^{-7}	6.4×10^{1}	155
^{35}S	87.1	8.0×10^{-3}	1.5×10^{6}	170
^{131}I	8.1	8.2×10^{-2}	1.5×10^{7}	820
^{32}P	14.3	4.8×10^{-2}	9.1×10^{6}	1700

is presented in Table A. 3.II (from Ada *et al.*, 1966). The relationship between disintegration patterns, emergent electrons, and grain formation has been described elsewhere for "ideal" situations such as point sources of radiation or radiation sources in very thin films. It is difficult to make adjustments to situations which are met in biology, such as histological sections or isotopes present on the surface of cells present in a smear. Table A. 3.II reports the results of experiments which mimicked such situations. Artificial films with thicknesses similar to those of histological sections were prepared. Most experiments used Ilford L$_4$ emulsion but Kodak NTB$_2$ emulsion appeared to give similar results. Sections of 5 μ thickness are commonly used in histology and if the isotope is distributed fairly evenly through the section, many of the emitted electrons will be absorbed in the section before reaching the overlying emulsion. This is particularly so with ^{3}H. Grains appearing in the emulsion are therefore primarily due to the higher energy electrons emitted by this isotope. Because of this, the yield of grains per disinte-

TABLE A 3.II

Isotope	Section thickness	Photographic emulsion	Grains/ disintegration	Grains/ emergent electron
^{3}H	5.0 μ	Ilford L$_4$	0.018	0.62
^{125}I	5.0 μ	Ilford L$_4$	0.23	1.23

gration is low and is the product of the higher energy electrons reacting with the emulsion. Furthermore, the resolution expected with these isotopes, especially in tissue sections, is less precise than would have been expected. For sections of density 1.3, it has been calculated that the theoretical range of the higher energy tritium electrons (10–14 keV) is 2.16–4.1 μ while those of [125]I (22–34 keV) is about 9–15 μ. As there is very little emission at the highest energy, the resolution seen is better than the upper levels of these values would suggest.

Strictly comparable figures are not available for electron microscopical radioautography. Values will depend on the thickness of both the section and the emulsion. As a guide however, Salpeter and Bachmann (1964) find values of 0.04 grain/disintegration for [3]H. This high figure is obtained because fewer electrons will be absorbed in these sections compared to standard sections. In contrast to ^{3}H, which exhibits a continuous spectrum of electron energies, ^{125}I emits electrons exhibiting several discrete activities. While it is generally assumed that the efficiencies of ^{3}H and ^{125}I in electron microscopic radioautography are similar we are not aware of any quantitative experiments on the point.

A knowledge of the grain yield per β or γ disintegration is necessary before the relationship between isotopes present in a cell or tissue section and grains in the emulsion can be evaluated. This information, together with a knowledge of the half-life of the isotope used and the extent of substitution of isotopes in the substance under study, enables the concentration of protein in the section or cell to be calculated.

REFERENCES

Abdou, N. I., and Ritcher, M., (1969). Cells involved in the immune response. X. The transfer of antibody-forming capacity to irradiated rabbits by antigen-reactive cells isolated from normal allogeneic rabbit bone marrow after passage through antigen-sensitized glass bead columns. *J. Exp. Med.* **130**, 141.

Ackerman, G. A., and Knouff, R. A., (1964). Lymphocytopoietic activity in the bursa of Fabricius. *In* "The Thymus in Immunobiology. Structure, Function and Disease" (R. A. Good and A. E. Gabrielsen, eds.), p. 123. Harper (Hoeber), New York.

Ada, G. L., and Byrt, P., (1969). Specific inactivation of antigen reactive cells with ^{125}I-labelled antigen. *Nature (London)* **222**, 1291.

Ada, G. L., and Lang, P. G., (1966). Antigen in tissues. II. State of antigen in lymph nodes of rats given isotopically labelled flagellin, haemocyanin or serum albumin. *Immunology* **10**, 431.

Ada, G. L., and Parish, C. R., (1968). Low zone tolerance to located flagellin in adult rats. A possible role for antigen localized in lymphoid follicles. *Proc. Nat. Acad. Sci. U.S.* **61**, 556.

Ada, G. L., and Williams, J. M., (1966). Antigens in tissues. I. State of bacterial flagella in lymph nodes of rats injected with isotopically labelled flagella. *Immunology* **10**, 417.

Ada, G. L., Nossal, G. J. V., Pye, J., and Abbot, A. (1964a). Antigens in immunity. I. Preparation and properties of flagellar antigens from *Salmonella adelaide*. *Aust. J. Exp. Biol. Med. Sci.* **42**, 267.

Ada, G. L., Nossal, G. J. V., and Pye, J., (1964b). Antigens in immunity. III. Distribution of iodinated antigens following injection into rats via the hind footpads. *Aust. J. Exp. Biol. Med. Sci.* **42**, 295.

Ada, G. L., Nossal, G. J. V., and Austin, C. M., (1964c). Antigens in immunity. V. The ability of cells in lymphoid follicles to recognize foreignness. *Aust. J. Exp. Biol. Med. Sci.* **42**, 331.

Ada, G. L., Nossal, G. J. V., and Pye, J., (1965). Antigens in immunity. XI. The uptake of antigen in animals previously rendered immunologically tolerant. *Aust. J. Exp. Biol. Med. Sci.* **43**, 337.

Ada, G. L., Askonas, B. A., Humphrey, J. H., McDevitt, H .O., and Nossal, G. J. V., (1966). Correlation of grain counts with radioactivity (iodine-125 and tritium) in autoradiography. *Exp. Cell. Res.* **41**, 557.

Ada, G. L., Parish, C. R., and Nossal, G. J. V., and Abbot, A., (1967). The tissue localization, immunogenic and tolerance-inducing properties of antigens and antigen-fragments. *Cold Spring Harbor Symp. Quant. Biol.* **32**, 381.

Ada, G. L., Lang, P. G., and Plymin, G., (1968). Antigen tissues. V. Effect of endotoxin on the fate of, and on the immune response to, serum albumin and to albumin-antibody complexes. *Immunology*, **14**, 825.

Ada, G. L., Byrt, P., Cooper, M. G., and Langman R., (1970). The reaction between labelled antigens and lymphocytes from normal, immunized and tolerant rats. *Proc. Aust. Biochem Soc.* **3**, 57.

Ada, G. L., Byrt, P., Mandel, T., and Warner, N. L., (1971, in press.). A specific reaction between antigen labelled with radioactive iodide and lymphocyte-like cells from normal, tolerant and immunized mice or rats. *In* "Developmental Aspects of Antibody Formation and Structure" (J. Sterzl and M. Riha, eds.). Academic Press, New York.

Adler, F. L., Fishman, M., and Dray, S., (1966). Antibody formation initiated *in vitro*. III. Antibody formation and allotypic specificity directed by ribonucleic acid from peritoneal exudate cells. *J. Immunol.* **97**, 554.

Albright, E. C., Larson, F. C., and Tust, R. H., (1954). *In vitro* conversion of thyroxin to triiodothyronine by kidney slices. *Proc. Soc. Exp. Biol. Med.* **86**, 137.

Anderer, F. A. (1963). Versuche zur Bestimmung den serologisch determinanten Gruppen des Tabak mosaikvirus. *Z. Naturforsch.* **18b**, 1010.

Anderer, F. A. and Schlumberger, H. D. (1965). Properties of different artificial antigens immunologically related to tobacco mosaic virus. *Biochim. Biophys. Acta* **97**, 503.

Anderer, F. A. and Schlumberger, H. D. (1966). Cross-reactions of antisera against the terminal amino acid and dipeptide of tobacco mosaic virus *Biochim. Biophys. Acta* **115**, 222.

Andreasen, E. (1943). Studies on thymolymphatic system; quantitative investigations on thymolymphatic systems in normal rats at different ages, under normal conditions and during inanition and restitution after starvation. *Acta Pathol. Microbiol. Scand.* **49**, 1.

Archer, G. T. (1968). The function of the eosinophil. *in* "11th Congress of the International Society of Blood Transfusion" (L. Holländer, ed.), p. 71. S. Karger, Basel.

Archer, G. T. and Hirsh, J. G. (1963). Motion picture studies on degranulation of horse eosinophils during phagocytosis. *J. Exp. Med.* 118, 287.

Argyris, B. F. (1968). Role of macrophages in immunological maturation. *J. Exp. Med.* 128, 459.

Argyris, B. F. and Askonas, B. A. (1968). Mouse peritoneal cells. Their ability to elicit or produce antibody after exposure to antigen. *Immunology* 14, 379.

Armstrong, W. D. and Diener, E. (1969). A new method for the enumeration of antigen reactive cells using a pure protein antigen. *J. Exp. Med.* 129, 371.

Arnon, R. and Sela, M. (1969). Antibodies to a unique region in lysozyme provoked by a synthetic antigen conjugate. *Proc. Nat. Acad. Sci. U.S.* 62, 163.

Arnon, R., Sela, M., Rachaman, E. S., and Shapiro, D. (1967). Cytolipin H-specific antibodies obtained with a synthetic polypeptide conjugate. *Eur. J. Biochem.* 2, 79.

Ashman, R. F., and Metzger, H. (1969). A Waldenström macroglobulin which binds nitrophenyl ligands. *J. Biol. Chem.* 244, 3405.

Askonas, B. A. and Humprey, J. H. (1958). Formation of specific antibodies and γ-globulin *in vitro*. A study of the synthetic ability of various tissues from rabbits immunized by different methods. *Biochem. J.* 68, 252.

Askonas, B. A. and Jaroskova, L. (1971). Macrophages as helper cells in antibody induction. *in* "Developmental Aspects of Antibody Formation and Structure" (J. Sterzl and M. Riha, eds.), Vol. 2. Publ. House Czech. Acad. Sci. Prague.

Askonas, B. A. and Rhodes, J. M. (1965). Immunogenicity of antigen containing ribonucleic acid preparations from macrophages. *Nature (London)* 205, 470.

Askonas, B. A., Auzins, I., and Unanue, E. R. (1968). Role of macrophages in the immune response. *Bull. Soc. Chim. Biol.* 50, 1113.

Atassi, M. Z. (1967). Periodate oxidation of sperm-whale myoglobin and the role of the methionine residues in the antigen-antibody reaction *Biochem. J.* 102, 478.

Atassi, M. Z. (1968a). Role of the amino groups and C-terminal of sperm-whale myoglobin in the antigen-antibody reaction. *Nature (London)* 209, 1209.

Atassi, M. Z. (1968b). Immunochemistry of sperm-whale myoglobin. III. Modification of the three tyrosine residues, and their role in the conformation and differentiation of their roles in the antigenic reactivity. *Biochemistry* 7, 3078.

Atassi, M. Z. and Caruso, D. R. (1968). Immunochemistry of sperm-whale myoglobin. II. Modification of the two tryptophan residues and their role in the conformation and antigen-antibody reaction. *Biochemistry* 7, 699.

Atassi, M. Z. and Saplin, B. J. (1968). Immunochemistry of sperm-whale myoglobin. I. The specific interaction of some tryptic peptides and of peptides containing all the reactive regions of the antigen. *Biochemistry* 7, 688.

Attardi, G., Cohn, M., Horibata, K., and Lennox, E. S. (1959). Symposium on the biology of cells modified by viruses or antigens. II. On the analysis of antibody synthesis at the cellular level. *Bacteriol. Rev.* 23, 213.

Auerbach, R. (1961). Experimental analysis of the origin of cell types in the development of the mouse thymus. *Develop. Biol.* 3, 336.

Auerbach, R. (1970). Toward a developmental theory of antibody formation: The germinal theory of immunity. *in* "Developmental Aspects of Antibody Formation and Structure" (J. Sterzl and M. Riha, eds.), Vol. 1, p. 23. Czech. Acad. Sci., Prague.

Austin, C. M. (1968). Patterns of migration of lymphoid cells. *Aust. J. Exp. Biol. Med. Sci.* **46**, 581.

Austin, C. M. and Nossal, G. J. V. (1966). Mechanism of induction of immunological tolerance. III. Cross-tolerance amongst flagellar antigens. *Aust. J. Exp. Biol. Med. Sci.* **44**, 341.

Ax, W., Kaboth, U., and Fischer, H. (1966). Immunologische studien am omentum. I. Mitt. Mikrokinematographische Beobachtungen an kultivierten Mäuse-Omenten; Nachweis gebildeter Anti-körper. *Z. Naturforsch*, **21b**, 782.

Azar, M. M. (1967). Studies on immunological tolerance to soluble proteins. I. Organ distribution of antigen in the adult mouse. *Proc. Soc. Exp. Biol. Med.* **125**, 849.

Baker, P. J., Bernstein, M., Pasanen, V., and Landy, M. (1966). Detection and enumeration of antibody producing cells by specific adherence of antigen-coated bentonite particles. *J. Immunol.* **97**, 767.

Bauer, H., Paronetto, F., Burns, W. A., and Einheber, A. (1966). The enhancing effect of the microbial flora on macrophage function and the immune response. *J. Exp. Med.* **123**, 1013.

Benacerraf, B. (1968). Cytophilic immunoglobulins and delayed hypersensitivity. *Fed. Proc.* **27**, 46.

Benacerraf, B., Ovary, Z., Bloch, K. J., and Franklin, E. C. (1963). Properties of guinea pig 7S antibodies. 1. Electrophoretic separation of two types of guinea pig 7S antibodies. *J. Exp. Med.* **117**, 937 (1963).

Benacerraf, B., Green, I., and Paul, W. E. (1967). The immune response of guinea pigs to hapten–poly-L-lysine conjugates as an example of the genetic control of the recognition of antigenicity. *Cold Spring Harbor Symp. Quant. Biol.* **32**, 56a.

Bendinelli, M. (1968). Haemolytic plaque formation by mouse peritoneal cells, and the effect on it of Friend virus infection. *Immunology* **14**, 837.

Bendinelli, M. and Wedderburn, N. (1967). Haemolytic plaque formation by unimmunized mouse peritoneal lymphocytes. *Nature* (*London*) **215**, 157.

Bennett, H. S., Luft, J. H., and Hampton, J. C. (1959). Morphological classification of vertebrate blood capillaries. *Amer. J. Physiol.* **196**, 381.

Benjamini, E., Young, J. D., Shimizu, M., and Leung, C. Y. (1964). Immunochemical studies on the tobacco mosaic virus protein. I. The immunological relationship of the tryptic peptides of tobacco mosaic virus protein to the whole protein. *Biochemistry* **3**, 1115.

Benjamini, E., Shimizu, M., Young, J. D., and Leung, C. Y. (1969). Immunochemical studies on tobacco mosaic virus protein. IX. Investigations on binding and antigenic specificity of antibodies to an antigenic area of tobacco mosaic virus protein. *Biochemistry* **8**, 2242.

Berenbaum, M. C. (1959). The autoradiographic localization of intracellular antibody. *Immunology* **2**, 71.

Berken, A. and Benacerraf, B. (1966). Properties of antibodies cytophilic for macrophages. *J. Exp. Med.* **123**, 119.

Bernier, G. M. and Cebra, J. J. (1964). Polypeptide chains of human gamma globulin: Cellular localization by fluorescent antibody. *Science* **144**, 1590.

Bernstein, I. D. and Ovary, Z. (1968). Absorption of antigens from the gastrointestinal tract. *Int. Arch. Allergy* **33**, 521.

Billingham, R. E., Brent, L., and Medawar, P. B. (1953). Actively acquired tolerance of foreign cells. *Nature* (*London*) 172, 603.

Biozzi, G., Stiffel, C., Mouton, D., Liacopoulos-Briot, M., Decreusefond, C., and Bouthillier, Y. (1966). Etude de phénomène de l'immuno-cyto-adhérence au cours de l'immunisation. *Ann. Inst. Pasteur* Paris. Suppl. au No. 3, 110, 7.

Bishop, D. C. and Abramoff, P. (1967). Analysis of normal and "immunogenic RNA" in peritoneal macrophage cells. *J. Reticuloendothelial Soc.* 4, 441.

Bishop, D. C., Pisciotta, A. V., and Abramoff, P. (1967). Synthesis of normal and "immunogenic RNA" by peritoneal macrophage cells. *J. Immunol.* 99, 751.

Blau, J. N. (1967). Antigen and antibody localization in Hassall's corpuscles. *Nature* 215, 1073.

Blau, J. N. and Veall, N. (1967). The uptake and localization of proteins, Evans Blue and carbon black in the normal and pathological thymus of the guinea pig. *Immunology* 12, 363.

Bloom, W. ed. (1948). "Histopathology of Irradiation from External and Internal Sources," p. 808. McGraw-Hill, New York.

Bos, W. H. (1967). Recirculatie en transformatie van lymphocyten. Doctorate degree, University of Groningen, Drukkerij van Denderen, Groningen.

Bouma, J. M. W. and Gruber, M. (1964). The distribution of cathepsins B and C in rat tissues. *Biochim. Biophys. Acta* 89, 545.

Bouma, J. M. W. and Gruber, M. (1966). The intracellular distribution of cathepsin B and cathepsin C in rat liver. *Biochim. Biophys. Acta* 113, 350.

Bowers, W. E., Finkenstaedt, J. T., and de Duve, C. (1967). Lysosomes in lymphoid tissue. I. The measurement of hydrolytic activities in whole homogenates. *J. Cell Biol.* 32, 325.

Bowers, W. E. and de Duve, C. (1967a). Lysosomes in lymphoid tissue. II. Intracellular distribution of acid hydrolases. *J. Cell Biol.* 32, 339.

Bowers, W. E. and de Duve, C. (1967b). Lysosomes in lymphoid tissue. III. Influence of various treatments of the animals on the distribution of acid hydrolases. *J. Cell Biol.* 32, 349.

Boyden, S. (1964). Cytophilic antibody in guinea pigs with delayed type hypersensitivity. *Immunology* 7, 474.

Boyden, S. (1965). The occurrence and significance of natural antibodies. *in* "Molecular and Cellular Basis of Antibody Formation" (J. Sterzl, ed.). Czech. Acad. Sci., Prague.

Boyden, S. and Sorkin, E. (1961). The adsorption of antibody and antigen by spleen cells *in vitro*. Some further experiments. *Immunology* 4, 244.

Boyer, G. S. (1960). Chorioallantoic membrane lesions produced by inoculation of adult fowl leukocytes. *Nature* 185, 327.

Braun, W. and Lasky, L. J. (1967). Antibody formation in new born mice initiated through adult macrophages. *Fed. Proc.* 26, 642.

Bretscher, P. A. and Cohn, M. (1968). Minimal model for the mechanism of antibody induction and paralysis by antigen. *Nature* 220, 444.

Britton, S. (1968). Induction of immunological paralysis *in vivo* and *in vitro*. *Acta Pathol. microbiol. Scand.* 72, 455.

Britton, S. and Möller, G. (1965). Immunity and tolerance to a bacterial lipopolysaccharide antigen. Studied at the cellular level, p. 213. *Mendel Mem. Symp. Czech. Acad. Sci. Prague*.

Britton, S., Wepsic, T., and Möller, G. (1968). Persistence of immunogenicity of two complex antigens retained *in vivo*. *Immunology* **14**, 491.

Brody, N. I., Walker, J. G., and Siskind, G. W. (1967). Studies on the control of antibody synthesis. Interaction of antigenic competition and suppression of antibody formation by passive antibody on the immune response. *J. Exp. Med.* **126**, 81.

Burnet, F. M. (1957). A modification of Jerne's theory of antibody production using the concept of clonal selection. *Aust. J. Sci.* **20**, 67.

Burnet, F. M. (1959). "The Clonal Selection Theory of Acquired Immunity." Vanderbilt Univ. Press, Nashville, Tennessee.

Burnet, F. M. (1965). Mast cells in the thymus of NZB mice. *J. Pathol. Bacteriol.* **89**, 271.

Burnet, F. M. (1967). The impact on ideas of immunology. *Cold Spring Harbor Symp. Quant. Biol.* **32**, 1.

Burnet, F. M. (1969). "Cellular Immunology" Books 1 and 2. Melbourne Univ. Press, Melbourne and Cambridge Univ. Press, London.

Burnet, F. M. and Fenner, F. (1949). "The Production of Antibodies" 2nd Ed. Macmillan, New York.

Bussard, A. E. (1963). "Définitions et critères de la tolérance immunologique." *in* "La tolérance acquise et la tolérance naturelle a l'égard de substances antigéniques défines." *Colloq. Int. Centre Nat. Rech. Sci.* No. 116.

Bussard, A. E. (1966). Antibody formation in nonimmune mouse peritoneal cells after incubation in gum containing antigen. *Science* **153**, 887.

Bussard, A. E. (1967). Primary antibody response induced *in vitro* among cells from normal animals. *Cold Spring Harbor Symp. Quant. Biol.* **32**, 465.

Bussard, A. E. and Hannoun, C. (1966). Antibody production by cells in tissue culture. II. Qualitative and quantitative aspects of antibody production (local hemolysis in gum) by cells obtained from long term culture. *J. Exp. Med.* **123**, 1047.

Bussard, A. E. and Lurie, M. (1967). Primary antibody response *in vitro* in peritoneal cells. *J. Exp. Med.* **125**, 873.

Bussard, A. E., Nossal, G. J. V., Mazie, J. C., and Lewis, H. (1971, in press). Formation of haemolytic plaques by peritoneal cells *in vitro*. II. Cell-to-cell interactions, effect of inhibitors and theoretical considerations. *in* "Developmental Aspects of Antibody Formation and Structure" (J. Sterzl and M. Riha, eds.), Vol. 2. Czech. Acad. Sci., Prague.

Buyukozer, I., Mutlu, K. S., and Pepe, F. A. (1965). Antigen (ferritin) and antibody distribution in the rat lymph node after primary and secondary responses and after prolonged stimulation. *Amer. J. Anat.* **117**, 385.

Byers, V. S. and Sercarz, E. (1971, in press). *In vitro* sensitivity and the antibody response to antigen and antibody. *in* "Developmental Aspects of Antibody Formation and Structure" (J. Sterzl and M. Riha, eds.), Vol. 2. Academic Press, New York.

Byrt, P. and Ada, G. L. (1969). An *in vitro* reaction between labelled flagellin or haemocyanin and lymphocyte-like cells from normal animals. *Immunology* **17**, 503.

Campbell, D. H. and Garvey, J. S. (1963). Nature of retained antigen and its role in immune mechanisms. *Advan. Immunol.* **3**, 261.

Cahnmann, H. J., Arnon, R., and Sela, M. (1966). Isolation and characterization of active fragments obtained by cleavage of immunoglobulin G with cyanogen bromide. *J. Biol. Chem.* **241**, 3247.

Cairns, J. (1962). The application of autoradiography to the study of DNA viruses. *Cold Spring Harbor Symp. Quant. Biol.* **27**, 311.

Carpenter, C. B., Gill, T. J., III, and Mann, L. T. (1967). Synthetic polypeptide metabolism. III. Degradation and organ localization of isomeric synthetic polypeptide antigens *J. Immunol.* **98**, 236.

Cayeux, P., Panijel, J., Cluzan, R., and Levillain, R. (1966). Streptococcal arthritis and cardiopathy experimentally induced in white mice. *Nature* **212**, 688.

Cebra, J. J. (1967). Common peptides comprising the N-terminal half of heavy chain from rabbit IgG and specific antibodies. *Cold Spring Harbor Symp. Quant. Biol.* **32**, 65.

Cerottini, J. C., McConahey, P. J., and Dixon, F. J. (1969). Specificity of the immunosuppression caused by passive administration of antibody. *J. Immunol.* **103**, 268.

Chiappino, G. and Pernis, B. (1964). Demonstration with immuno-fluorescence of 19 S macroglobulins and 7 S gamma globulins in different cells of the human spleen. *Pathol. Microbiol. (Basel)* **27**, 8.

Cinader, B. and Dubert, J. M. (1955). Acquired immune tolerance to human albumin and response to subsequent injections of diazo human albumin, *Brit. J. Exp. Pathol.* **36**, 515.

Claman, H. N. (1971, in press). Cellular interaction in the immune response. *in* "Developmental Aspects of Antibody Formation and Structure" (J. Sterzl and M. Riha, eds.), Vol. 2. Czech. Acad. Sci., Prague.

Claman, H. N., Chaperon, E. A., and Triplett, R. F. (1966). Thymus-marrow cell combinations—synergism in antibody production. *Proc. Soc. Exp. Biol. Med.* **122**, 1167.

Clark, S. L. (1962). The reticulum of lymph nodes in mice studied with the electron microscope. *Amer. J. Anat.* **110**, 217.

Clark, S. L. (1964a). "The Thymus," Wistar Inst. Symp. Monogr. No. 2 (V. Defendi and D. Metcalf, eds.), p. 9. Wistar Inst. Press, Philadelphia, Pennsylvania.

Clark, S. L. (1964b). Electron microscopy of the thymus in mice of strain 12a/J. *in* "The Thymus in Immunobiology. Structure, Function and Role in Disease" (R. A. Good and A. E. Gabrielsen, eds.), p. 85. Harper (Hoeber), New York.

Clark, S. L. (1966). Cytological evidences of secretion in the thymus. *in* "The Thymus—Experimental and Clinical Studies" (G. E. W. Wolstenholme, and R. Porter, eds.), p. 3. Churchill, London.

Coffey, J. W. and de Duve, C. (1968). Digestive activity of lysosomes. II. The digestion of proteins by extracts of rat liver lysosomes. *J. Biol. Chem.* **243**, 3255.

Cohen, E. P. (1967a). Conversion of non-immune cells into antibody-forming cells by RNA. *Nature (London)* **213**, 462.

Cohen, E. P. (1967b). The appearance of a new species of RNA in the mouse spleen after immunization as detected by molecular hybridization. *Proc. Nat. Acad. Sci. U.S.* **57**, 673.

Cohen, E. P. and Raska, K. Jr. (1968). Unique species of RNA in peritoneal cells exposed to different antigens. *in* "Nucleic Acids in Immunology" (O. Plescia and W. Braun, eds.), p. 573. Springer-Verlag, New York.

Cohen, S., Holloway, R. C., Matthews, C., and McFarlane, A. (1956). Distribution and elimination of ¹³¹I- and ¹⁴C-labelled plasma proteins in the rabbit. *Biochem. J.* **62**, 143.

Cohn, Z. A. (1962). Influence of rabbit polymorphonuclear leucocytes and macrophages on the immunogenicity of *Escherichia coli*. *Nature* **196**, 1066.

Cohn, Z. A. (1964). The fate of bacteria within phagocytic cells. III. Destruction of an *Escherichia coli* agglutinogen within polymorphonuclear leucocytes and macrophages. *J. Exp. Med.* **120**, 869.

Cohn, Z. A. (1966). The regulation of pinocytosis in mouse macrophages. I. Metabolic requirements as defined by the use of inhibitors. *J. Exp. Med.* **124**, 557.

Cohn, Z. A. and Benson, B. (1965a). The differentiation of mononuclear phagocytes. Morphology, cytochemistry and biochemistry. *J. Exp. Med.* **121**, 153.

Cohn, Z. A. and Benson, B. (1965b). The in vitro differentiation of mononuclear phagocytes. I. The influence of inhibitors and the results of autoradiography *J. Exp. Med.* **121**, 279.

Cohn, Z. A. and Benson, B. (1965c). The in vitro differentiation of mononuclear phagocytes. II. The influence of serum on granule formation, hydrolase production, and pinocytosis. *J. Exp. Med.* **121**, 835.

Cohn, Z. A. and Benson, B. (1965d). The in vitro differentiation of mononuclear phagocytes. III. The reversibility of granule and hydrolytic enzyme formation and the turnover of granule constituents. *J. Exp. Med.* **122**, 455.

Cohn, Z. A. and Parks, E. (1967a). The regulation of pinocytosis in mouse macrophages. II. Factors inducing vesicle formation. *J. Exp. Med.* **125**, 213.

Cohn, Z. A. and Parks, E. (1967b). The regulation of pinocytosis in mouse macrophages. III. The induction of vesicle formation by nucleosides and nucleotides. *J. Exp. Med.* **125**, 457.

Cohn, Z. A. and Parks, E. (1967c). The regulation of pinocytosis in mouse macrophages. IV. The immunological induction of pinocytic vesicles, secondary lysosomes, and hydrolytic enzymes. *J. Exp. Med.* **125**, 1091.

Cohn, Z. A., Fedorko, M. E., and Hirsch, J. G. (1966). The in vitro differentiation of mononuclear phagocytes. V. The formation of macrophage lysosomes. *J. Exp. Med.* **123**, 757 (1966).

Cole, L. J. and Garver, R. M. (1961). Homograft-reactive large mononuclear leucocytes in peripheral blood and peritoneal exudates. *Amer. J. Physiol.* **200**, 147.

Cole, G. J. and Morris, B. (1970). The effects of thymectomy in the sheep. II. The response to antigen. *Aust. J. Exp. Biol. Med. Sci.*, in press.

Conchie, J., Hay, A. J., and Levvy, G. A. (1961). Mammalian glycosidases. III. The intracellular localization of β-glucuronidase in different mammalian tissues. *Biochem. J.* **79**, 324.

Coons, A. H., Creech, H. J., Jones, R. N., and Berliner, E. (1942). The demonstration of pneumococcal antigen in tissues by the use of fluorescent antibody. *J. Immunol.* **45**, 159.

Cooper, G. N. and Thonard, J. C. (1967). Serum antibody responses to intestinal implantation of antigens in rats. *J. Pathol. Bacteriol.* **93**, 213.

Cooper, G. N. and Turner, K. (1967). Immunological responses in rats following antigenic stimulation of Peyer's patches. I. Characteristics of the primary response. *Aust. J. Exp. Biol. Med. Sci.* **45**, 363 (1967).

Cooper, G. N. and Turner, K. (1968). Immunological responses in rats following antigenic stimulation of Peyer's patches. III. Local and general sequelae. *Aust. J. Exp. Biol. Med. Sci.* **46**, 415.

Cooper, G. N., Halliday, W. J., and Thonard, J. C. (1967). Immunological reactivity associated with antigens in the intestinal tract of rats. *J. Pathol. Bacteriol.* **93**, 223.

Coulson, A. S., Gurner, B. W., and Coombs, R. A. A. (1967). Macrophage-like properties of some guinea pig transformed cells. *Int. Arch. Allergy* **32**, 264.

Crumpton, M. J. (1967). "The molecular basis of the serological specificity of proteins, with particular reference to sperm whale myoglobin. *in* "Antibodies to Biologically Active Molecules" (B. Cinader, ed.), Vol. I, p. 61. Pergamon, New York.

Crumpton, M. J. and Wilkinson, J. M. (1965). The immunological activity of some of the chymotyptic peptides of sperm whale myoglobin. *Biochem. J.* **94**, 545 (1965).

Cunningham, A. J. (1969a). The development of clones of antibody-forming cells in the spleens of irradiated mice. I. Detection of plaque-forming cell colonies. *Aust. J. Exp. Biol. Med. Sci.* **47**, 485.

Cunningham, A. J. (1969b). The development of clones of antibody-forming cells in the spleens of irradiated mice. II. Some properties of plaque-forming cell colonies, and evidence for their clonal nature. *Aust. J. Exp. Biol. Med. Sci.* **47**, 493.

Cunningham, A. J. (1970). Presented at *Aust. Soc. Immunol. Meeting, Adelaide, Australia, December, 1969.*

Cunningham, A. J., Smith, J. B., and Mercer, E. H. (1966). Antibody formation by single cells from lymph nodes and efferent lymph of sheep. *J. Exp. Med.* **124**, 701.

Davey, M. J. and Asherson, G. L. (1967). Cytophilic antibody. I. Nature of the macrophage receptor. *Immunology* **12**, 13.

David, J. R., Al-Askari, S., Lawrence, H. S., and Thomas, L. (1964). Delayed hypersensitivity *in vitro.* I. The specificity of the inhibition of cell migration by antigens. *J. Immunol.* **93**, 264.

Davies, A. J. S., Leuchars, E., Wallis, V., Marchant, R., and Elliott, E. V. (1967). The failure of thymus-derived cells to produce antibody. *Transplantation* **5**, 222.

de Duve, C. and Wattiaux, R. (1966). Functions of lysosomes. *Ann. Rev. Physiol.* **28**, 435.

Deichmiller, M. P., and Dixon, F. J. (1960). The metabolism of serum proteins in neonatal rabbits. *J. Gen. Physiol.* **43**, 1047.

De Petris, S. (1967). Polyribosomes in thin sections of 5563 plasmacytoma cells. *J. Mol. Biol.* **23**, 215.

De Petris, S. and Karlsbad, G. (1965). Localization of antibodies by electron microscopy in developing antibody-producing cells. *J. Cell Biol.* **26**, 759.

Diener, E. (1968). A new method for the enumeration of single antibody forming cells. *J. Immunol.* **100**, 1062.

Diener, E. and Armstrong, W. D. (1967). Induction of antibody formation and tolerance *in vitro* to a purified protein antigen. *Lancet* **ii**, 1281.

Diener, E. and Armstrong, W. D. (1969). Immunological tolerance *in vitro;* kinetic studies at the cellular level. *J. Exp. Med.* **129**, 591.

Diener, E. and Feldmann, M. (1970). Antibody mediated suppression of the immune response *in vitro*. II. A new approach to a phenomenon of immunological tolerance. *J. Exp. Med.*, **132**, 31.

Diener, E. and Nossal, G. J. V. (1966). Phylogenetic studies on the immune response. I. Localization of antigens and immune response in the toad, *Bufo marinus*. *Immunology* **10**, 535.

Diener, E., Ealey, E. H. M., and Legge, J. (1967). Phylogenetic studies on the immune response. III. Autoradiographic studies on the lymphoid system of the Australian echidna *Tachyglossus aculeatus*. *Immunology* **13**, 339.

Diener, E., Shortman, K., and Russell, P. (1970). Induction of immunity and tolerance *in vitro* in the absence of phagocytic cells. *Nature (London)* **225**, 731.

Dixon, F. J. and McConahey, P. J. (1971, in press). The effect of antibody on antibody formation. *in* "Developmental Aspects of Antibody Formation and Structure" (J. Sterzl and M. Riha, eds.). Czech. Acad. Sci., Prague.

Dixon, F. J., Jacot-Guillarmod, H., and McConahey, P. J. (1967). The effect of passively administered antibody on antibody synthesis. *J. Exp. Med.* **125**, 1119.

Dresser, D. W. (1961a). Effectiveness of lipid and lipidophilic substances as adjuvants. *Nature (London)* **191**, 1169.

Dresser, D. W. (1961b). Acquired immunological tolerance to a fraction of bovine gamma globulin. *Immunology* **4**, 13.

Dresser, D. W. (1962a). Specific inhibition of antibody production. I. Protein-overloading paralysis. *Immunology* **5**, 161.

Dresser, D. W. (1962b). Specific inhibition of antibody production. II. Paralysis induced in adult mice by small quantities of protein antigen. *Immunology* **5**, 378.

Dresser, D. W. and Mitchison, N. A. (1968). The mechanism of immunological paralysis. *Advan. Immunol.* **8**, 129.

Dutton, R. W. (1967). *In vitro* studies of immunological responses of lymphoid cells. *Advan. Immunol.* **6**, 253.

Dutton, R. W. and Eady, J. D. (1964). An *in vitro* system for the study of the mechanism of antigenic stimulation in the secondary response. *Immunology* **7**, 40.

Dutton, R. W., McCarthy, M. M., Mishell, R. I., and Raidt, D. J. (1970). Cell components in the immune response. 4. Relationships and possible interactions. *Cell Immunol.* **1**, 196.

Dutton, R. W. and Mishell, R. I. (1967a). Cellular events in the immune response. The *in vitro* response of normal spleen cells to erythrocyte antigens. *Cold Spring Harbor Symp. Quant. Biol.* **32**, 407.

Dutton, R. W. and Mishell, R. I. (1967b). Cell populations and cell proliferation in the *in vitro* response of normal mouse spleen to heterologous erythrocytes. *J. Exp. Med.* **126**, 443.

Dwyer, J. and Mackay, I. R. (1970). Antigen binding lymphocytes in human blood. *Lancet* **i**, 164.

Edelman, G. M. (1964). Formation of active 7 S antibody molecules by reassociation of L and H polypeptide chains. *in* "Molecular and Cellular Basis of Antibody Formation" (J. Sterzl, ed.), p. 113. Publ. House Czech. Acad. Sci., Prague.

Edelman, G. M. and Gall, W. E. (1969). The antibody problem. *Ann. Rev. Biochem.* **38**, 415.

Edmundson, A. B. (1965). Amino acid sequence of sperm whale myoglobin. *Nature (London)* **205**, 883.

Ehrenreich, B. A. and Cohn, Z. A. (1968a). Fate of hemoglobin pinocytosed by macrophages *in vitro*. *J. Cell Biol.* **38**, 244.

Ehrenreich, B. A. and Cohn, Z. A. (1968b). Pinocytosis by macrophages. *J. Reticuloendothel. Soc.* **5**, 230.

Fagraeus, A. (1948). Antibody production in relation to development of plasma cells *in vivo* and *in vitro* experiments. *Acta Med. Scand.* **130** (Suppl. 204), 3.

Fahey, J. L. and Finegold, I. (1967). Synthesis of immunoglobulins in human lymphoid cell lines. *Cold Spring Harbor Symp. Quant. Biol.* **32**, 283.

Fahey, J. L., Finegold, I., Rabson, A. S., and Manaker, R. A. (1966). Immunoglobulin synthesis *in vitro* by established human cell lines. *Science* **152**, 1259.

Fazekas de St. Groth, S. (1967). Cross-recognition and cross-reactivity. *Cold Spring Harbor Symp. Quant. Biol.* **32**, 525.

Feldmann, M. and Diener, E. (1970). Antibody-mediated suppression of the immune response *in vitro*. I. Evidence for a central effect. *J. Exp. Med.* **131**, 247.

Felton, L. D. (1949). The significance of antigen in animal tissues. *J. Immunol.* **61**, 107.

Felton, L. D., Prescott, B., Kauffmann, G., and Ottinger, B. (1955). Pneumococcal antigenic polysaccharide substances from animal tissues. *J. Immunol.* **74**, 205.

Fenner, F. J. (1968). The biology of animal viruses. II. "The Pathogenesis and Ecology of Viral Infections." Academic Press, New York.

Fetherstonhaugh, P. (1970). The immunogenicity and tolerance-inducing ability of soluble extracts of sheep red blood cell membranes. *Int. Arch. Allergy* **39**, 310.

Finn, R., Clarke, C. A., Donohoe, W. T., McConnell, R. B., Sheppard, P. M., Lehane, D., and Kulke, W. (1961). Experimental studies on the prevention of Rh haemolytic disease. *Brit. Med. J.* **i**, 1486.

Fishman, M. (1959). Antibody formation in tissue culture. *Nature* **183**, 1200.

Fishman, M. (1961). Antibody formation *in vitro*. *J. Exp. Med.* **114**, 837.

Fishman, M. (1969). Induction of antibodies *in vitro*. *Ann. Rev. Microbiol.* **23**, 199.

Fishman, M. and Adler, F. L. (1963). Antibody formation initiated *in vitro*. II. Antibody synthesis in X-irradiated recipients of diffusion chambers containing nucleic acid derived from macrophages incubated with antigen. *J. Exp. Med.* **117**, 595.

Fishman, M., van Rood, J. J., and Adler, F. L. (1965). The initiation of antibody formation by ribonucleic acid from specifically stimulated macrophages. *in* "Molecular and Cellular Basis of Antibody Formation" (J. Sterzl, ed.), p. 491. Czech. Acad. Sci., Prague.

Fishman, M., Adler, F. L. and Holub, M. (1968). Antibody formation initiated *in vitro* with RNA and RNA-antigen complexes. *in* "Nucleic Acids in Immunology" (O. Plescia and W. Braun, eds.), p. 439. Springer-Verlag, Berlin.

Fitch, F. W. and Rowley, D. A. (1968). Quoted Uhr, J. W. and Möller, G. *Advan. Immunol.* **8**, 81.

Fleischman, J. B., Pain, R. H., and Porter, R. R. (1962). Reduction of γ-globulins. *Arch. Biochem. Biophys. Suppl.* **1**, 174.

Ford, C. E. (1966). Traffic of lymphoid cells in the body. *in* "The Thymus—Experimental and Clinical Studies" (G. E. W. Wolstenholme and R. Porter, eds.), p. 131. Churchill, London.

Ford, W. L. and Gowans, J. L. (1967). The role of lymphocytes in antibody formation. II. The influence of lymphocyte migration on the initiation of antibody formation in the isolated perfused spleen. *Proc. Roy. Soc. B* **168**, 244.

Ford, W. L., Gowans, J. L., and McCullagh, P. J. (1966). The origin and function of lymphocytes. in "The Thymus—Experimental and Clinical Studies" (G. E. W. Wolstenholme and R. Porter, eds.), p. 58. Churchill, London.

Frank, M. M. and Humphrey, J. H. (1968). The subunits in rabbit anti-Forssman IgM antibody. *J. Exp. Med.* **127**, 967.

Franzl, R. E. (1962). Immunogenic sub-cellular particles obtained from spleens of antigen-injected mice. *Nature (London)* **195**, 457.

Freda, V. J., Gorman, J. G., and Pollack, W. (1964). Successful prevention of experimental Rh sensitization in man with an anti-Rh gamma 2-globulin antibody preparation: a preliminary report. *Transfusion* **4**, 26.

Frei, P. C., Benacerraf, B., and Thorbecke, G. J. (1965). Phagocytosis of the antigen, a crucial step in the induction of the primary response. *Proc. Nat. Acad. Sci. U.S.* **53**, 20.

Friedman, H. P., Stavitsky, A. B., and Solomon, J. M. (1965). Induction *in vitro* of antibodies to phage T2. Antigens in the RNA extract employed. *Science* **149**, 1106.

Gabathuler, M. P. and Ryser, H. J. P. (1967). Fate of serum albumin ingested by sarcoma cells in suspension culture. *The Pharmacologist* **9**, 240.

Gallily, R. and Feldman, M. (1967). The role of macrophages in the induction of antibody in X-irradiated animals. *Immunology* **12**, 197.

Garvey, J. S. (1968). On the role of antigen fragments and RNA in the immune response of rabbits to a soluble antigen. in "Nucleic Acids in Immunology" (O. Plescia and W. Braun, eds.), p. 487. Springer-Verlag, New York.

Garvey, J. S. and Campbell, D. H. (1957). The retention of ^{35}S-labelled bovine serum albumin in normal and immunized rabbit liver tissue. *J. Exp. Med.* **105**, 361.

Gell, P. G. H., Kelus, A. S., Coombs, R. R. A., Gurner, B. W., Janeway, C. A., and Wilson, A. B. (1971, in press). Immunoglobulin determinants on the lymphocytes of normal rabbits. in "Developmental Aspects of Antibody Formation and Structure" (J. Sterzl and M. Riha, eds.), Vol. 1, p. 2671. Publ. House Czech. Acad. Sci., Prague.

Gerlings-Petersen, B. T. and Pondman, K. W. (1965). The relationship between complement, the heterogeneity of antibody and phagocytosis. *Bibl. Haematol.* **28**, 829.

Gerritsen, T. (1969). "Modern Separation Methods of Macromolecules and Particles in Progress in Separation and Purification" (T. Gerritsen, ed.), Vol. 2. Wiley (Interscience), New York.

Gill, T. J., III, Kunz, H. W., Gould, H. J., and Doty, P. (1964). Studies on synthetic polypeptide antigens. XI. The antigenicity of optically isomeric synthetic polypeptides. *J. Biol. Chem.* **239**, 1107.

Gill, T. J., Papermaster, D. S., and Mowbray, J. F. (1965). Synthetic polypeptide metabolism. I. The metabolic fate of enantiomorphic polymers. *J. Immunol.* **95**, 794.

Givol, D. (1967). The cleavage of rabbit immunoglobulin G by trypsin after mild reduction and aminoethylation. *Biochem. J.* **104**, 39c.

Givol, D. and DeLorenzo, F. (1968). The position of various cleavages of rabbit immunoglobulin G. *J. Biol. Chem.* **243**, 1886.

Givol, D. and Sela, M. (1964). Isolation and fragmentation of antibodies to polytyrosyl gelatin. *Biochemistry* **3**, 444.

Glenny, A. T. and Hopkins, B. E. (1932). Duration of passive immunity. *J. Hyg.* **22**, 12.

Globerson, A. and Auerbach, R. (1965). Primary immune reactions in organ cultures. Science 149, 991.

Globerson, A. and Auerbach, R. (1966). Primary antibody response in organ cultures. J. Exp. Med. 124, 1001.

Golub, E. S., Mishell, R. I., Weigle, W. O., and Dutton, R. W. (1968). A modification of the hemolytic plaque assay for use with protein antigens. J. Immunol. 100, 133.

Goldschneider, I. and McGregor, D. D. (1968). Migration of lymphocytes and thymocytes in the rat. I. The route of migration from blood to spleen and lymph nodes. J. Exp. Med. 127, 155.

Good, R. A. and Gabrielsen, A. E. (1964). in "The Thymus in Immunology. Structure, Function and Role in Disease" (R. A. Good and A. E. Gabrielsen, eds.), p. 314. Harper (Hoeber), New York.

Gordon, G. B., Miller, L. R., and Bensch, K. G. (1965). Studies on the intracellular digestive process in mammalian tissue culture cells. J. Cell Biol. 25, 41.

Gottlieb, A. A. (1968). The antigen-RNA complex of macrophages. in "Nucleic Acids in Immunology" (O. Plescia and W. Braun, eds.), p. 471. Springer-Verlag, New York.

Gottlieb, A. A. (1969a). Studies on the binding of soluble antigens to a unique ribonucleoprotein fraction of macrophage cells. Biochemistry 8, 2111.

Gottlieb, A. A. (1969b). Macrophage ribonucleoprotein: nature of the antigenic fragment 592. Science 165, 597.

Gottlieb, A. A. and Straus, D. S. (1969). Physical studies on the light density ribonucleoprotein complex of macrophage cells. J. Biol. Chem. 244, 3324.

Gottlieb, A. A., Glisin, V. R., and Doty, P. (1967). Studies on macrophage RNA involved in antibody production. Proc. Nat. Acad. Sci. U.S. 57, 1849.

Gowans, J. L. (1959). The recirculation of lymphocytes from blood to lymph in the rat. J. Physiol. (London) 146, 54.

Gowans, J. L. (1962). The fate of parental strain small lymphocytes in F1 hybrid rats. Ann. N.Y. Acad. Sci. 99, 432.

Gowans, J. L. and McGregor, D. D. (1965). The immunological activities of lymphocytes. Progr. Allergy 9, 1.

Granger, G. A. and Weiser, R. S. (1966). Homograft target cells: contact destruction in vitro by immune macrophages. Science 151, 97.

Greenwood, F. C., Hunter, W. M., and Glover, J. S. (1963). The preparation of ^{131}I-labelled human growth hormone of high specific radioactivity. J. Biochem. 89, 114.

Habicht, G. S., Chiller, J. M., and Weigle, W. O. (1971, in press). Absence of plaque-forming cells in animals immunologically unresponsive to protein antigens. in "Developmental Aspects of Antibody Formation and Structure" (J. Sterzl and M. Riha, eds.), Vol. 2. Czech. Acad. Sci., Prague.

Hall, J. G. and Morris, B. (1962). The output of cells in lymph from the popliteal node of sheep. Quart. J. Exp. Physiol. 47, 360.

Hall, J. G. and Morris, B. (1965). The origin of the cells in the efferent lymph from a single lymph node. J. Exp. Med. 121, 901.

Han, S. (1961). The ultrastructure of the mesenteric lymph node of the rat. Amer. J. Anat. 109, 183.

Hanan, R. and Oyama, J. (1954). Inhibition of antibody formation in mature rabbits by contact with the antigen at an early age. J. Immunol. 73, 49.

Hanna, M. G., Jr. (1965). Germinal center changes and plasma cell reaction during the primary immune response. *Int. Arch. Allergy* **26**, 230.

Hanna, M. G., Jr., and Szakal, A. K. (1968). Localization of ^{125}I-labeled antigen in germinal centers of mouse spleen. Histologic and ultrastructural autoradiographic studies of the secondary immune reaction. *J. Immunol.* **101**, 949.

Hanna, M. G., Jr., Makinodan, T., and Fisher, W. D., (1967). Lymphatic tissue germinal center localisation of I^{125}-labeled heterologous and isologous macroglobulins. *in* "Germinal Centers in Immune Responses" (H. Cottier, N. Odartchenko, R. Schindler, and C. C. Congdon, eds.), p. 86. Springer-Verlag, New York.

Hanna, M. G., Jr., Francis, M. W., and Peters, L. C. (1968). Localization of ^{125}I-labelled antigen in germinal centres of mouse spleen: effects of competitive injection of specific or non-cross-reacting antigen. *Immunology* **15**, 75.

Hanna, M. G., Jr., Nettesheim, P., and Walburg, H. E., Jr. (1969a). A comparative study of immune reaction in germfree and conventional mice. *in* "Advances in Experimental Medicine and Biology" (E. A. Mirand and N. Back, eds.), Vol. 3, "Germfree Biology." Plenum, New York.

Hanna, M. G., Jr., Szakal, A. K., Nettesheim, P., and Walburg, H. E., Jr. (1969b). The relation of antigen localization to the development and growth of lymphoid germinal centers. *in* "Lymphatic Tissue and Germinal Centers in Immune Response. Advances in Experimental Medicine and Biology" (L. Fiore-Donati and M. G. Hanna, Jr., eds.), Vol. 5, p. 149. Plenum, New York.

Hannoun, C. and Bussard, A. E. (1966). Antibody production by cells in tissue culture. 1. Morphological evolution of lymph node and spleen cells in culture. *J. Exp. Med.* **123**, 1035.

Hartmann, K., Dutton, R. W., McCarthy, M. M., and Mishell, R. I. (1970). Cell components in the immune response. II. Cell attachment separation of immune cells. *Cell Immunol.* **1**, 182.

Hašek, M. Lengerová, A., and Vojtiškova, M., eds. (1962). "Symposium on Mechanisms of Immunological Tolerance." Czech. Acad. Sci., Prague.

Haskill, J. S. (1969). Density distribution analysis of antigen-sensitive cells in the rat. *J. Exp. Med.* **130**, 877.

Haskill, J. S., Byrt, P., and Marbrook, J. (1970). *In vitro* and *in vivo* studies of the immune response to sheep erythrocytes using partially purified cell preparations. *J. Exp. Med.* **131**, 57.

Heimer, R. and Schnoll, S. (1968). Fc-like fragments in peptic digests of human immunoglobulin G. *J. Immunol.* **100**, 231.

Heimer, R., Schnoll, S., and Primack, A. (1967). Products of the peptic digestion of human γ G-immunoglobulin. *Biochemistry* **6**, 127.

Heineke, H. (1904–1905). Experimentelle Untersuchungen über die einwirkung der Röntenstrahlen auf innere Organe. *Mitt. Grensg. Med. Chir.* **14**, 21.

Heise, E. R. and Myrvik, Q. N. (1967). Secretion of lysozyme by rabbit alveolar macrophages in vitro. *J. Reticuloendothelial Soc.* **4**, 510.

Heller, J. H. (1958). Measurement of the function of the reticuloendothelium. *Ann. N.Y. Acad. Sci.* **73**, 212.

Hellman, T. (1914). The normal amount of lymphoid tissue in rabbits at different post-fetal ages. Inaug. Dissertation, Upsala, Akademiska Boktryckeriet, Edv. Berling.

Henry, C. and Jerne, N. K. (1967). The depressive effect of 7 S antibody and the enhancing effect of 19 S antibody in the regulation of the primary immune response. *in* "Nobel Symposium 3 on Gamma Globulins" (J. Killander, ed.), p. 421. Almqvist & Wiksell, Stockholm.

Henry, C. and Jerne, N. K. (1968). Competition of 19 S and 7 S antigen receptors in the regulation of the primary immune response. *J. Exp. Med.* **128**, 133.

Herd, Z. L. and Ada, G. L. (1969a). The retention of ^{125}I-immunoglobulin, IgG subunits and antigen-antibody complexes in rat footpads and draining lymph nodes. *Aust. J. Exp. Biol. Med. Sci.* **47**, 63.

Herd, Z. L. and Ada, G. L. (1969b). Distribution of ^{125}I-immunoglobulins, IgG subunits and antigen-antibody complexes in rat lymph nodes. *Aust. J. Exp. Biol. Med. Sci.* **47**, 73.

Hill, W. C. and Cebra, J. J. (1965). Horse and S1 immunoglobulins. I. Properties of γM antibody. *Biochemistry* **4**, 2575.

Hirst, J. A. and Dutton, R. W. (1970). Cell components in the immune response. III. Neonatal thymectomy: restoration in culture. *Cell Immunol.* **1**, 190.

Holter, H. (1959). Pinocytosis. *Intern. Rev. Cytol.* **8**, 481.

Holub, M., Ax, W., Fischer, H., Freund-Mölbert, E., Krüsmann, W. F., Maltheo, M. L., Říha, I., Sulc, J., and Tlaskalová, H. (1971, in press). The relations of reticulohistiocytic and lymphoid cells in the development of tissue structure connected with antibody formation. *in* "Developmental Aspects of Antibody Formation and Structure" (J. Sterzl and M. Riha, eds.), Vol. 2. Publ. House Czech. Acad. Sci., Prague.

Horiuchi, A. and Waksman, B. H. (1968). Role of the thymus in tolerance. VI. Tolerance to bovine γ-globulin in rats given a low dose of irradiation and injection of nonaggregated or aggregated antigen into the shielded thymus. *J. Immunol.* **100**, 974.

Horiuchi, A., Gery, I., and Waksman, B. H. (1968). Role of the thymus in tolerance. VII. Distribution of nonaggregated and heat-aggregated bovine gamma globulin in lymphoid organs of normal newborn and adult rats. *Yale J. Biol. Med.* **41**, 13.

Howard, J. G. and Benacerraf, B. (1966). Properties of macrophage receptors for cytophilic antibodies. *Brit. J. Exp. Pathol.* **47**, 193 (1966).

Howard, J. G., Boak, J. L., and Christie, G. H. (1966). Further studies on the transformation of thoracic duct cells into liver macrophages. *Ann. N.Y. Acad. Sci.* **129**, 327.

Huber, H. and Fudenberg, H. H. (1968). Receptor sites of human monocytes for IgG. *Int. Arch. Allergy* **34**, 18.

Huber, H., Douglas, S. D., and Fudenberg, H. H. (1969). The IgG receptor: an immunological marker for the characterization of mononuclear cells. *Immunology* **17**, 7.

Hummeler, K., Harris, T. N., Tomassini, N., Hechtel, M., and Farber, M. B. (1966). Electron microscopic observations on antibody-producing cells in lymph and blood. *J. Exp. Med.* **124**, 255.

Humphrey, J. H. (1961). The metabolism of homologous and heterologous serum proteins in baby rabbits. *Immunology* **4**, 380.

Humphrey, J. H. (1969). The fate of antigen and its relationship to the immune response. The complexity of antigens. *Antibiot. Chemother.* **15**, 7.

Humphrey, J. H. and Frank, M. M. (1967). The localization of non-microbial antigens in the draining lymph nodes of tolerant, normal and primed rabbits. *Immunology* **13**, 87.

Humphrey, J. H. and Keller, H. U. (1971, in press). Some evidence for specific interaction between immunologically competent cells and antigen. *in* "Developmental Aspects of Antibody Formation and Structure" (J. Sterzl and M. Riha, eds.), Vol. 2. Academic Press, New York.

Humphrey, J. H. and Turk, J. L. (1961). Immunological unresponsiveness in guinea pigs. Immunological unresponsiveness to heterologous serum proteins. *Immunology* **4**, 301.

Humphrey, J. H. and White, R. G. (1964). "Immunology for Students of Medicine," p. 201. Blackwell, Oxford.

Humphrey, J. H., Parrott, D. M. V., and East, J. (1964). Studies on globulin and antibody production in mice thymectomized at birth. *Immunology* **7**, 419.

Humphrey, J. H., Askonas, B. A., Auzins, I., Schechter, I., and Sela, M. (1967). The localization of antigen in lymph nodes and its relation to specific antibody-producing cells. II. Comparison of iodine-125 and tritium labels. *Immunology* **13**, 71.

Ingraham, J. S. and Bussard, A. E. (1964). Application of a localized hemolysin reaction for specific detection of individual antibody forming cells. *J. Exp. Med.* **119**, 667.

Isliker, H., Jacot-Guillarmod, H., and Jaton, J. C. (1965). The structure and biological activity of immunoglobulins and their sub-units. *Ergeb. Physiol. Biol. Chem. Exp. Pharmakol.* **56**, 67.

Jacobson, L. O. (1952). Evidence for humoral factor (or factors) concerned in recovery from radiation injury. *Cancer Res.* **12**, 315.

Janeway, C. A., Jr., and Humphrey, J. H. (1968). Synthetic antigens composed exclusively of L- or D-amino acids. II. Effect of optical configuration on the metabolism and fate of synthetic polypeptide antigens in mice. *Immunology* **14**, 225.

Janeway, C. A., Jr., and Humphrey, J. H. (1969). The fate of a D-amino acid polypeptide. [p(D-Tyr, D-Glu, D-Ala), 247] in newborn and adult mice. Relationship to the induction of tolerance. *Israel J. Med. Sci.* **5**, 185.

Janeway, C. A., Jr., and Sela, M. (1967). Synthetic antigens composed exclusively of L- or D-amino acids. I. Effect of optical configuration on the immunogenicity of synthetic polypeptides in mice. *Immunology* **13**, 29.

Jaroslow, B. N. and Nossal, G. J. V. (1966). The effects of X-irradiation on antigen localization in lymphoid follicles. *Aust. J. Exp. Biol. Med. Sci.* **44**, 609.

Jerne, N. K. (1969). The complete solution of immunology. *Aust. Ann. Med.* **18**, 345.

Jerne, N. K. (1970). The generation of self-tolerance and of antibody diversity. *Proc. Nat. Acad. Sci. U.S.*, in press.

Jerne, N. K. and Nordin, A. A. (1963). Plaque formation in agar by single antibody producing cells. *Science* **140**, 405.

Kabat, E. A. (1966). The nature of an antigenic determinant. *J. Immunol.* **97**, 1.

Kaboth, U., Ax, W., and Fischer, H. (1966). Immunologische Studien am Omentum. II. Mitteilung: Zur Immunmorphologie der "Plaquebildenden" Milchflecken im Mäuseomentum. *Z. Naturforsch B* **21**, 789.

Kaplan, M. H., Coons, A. H., and Deane, H. W. (1950). Localization of antigen in tissue cells. III. Cellular distribution of pneumococcal polysaccharides types II and III in the mouse. *J. Exp. Med.* **91**, 15.

Karnovsky, M. L. (1962). Metabolic basis of phagocytic activity. *Physiol. Rev.* **42**, 143.

Kendrew, J. C., Watson, H. C., Strandberg, B. E., Dickerson, R. E., Phillips, D. C., and Shore, V. C. (1961). The amino acid sequence of sperm whale myoglobin. A partial determination by X-ray methods, and its correlation with chemical data. *Nature* (*London*) **190**, 666.

Kennedy, J. C., Till, J. E., Siminovitch, L., and McCulloch, E. A. (1965). Radiosensitivity of the immune response to sheep red cells in the mouse, as measured by the hemolytic plaque method. *J. Immunol.* **94**, 715.

Kennedy, J. C., Till, J. E., Siminovitch, L., and McCulloch, E. A. (1966). The proliferative capacity of antigen sensitive precursors of hemolytic plaque-forming cells. *J. Immunol.* **96**, 973.

Kishimoto, T., Onoue, K., and Yamamura, Y. (1968). Structure of human immunoglobulin M. III. Pepsin fragmentation of IgM. *J. Immunol.* **100**, 1032.

Kobayashi, T., Rinker, J. N., and Koffler, H. (1959). Purification and chemical properties of flagellin. *Arch. Biochem. Biophys.* **84**, 342.

Kölsch, E. and Mitchison, N. A. (1968). The subcellular distribution of antigen in macrophages. *J. Exp. Med.* **128**, 1059.

Kossard, S. and Nelson, D. S. (1968a). Studies on cytophilic antibodies. III. Sensitization of homologous and heterologous macrophages by cytophilic antibodies; inhibition of sensitization by normal serum. *Aust. J. Exp. Biol. Med. Sci.* **46**, 51.

Kossard, S. and Nelson, D. S. (1968b). Studies on cytophilic antibodies. IV. The effects of proteolytic enzymes (trypsin and papain) on the attachment to macrophages of cytophilic antibodies. *Aust. J. Exp. Biol. Med. Sci.* **46**, 63.

Lamm, M. E. (1969). Further comparison of guinea pig γ1- and γ2-immunoglobulins. Amino acid compositions of the polypeptide chains and papain fragments. *Immunochemistry* **6**, 235.

Lamm, M. E., Lisowska-Bernstein, B., and Nussenzweig, V. (1967). Comparison of guinea pig γ1- and γ2-immunoglobulins by peptide mapping. *Biochemistry* **6**, 2819.

Lamoureux, G., McPherson, T. A., Carnegie, P. R., and Mackay, I. R. (1968). Lymph node localisation and whole body distribution of radioiodinated encephalitogenic polypeptide in guinea pigs. *Clin. Exp. Immunol.* **3**, 25.

Landsteiner K. (1946). "The Specificity of Serological Reactions," 2nd ed. Harvard Univ. Press, Cambridge, Massachusetts.

Landy, M. and Braun, W. (eds.) (1969). "Immunological Tolerance—A Reassessment of Mechanisms of the Immune Response" Academic Press, New York.

Lang, P. G. and Ada, G. L. (1967a). Antigen in tissues. IV. The effect of antibody on the retention and localization of antigen in rat lymph nodes. *Immunology* **13**, 523.

Lang, P. G. and Ada, G. L. (1967b). The localization of heat denatured serum albumin in rat lymph nodes. *Aust. J. Exp. Biol. Med. Sci.* **45**, 445.

Lang, W., Nase, S., and Rajewsky, K. E. (1969). Inhibition of the immune response *in vitro* to sheep red blood cells by passive antibody. *Nature* (*London*) **223**, 949.

Lapresle, C. and Webb, T. (1965). Isolation and study of a fragment of human serum albumin containing one of the antigenic sites of the whole molecule. *Biochem. J.* **95**, 245.

Laws, J. O. (1952). The degradation of proteins labelled with radioactive iodine in control and sensitized rabbits. *Brit. J. Exp. Pathol.* **33**, 354.

Leduc, E. H., Coons, A. H., and Connolly, J. M. (1955). Studies on antibody production II; the primary and secondary responses in popliteal lymph node of rabbit. *J. Exp. Med.* **102**, 61.

Levine, B. B. and Benacerraf, B. (1964). Studies in antigenicity. The relationship between *in vivo* and *in vitro* enzymatic degradability of hapten-polylysine conjugates and their antigenicities in guinea pigs. *J. Exp. Med.* **120**, 955.

Levvy, G. A. and Conchie, J. (1964). The subcellular localization of the "lysosomal" enzymes and its biological significance. *Progr. Biophys. Mol. Biol.* **14**, 105.

Lewis, H., Mitchell, J., and Nossal, G. J. V. (1969). Subpopulations of rat and mouse thoracic duct small lymphocytes in the *Salmonella* flagellar antigen system. *Immunology* **17**, 955.

Lind, P. E. (1968). Cellular localization of ^{125}I-labelled *Salmonella adelaide* flaggelin following injection into the rat in the presence of Freund's complete adjuvant. *Aust. J. Exp. Biol. Med. Sci.* **46**, 189.

Lind, P. E. (1970). Influence of neonatal thymectomy on antibody production in the Lewis rat. *Int. Arch. Allergy* **37**, 258.

Linscott, W. D. and Weigle, W. O. (1965). Anti-bovine serum albumin specificity and binding affinity after termination of tolerance to bovine serum albumin. *J. Immunol.* **95**, 546.

Litt, M. (1964). Eosinophils and antigen-antibody reactions. *Ann. N.Y. Acad. Sci.* **116**, 964.

Litt, M. (1967). Studies of the latent period. I. Primary antibody in guinea pig lymph nodes 7½ minutes after introduction of chicken erythrocytes. *Cold Spring Harbor Symp. Quant. Biol.* **32**, 477.

Loutit, J. F. (1960). Biocycles in the reticuloendothelial system. *Ann. N.Y. Acad. Sci.* **88**, 122.

Lowy, J. and Hanson, J. (1965). Electron microscope studies of bacterial flagella. *J. Mol. Biol.* **11**, 293.

McConahey, P. J. and Dixon, F. J. (1966). A method of trace iodination of proteins for immunologic studies. *Int. Arch. Allergy* **29**, 185.

McConahey, P. J., Cerottini, J. C., and Dixon, F. J. (1968). An approach to the quantitation of immunogenic antigen. *J. Exp. Med.* **127**, 1003.

McDevitt, H. O. and Benacerraf, B. (1970). Genetic control of specific immune responses. *Advan. Immunol.* **11**, 31.

McDevitt, H. O. and Sela, M. (1965). Genetic control of the antibody response. I. Demonstration of determinant-specific differences in response to synthetic polypeptide antigens in two strains of inbred mice. *J. Exp. Med.* **122**, 517.

McDevitt, H. O., Askonas, B. A., Humphrey, J. H., Schechter, I., and Sela, M. (1966). Localization of antigen in relation to specific antibody-producing cells. I. Use of a synthetic polypeptide [(T, G)-A-L] labelled with iodine-125. *Immunology* **11**, 337.

McDonough, M. W. (1965). Amino acid composition of antigenically distinct *Salmonella* flagellin proteins. *J. Mol. Biol.* **12**, 342.

Mäkelä, O. (1965). Single lymph node cells producing heteroclitic bacteriophage antibody. *J. Immunol.* **95**, 378.

Mäkelä, O. (1967). The specificity of antibodies produced by single cells. *Cold Spring Harbor Symp. Quant. Biol.* **32**, 423.

Mäkelä, O. and Cross, A. M. (1970). The diversity and specialization of immunocytes. *Progr. Allergy* (in press).

Mäkelä, O. and Nossal, G. J. V. (1961). Bacterial adherence: A method for detecting antibody production by single cells. *J. Immunol.* **87**, 447.

Mäkelä, O. and Nossal, G. J. V. (1962). Autoradiographic studies on the immune response. II. DNA synthesis amongst single antibody-producing cells. *J. Exp. Med.* **115**, 231.

Mandel, T. (1969). Epithelial cells and lymphopoiesis in the cortex of guinea pig thymus. *Aust. J. Exp. Biol. Med. Sci.* **47**, 153.

Mandel, T., Byrt, P., and Ada, G. L. (1970). A morphological examination of antigen reactive cells from mouse spleen and peritoneal cavity. *Exp. Cell Res.* **58**, 179.

Mandy, W. J., Fudenberg, H. H., and Lewis, F. B. (1966). A new serum factor in normal rabbits. I. Identification and characterization. *J. Immunol.* **95**, 501.

Marbrook, J. (1967). Primary immune response in cultures of spleen cells. *Lancet* **ii**, 1279.

Marchalonis, J. J. (1969). An enzymatic method for the trace iodination of immunoglobulins and other proteins. *J. Biochem.* **113**, 299.

Marchalonis, J. J. and Edelman, G. M. (1968). Phylogenetic origins of antibody structure. III. Antibodies in the primary immune response of the sea lamprey, *Petitomyzon marinus. J. Exp. Med.* **127**, 981.

Marchalonis, J. J. and Gledhill, V. X. (1968). An elementary stochastic model for the induction of immunity and tolerance. *Nature (London)* **220**, 608.

Marchalonis, J. J. and Nossal, G. J. V. (1968). Electrophoretic analysis of antibody produced by single cells. *Proc. Nat. Acad. Sci. U.S.* **61**, 860.

Marchesi, V. T. and Gowans, J. L. (1964). The migration of lymphocytes through the endothelium of venules in lymph nodes: an electron microscope study. *Proc. Roy. Soc. B* **159**, 283.

Marshall, A. H. E. and White, R. G. (1961). The immunological reactivity of the thymus. *Brit. J. Exp. Pathol.* **42**, 379.

Maurer, P. H. (1964). Use of synthetic polymers of amino acids to study the basis of antigenicity. *Progr. Allergy* **8**, 1.

Mego, J. L. and McQueen, J. D. (1965). The uptake and degradation of the injected labeled proteins by mouse liver particles. *Biochim. Biophys. Acta* **100**, 136.

Mego, J. L., Bertini, F., and McQueen, J. D. (1967). The use of formaldehyde treated ^{131}I-albumin in the study of digestive vacuoles and some properties of these particles from mouse liver. *J. Cell Biol.* **32**, 699.

Mellors, R. C. and Brzosko, W. J. (1962). Studies in molecular pathology I. Localization and pathogenic role of heterologous immune complexes. *J. Exp. Med.* **115**, 891.

Mellors, R. C. and Korngold, L. (1963). The cellular origin of human immunoglobulins. *J. Exp. Med.* **118**, 387.

Merchant, B. and Hraba, T. (1966). Lymphoid cells producing antibody against simple haptens: detection and enumeration. *Science* **152**, 1378.

Merler, E. and Janeway, C. A. (1968). Immunochemical identification of cytophilic antibody in human lymphocytes. *Proc. Nat. Acad. Sci. U.S.* **59**, 393.

Metcalf, D. (1965). Delayed effect of thymectomy in adult life on immunological competence. *Nature (London)* **208**, 1336.

Metcalf, D. (1966). "The Thymus—Its Role in Immune Responses, Leukaemia Development and Carcinogenesis." Springer-Verlag, Heidelberg.

Metcalf, D. and Ishidate, M., Jr. (1962). PAS positive reticulin cells in the thymus cortex of high and low leukaemia strains of mice. *Aust. J. Exp. Biol. Med. Sci.* **40**, 57.

Metcalf, D. and Wiadrowski, M. (1966). Autoradiographic analysis of lymphocyte proliferation in the thymus and in thymic lymphoma tissue. *Cancer Res.* **26**, 483.

Micklem, H. S., Ford, C. E., Evans, E. P., and Gray, J. (1966). Interrelationships of myeloid and lymphoid cells: Studies with chromosome marked cells transfused into lethally irradiated mice. *Proc. Roy. Soc. B* **165**, 78.

Mihaesco, C. and Seligmann, M. (1968). Papain digestion fragments of human IgM globulins. *J. Exp. Med.* **127**, 431.

Miller, F. and Metzger, H. (1966). Characterization of a human macroglobulin. III. The products of tryptic digestion. *J. Biol. Chem.* **241**, 1732.

Miller, J. F. A. P. (1961). Immunological function of the thymus. *Lancet* **ii**, 748.

Miller, J. F. A. P. (1965). Effect of thymectomy in adult mice on immunological responsiveness. *Nature (London)* **208**, 1337.

Miller, J. F. A. P. (1967). The thymus, yesterday, today and tomorrow. *Lancet* **ii**, 1299.

Miller, J. F. A. P. and Martin, W. J. Unpublished data.

Miller, J. F. A. P. and Mitchell, G. F. (1967). The thymus and the precursors of antigen reactive cells. *Nature (London)* **216**, 659.

Miller, J. F. A. P. and Mitchell, G. F. (1968). Cell to cell interaction in the immune response. I. Hemolysin-forming cells in neonatally thymectomized mice reconstituted with thymus or thoracic duct lymphocytes. *J. Exp. Med.* **128**, 801.

Miller, J. F. A. P. and Mitchell, G. F. (1969). Thymus and antigen-reactive cells. *Transplant. Rev.* **1**, 3.

Miller, J. F. A. P. and Osoba, D. (1967). Current concepts of the immunological function of the thymus. *Physiol. Rev.* **47**, 437.

Miller, J. F. A. P., Dukor, P., Grant, G., Sinclair, N. R. S. C., and Sacquet, E. (1967). The immunological responsiveness of germfree mice thymectomized at birth. I. Antibody production and skin homograft rejection. *Clin. Exp. Immunol.* **2**, 531.

Miller, J. F. A. P., DeBurgh, M., Dukor, P., Grant, G., Allman, V., and House, W. (1966). Regeneration of thymus grafts. II. Effects on immunological capacity. *Clin. Exp. Immunol.* **1**, 61.

Miller, J. J., III (1964a). An autoradiographic study of plasma cell and lymphocyte survival in rat popliteal lymph nodes. *J. Immunol.* **92**, 673.

Miller, J. J., III, (1964b). Studies of lymph node cells. Doctorate Thesis, University of Melbourne, Melbourne, Australia.

Miller, J. J., III, and Nossal, G. J. V. (1964). Antigens in immunity. VI. The phagocytic reticulum of lymph node follicles. *J. Exp. Med.* **120**, 1075.

Miller, J. J., III, Johnsen, D. O., and Ada, G. L. (1968). Differences in localization of *Salmonella* flagella in lymph node follicles of germ-free and conventional rats. *Nature (London)* **217**, 1059.

Mishell, R. I. and Dutton, R. W. (1966). Immunization of normal mouse spleen cell suspensions *in vitro*. *Science* **153**, 1004.

Mishell, R. I. and Dutton, R. W. (1967). Immunization of dissociated spleen cell cultures from normal mice. *J. Exp. Med.* **126**, 423.

Mishell, R. I., Dutton, R. W., and Raidt, D. J. (1970). Cell components in the immune response. I. Gradient separation of immune cells. *Cell Immunol.* **1**, 175.

Mitchell, G. F. and Miller, J. F. A. P. (1968). Cell to cell interaction in the immune response. II. The source of hemolysin-forming cells in irradiated mice given bone marrow and thymus or thoracic duct lymphocytes. *J. Exp. Med.* **128**, 821.

Mitchell, J. and Nossal, G. J. V. (1966). Mechanism of induction of immunological tolerance. I. Localization of tolerance-inducing antigen. *Aust. J. Exp. Biol. Med. Sci.* **44**, 211.

Mitchison, N. A. (1964). Induction of immunological paralysis in two zones of dosage. *Proc. Roy. Soc. B* **161**, 275.

Mitchison, N. A. (1967). Antigen recognition responsible for the induction *in vitro* of the secondary response. *Cold Spring Harbor Symp. Quant. Biol.* **32**, 431.

Mitchison, N. A. (1969). in "Immunological Tolerance—A Reassessment of Mechanisms of the Immune Response" (M. Landy and W. Braun, eds.), p. 149. Academic Press, New York.

Mitchison, N. A., Rajewsky, K., and Taylor, R. B. (1971, in press). Cooperation of autogenic determinants and of cells in the induction of antibodies. in "Developmental Aspects of Antibody Formation and Structure" (J. Sterzl and M. Riha, eds.), Vol. 2. Publ. House Czech. Acad. Sci., Prague.

Moe, R. E. (1964). Electron microscopic appearance of the parenchyma of lymph nodes. *Amer. J. Anat.* **114**, 341.

Möller, G. (1968). Regulation of cellular antibody synthesis. Cellular 7 S production and longevity of 7 S antigen-sensitive cells in the absence of antibody feedback. *J. Exp. Med.* **127**, 291.

Möller, G. and Wigzell, H. (1965). Antibody synthesis at the cellular level. Antibody-induced suppression of 19 S and 7 S antibody response. *J. Exp. Med.* **121**, 969.

Möller, G., Zukoski, C., Lundgren, G., Beckman, V., and Möller, E. (1968). *In vitro* cytotoxicity by non-immune lymphoid cells: Differential mechanism of action between various cell types. in "Advance in Transplantation" (J. Dausset, J. Hamburger, and G. Mathé, eds.), p. 67. Munksgaard, Copenhagen.

Moore, M. A. S. (1967). Experimental studies on the development of haemopoietic tissue. Thesis submitted for Ph.D., Magdalen College, Oxford, England.

Moore, M. A. S. and Owen, J. J. T. (1967a). Experimental studies on the development of the thymus. *J. Exp. Med.* **126**, 715.

Moore, M. A. S. and Owen, J. J. T. (1967b). Chromosome marker studies in the irradiated chick embryo. *Nature (London)* **215**, 1081.

Mosier, D. E. (1967). A requirement for two cell types for antibody formation *in vitro*. *Science* **158**, 1573.

Mosier, D. E. (1969). Cell interactions in the primary immune response *in vitro*: A requirement for specific cell clusters. *J. Exp. Med.* **129**, 351.

Mosier, D. E. and Cohen, E. P. (1968). Induction and rapid expression of an immune response *in vitro*. *Nature (London)* **219**, 969.

Mosier, D. E. and Coppleson, L. W. (1968). A three cell interaction required for the induction of the primary immune response *in vitro*. *Proc. Nat. Acad. Sci. U.S.* **61**, 542.

Mosier, D. E., Fitch, F. W., Rowley, D. A., and Davies, A. J. S. (1970). Cellular deficit in thymectomized mice. *Nature (London)* **225**, 276.

Munro, A. and Hunter, P. (1970). *In vitro* reconstitution of the immune response of thymus-deprived mice to sheep red blood cells. *Nature (London)* **225**, 277.

Muramatsu, S., Morita, T., and Sohmura, Y. (1966). Cellular kinetics of phagocytic cells in immunized X-irradiated mice. *J. Immunol.* **95**, 1134.

Nakamura, R. M., Spiegelberg, H. L., Lee, S., and Weigle, W. O. (1968). Relationship between molecular size and intra- and extravascular distribuiton of protein antigens. *J. Immunol.* **100**, 376.

Naor, D. and Sulitzeanu, D. (1967). Binding of radioiodinated bovine serum albumin to mouse spleen cells. *Nature (London)* **214**, 687.

Naor, D. and Sulitzeanu, D. (1968). Binding of radioiodinated bovine serum albumin to lymphoid cells of specifically primed or immunized mice *in vitro*. *Life Sci.* **7**, 377.

Naor, D. and Sulitzeanu, D. (1969). Binding of ^{125}I-BSA to lymphoid cells of tolerant mice. *Int. Arch. Allergy* **36**, 112.

Nelson, D. S. (1969). Macrophages and immunity. *in* "Frontiers of Biology" (A. Neuberger and E. L. Tatum, eds.). North Holland Publ. London.

Nelson, D. S. and Mildenhall, P. (1967). Studies on cytophilic antibodies. I. The production by mice of macrophage cytophilic antibodies to sheep erythrocytes; relationship to the production of other antibodies and the development of delayed type hypersensitivity. *Aust. J. Exp. Biol. Med. Sci.* **45**, 113.

Nelson, D. S., Kossard, S., and Cox, P. E. (1967). Heterogeneity of macrophage cytophilic antibodies in immunized mice. *Experientia* **23**, 490.

Nettesheim, P. and Makinodan, T. (1965). Differentiation of lymphocytes undergoing an immune response in diffusion chambers. *J. Immunol.* **94**, 868.

Neville, D. M. (1967). Fractionation of cell membrane protein by disc electrophoresis. *Biochim. Biophys. Acta* **133**, 168.

Nisonoff, A., Wissler, F. C., and Woernley, D. L. (1959). Mechanism of formation of univalent fragments of rabbit antibody. *Biochem. Biophys. Res. Commun.* **1**, 318.

Nossal, G. J. V. (1964). Studies on the rate of seeding of lymphocytes from the intact guinea pig thymus. *Ann. N.Y. Acad. Sci.* **120**, 171.

Nossal, G. J. V. (1969). Antigen dosage in relation to responsiveness and non-responsiveness. *in* "Immunological Tolerance—A Reassessment of Mechanisms of the Immune Response" (M. Landy and W. Braun, eds.), p. 53. Academic Press, New York.

Nossal, G. J. V. and Lederberg, J. (1958). Antibody production by single cells. *Nature* **181**, 1419.

Nossal, G. J. V. and Mäkelä, O. (1962a). Elaboration of antibodies by single cells. *Ann. Rev. Microbiol.* **16**, 53.

Nossal, G. J. V. and Mäkelä, O. (1962b). Autoradiographic studies on the immune response. I. The kinetics of plasma cell proliferation. *J. Exp. Med.* **115**, 209.

Nossal, G. J. V. and Mitchell, J. (1966). The thymus in relation to immunological tolerance. *in* "Thymus: Experimental and Clinical Studies" (G. E. W. Wolstenholme and R. Porter, eds.), p. 105. Churchill, London.

Nossal, G. J. V., Ada, G. L., and Austin, C. M. (1964a). Antigens in immunity. II. Immunogenic properties of flagella, polymerized flagellin and flagellin in the primary response. *Aust. J. Exp. Biol. Med. Sci.* **42**, 283.

Nossal, G. J. V., Ada, G. L., and Austin, C. M. (1964b). Antigens in immunity. IV. Cellular localization of ^{125}I- and ^{131}I-labelled flagella in lymph nodes. *Aust. J. Exp. Biol. Med. Sci.* **42**, 311.

Nossal, G. J. V., Szenberg, A., Ada, G. L., and Austin, C. M. (1964c). Single cell studies on 19 S antibody formation. *J. Exp. Med.* **119**, 485.

Nossal, G. J. V., Austin, C. M., and Ada, G. L., (1965a). Antigens in immunity. VII. Analysis of immunological memory. *Immunology* 9, 333.

Nossal, G. J. V., Ada, G. L., and Austin, C. M. (1965b). Antigens in immunity. VIII. Localization of ^{125}I-labeled antigens in the secondary response. *Immunology* 9, 349.

Nossal, G. J. V., Ada, G. L., and Austin, C. M. (1965c). Antigens in immunity. IX. The antigen content of single antibody-forming cells. *J. Exp. Med.* 121, 945.

Nossal, G. J. V., Ada, G. L., and Austin, C. M. (1965d). Antigens in immunity. X. Induction of immunological tolerance to *Salmonella adelaide* flagellin. *J. Immunol.* 95, 665.

Nossal, G. J. V., Austin, C. M., Pye, J., and Mitchell, J. (1966). Antigens in immunity. XII. Antigen-trapping in the spleen. *Int. Arch. Allergy Appl. Immunol.* 29, 368.

Nossal, G. J. V., Williams, G. M., and Austin, C. M. (1967). Antigens in immunity. XIII. The antigen content of single antibody-forming cells early in primary and secondary immune responses. *Aust. J. Exp. Biol. Med. Sci.* 45, 581.

Nossal, G. J. V., Abbot, A., and Mitchell, J. (1968a). Antigens in immunity. XIV. Electron microscopic-autoradiographic studies of antigen capture in the lymph node medulla. *J. Exp. Med.* 127, 263.

Nossal, G. J. V., Abbot, A., Mitchell, J., and Lummus, Z. (1968b). Antigens in immunity. XV. Ultrastructural features of antigen capture in primary and secondary lymphoid follicles. *J. Exp. Med.* 127, 277.

Nossal, G. J. V., Cunningham, A. J., Mitchell, G. F., and Miller, J. F. A. P. (1968c). Cell to cell interaction in the immune response. III. Chromosomal marker analysis of single antibody-forming cells in reconstituted, irradiated, or thymectomized mice. *J. Exp. Med.* 128, 839.

Nossal, G. J. V., Bussard, A. E., Lewis, H., and Mazie, J. C. (1971, in press). Formation of hemolytic plaques by peritoneal cells *in vitro*. I. A new technique enabling micromanipulation and yielding higher plaque numbers. *in* "Developmental Aspects of Antibody Formation and Structure" (J. Sterzl and M. Riha, eds.), Vol. 2. Publ. House, Czech. Acad. Sci., Prague.

Nussenzweig, V. and Benacerraf, B. (1964). Studies on the properties of fragments of guinea pig $\gamma 1$ and $\gamma 2$ antibodies obtained by papain and digestion and mild reduction. *J. Immunol.* 93, 1008.

Nussenzweig, V. and Benacerraf, B. (1967). Synthesis, structure and specificity of 7 S guinea pig immunoglobulins. *in* "Nobel Symposium 3 on Gamma Globulins" (J. Killander, ed.), p. 233. Almqvist & Wiksell, Stockholm.

O'Brien, T. F., Michaelides, M. C., and Coons, A. H. (1963). Studies on antibody production. VI. The course, sensitivity and histology of the secondary response *in vitro*. *J. Exp. Med.* 117, 1053.

Onoue, K., Yagi, Y., Grossberg, A. L., and Pressman, D. (1965). Number of binding sites of rabbit macroglobulin antibody and its subunits. *Immunochemistry* 2, 401.

Onoue, K., Kishimoto, T., and Yamamura, Y. (1968). Structure of human immunoglobulin M. II. Isolation of a high molecular weight Fc fragment of IgM composed of several Fc subunits. *J. Immunol.* 100, 238.

Oort, J. and Turk, J. L. (1965). A histological and autoradiographic study of lymph nodes during the development of contact sensitivity in the guinea pig. *Brit. J. Exp. Pathol.* 46, 147.

Osoba, D. (1969). Restriction of the capacity to respond to two antigens by single precursors of antibody-producing cells in culture. *J. Exp. Med.* 129, 141.

Osoba, D. and Miller, J. F. A. P. (1963). Evidence for a humoral thymus factor responsible for the maturation of immunological faculty. *Nature* (*London*) **199**, 653.

Oudin, J. and Michel, M. (1969). Idiotypy of rabbit antibodies. II. Comparison of idiotypy of various kinds of antibodies formed in the same rabbits against *Salmonella typhi. J. Exp. Med.* **130**, 619.

Ovary, Z. and Karush, F. (1961). Studies on the immunologic mechanism of anaphylaxis. II. Sensitizing and combining capacity *in vivo* of fractions separated from papain digests of anti-hapten antibody. *Immunology* **86**, 146.

Owen, R. D. (1945). Immunogenetic consequences of vascular anastomoses between bovine twins. *Science* **102**, 400.

Palmer, J. Unpublished data.

Panijel, J. and Cayeux, P. (1965). Arthrites et cardiopathies streptococciques (*Streptococcus pyrogènes*) obtenues expérimentalement chez la souris. *C. R. Acad. Sci.* (*Paris*) **261**, 607.

Panijel, J. and Cayeux P. (1968). Immunosuppressive effect of macrophage antiserum. *Immunology* **14**, 769.

Papermaster, D. S., Gill, T. J., III and Anderson, W. F. (1965). Synthetic polypeptide metabolism. II. The binding of synthetic polypeptides to serum proteins. *Immunology* **95**, 804.

Parish, C. R. (1969). Immunochemical studies of bacterial flagellin. Ph.D. Thesis, University of Melbourne, Melbourne, Australia.

Parish, C. R. and Ada, G. L. (1969a). Cleavage of bacterial flagellin with cyanogen bromide. Chemical and physical properties of the protein fragments. *J. Biochem.* **113**, 489.

Parish, C. R. and Ada, G. L. (1969b). The tolerance inducing properties in rats of bacterial flagellin cleaved at the methionine residues. *Immunology* **17**, 153.

Parish, C. R. and Fetherstonhaugh, P. (1971, in preparation). Oxidation of the methionine residues of bacterial flagellin during iodination with chloramine-T.

Parish, C. R., Wistar, R., Jr., and Ada, G. L. (1969). Cleavage of bacterial flagellin with cyanogen bromide. Antigenic properties of the protein fragments. *Biochem. J.* **113**, 501.

Parish, W. E. (1965). Differentiation between cytophilic antibody and opsonin by a macrophage phagocytic system. *Nature* (*London*) **208**, 594.

Parkhouse, R. M. E. and Dutton, R. W. (1966). Inhibition of spleen cell DNA synthesis by autologous macrophages. *J. Immunol.* **97**, 663.

Parrott, D. M. V. (1967). The integrity of the germinal center: An investigation of the differential localisation of labeled cells in lymphoid organs. *in* "Germinal Centers in Immune Responses" (H. Cottier *et al.*, eds.), p. 168. Springer-Verlag, Berlin.

Pearlman, D. S. (1966). The influence of antibodies on immunologic responses. *Fed. Proc.* **25**, 548.

Perey, D. Y. and Good, R. A. (1968). Experimental arrest and induction of lymphoid development in intestinal lymphoepithelial tissues of rabbits. *Lab. Invest.* **18**, 15.

Perey, D. Y., Cooper, M. D., and Good, R. A. (1967). Normal second set wattle homograft rejection in agammaglobulinemic chickens. *Transplantation* **5**, 615.

Perey, D. Y., Cooper, M. D., and Good, R. A. (1968). Lymphoepithelial tissues of the intestine and differentiation of antibody production. *Science* **161**, 265.

Perkins, E. H. and Makinodan, T. (1965). The suppressive role of mouse peritoneal phagocytes in agglutinin response. *J. Immunol.* **94**, 765.

Perkins, E. H., Morita, T., and Nettesheim, P. (1965). Effect of X-irradiation on the phagocytosis of foreign erythrocytes. *Fed. Proc.* **24**, 381.

Pernis, B. and Chiappino, G. (1964). Identification in human lymphoid tissues of cells that produce group 1 or group 2 gamma globulins. *Immunology* **7**, 500.

Pick, E. and Feldman, J. D. (1967). Autoradiographic plaques for the detection of antibody formation to soluble proteins by single cells. *Science* **156**, 964.

Pierce, C. W. (1967). The effects of endotoxin on the immune response in the rat. III. Elimination of ^{125}I-labeled bovine γ-globulin from the circulation of rats. *Lab. Invest.* **17**, 380.

Pierce, C. W. (1969a). Immune responses *in vitro*. I. Cellular requirements for the immune response by nonprimed and primed spleen cells *in vitro*. *J. Exp. Med.* **130**, 345.

Pierce, C. W. (1969b). Immune responses *in vitro*. II. Suppression of the immune response *in vitro* by specific antibody. *J. Exp. Med.* **130**, 365.

Pierce, C. W. and Benacerraf, B. (1969). Immune response *in vitro:* Independence of "Activated" lymphoid cells. *Science* **166**, 1002.

Pinchuck, P. and Maurer, P. H. (1968). Genetic control of aspects of the immune response. *in* "Regulation of the Antibody Response" (B. Cinader, ed.), p. 97. Thomas, Springfield, Illinois.

Pinchuck, P., Fishman, M., Adler, F. L., and Maurer, P. H. (1968). Antibody formation: Initiation in "nonresponder" mice by macrophage synthetic polypeptide RNA. *Science* **160**, 194.

Playfair, J. N. L., Papermaster, B. W., and Cole, L. J. (1965). Focal antibody production by transferred spleen cells in irradiated mice. *Science* **149**, 998.

Plotz, P. H. (1969). Specific inhibition of an antibody response by affinity labelling. *Nature (London)* **223**, 1373.

Porter, R. R. (1959). The hydrolysis of rabbit gamma globulin and antibodies with crystalline papain. *Biochem. J.* **73**, 119.

Porter, R. R. and Press, E. M. (1962). Immunochemistry. *Ann. Rev. Biochem.* **31**, 625.

Putnam, F. W. (1969). Immunoglobulin structure: variability and homology. *Science* **163**, 633.

Rabinovitch, M. (1967a). The role of antibodies in the ingestion of aldehyde-treated erythrocytes attached to macrophages. *J. Immunol.* **99**, 232.

Rabinovitch, M. (1967b). Studies on the immunoglobulins which stimulate the ingestion of glutaraldehyde-treated red cells attached to macrophages. *J. Immunol.* **99**, 1115.

Raidt, D. J., Mishell, R. I., and Dutton, R. W. (1968). Cellular events in the immune response. Analysis and *in vitro* response of mouse spleen cell populations separated by differential flotation in albumin gradients. *J. Exp. Med.* **128**, 681.

Rajewsky, K., Rottländer, E., Peltre, G., and Müller, B. (1967). The immune response to a hybrid protein molecule: specificity of secondary stimulation and of tolerance induction. *J. Exp. Med.* **126**, 581.

Rajewsky, K., Schirrmacher, V., Nase, S., and Jerne, N. K. (1969). The requirement of more than one antigenic determinant for immunogenicity. *J. Exp. Med.* **129**, 1131.

Rappaport, I. (1965). The antigenic structure of tobacco mosaic virus. *Advan. Virus Res.* **11**, 223.

Reade, P. C. and Casley-Smith, J. R. (1965). The functional development of the reticulo-endothelial system. II. The histology of blood clearance by the fixed macrophages of foetal rats. *Immunology* **9**, 61.

Reade, P. C. and Jenkin, C. R. (1965). The functional development of the reticulo-endothelial system. I. The uptake of intravenously injected particles by foetal rats. *Immunology* **9**, 53.

Reade, P. C., Turner, K. J., and Jenkin, C. R. (1965). The functional development of the reticulo-endothelial system. IV. Studies of serum opsonins to *Salmonella typhimurium* in foetal and natal rats. *Immunology* **9**, 75.

Reiss, E., Mertens, E., and Ehrich, W. E. (1950). Agglutination of bacteria by lymphoid cells *in vitro*. *Proc. Soc. Exp. Biol. Med.* **74**, 732.

Rhodes, J. M. and Lind, I. (1968). Antigen uptake *in vivo* by peritoneal macrophages from normal mice and those undergoing primary or secondary responses. *Immunology* **14**, 511.

Robbins, J., Eitzman, D. V., and Smith, R. T. (1963). The catabolism of protein antigens in the newborn and maturing rabbit. *J. Exp. Med.* **118**, 959.

Robbins, J., Kenny, K., and Suter, E. (1965). The isolation and biological activities of rabbit γM- and γG-anti-*Salmonella typhimurium* antibodies. *J. Exp. Med.* **122**, 385.

Roberts, A. N. (1964). Quantitative cellular distribution of tritiated antigen in immunized mice. *Amer. J. Pathol.* **44**, 411.

Roberts, A. N. (1966a). Rapid uptake of tritiated antigen by mouse eosinophils. *Nature* **210**, 266.

Roberts, A. N. (1966b). Cellular localization and quantitation of tritiated antigen in mouse lymph nodes during early primary immune response. *Amer. J. Pathol.* **49**, 889.

Roberts, A. N. and Haurowitz, F. (1962). Intracellular localization and quantitation of tritiated antigens in reticuloendothelial tissues of mice during secondary and hyperimmune responses. *J. Exp. Med.* **116**, 407.

Roelants, G. E. and Goodman, J. W. (1968). Immunochemical studies on the poly-γ-D-glutamyl capsule of *Bacillus anthracis*. IV. The association with peritoneal exudate cell ribonucleic acid of the polypeptide in immunogenic and non-immunogenic forms. *Biochemistry* **7**, 1432.

Roelants, G. E. and Goodman, J. W. (1970). Tolerance induction by a non-immunogenic molecule: A model for immune induction and tolerance. Submitted.

Roelants, G. E., Sinyk, G., and Goodman, J. W. (1969). Immunochemical studies on the poly-γ-D-glutamyl capsule of *Bacillus anthracis*. V. The *in vivo* fate and distribution in rabbits of the polypeptide in immunogenic and non-immunogenic forms. *Israel J. Med. Sci.* **5**, 196.

Roseman, J. (1969). X-ray resistant cell required for the induction of *in vitro* antibody formation. *Science* **165**, 1125.

Roser, B. J. (1965). The distribution of intravenously injected peritoneal macrophages in the mouse. *Aust. J. Exp. Biol. Med. Sci.* **43**, 553.

Rotman, B. (1961). Measurement of activity of single molecules of β-D-galactosidase. *Proc. Nat. Acad. Sci. U.S.* **47**, 1981.

Rowley, D. (1962). Phagocytosis. *Advan. Immunol.* **2**, 241.

Rowley, D. (1970). Genetic control of species susceptibility to infection. in "Developmental Aspects of Antibody Formation and Structure" (J. Sterzl and M. Riha, eds.), **1**, 207. Academic Press, New York.

Rowley, D. and Fitch, F. W. (1964). Homeostasis of antibody formation in the adult rat. *J. Exp. Med.* **120**, 987.

Rowley, D. and Turner, K. J. (1966). Number of molecules of antibody required to promote phagocytosis by one bacterium. *Nature (London)* **210**, 496.

Rowley, D., Thöni, M., and Isliker, H. (1965). Opsonic requirements for bacterial phagocytosis. *Nature (London)* **207**, 210.

Russell, P. and Roser, B. (1966). The distribution and behaviour of intravenously injected pulmonary alveolar macrophages in the mouse. *Aust. J. Exp. Biol. Med. Sci.* **44**, 629.

Ryser, H. (1963). Comparison of the incorporation of tyrosine and its iodinated analogs into the proteins of Ehrlich ascites tumour cells and rat-liver slices. *Biochim. Biophys. Acta.* **78**, 759.

Sage, H. J., Deutsch, G. F., Fasman, G. D., and Levine, L. (1964). The serological specificity of the poly-alanine immune system. *Immunochemistry* **1**, 133.

Saha, A., Garvey, J. S., and Campbell, D. H. (1964). The physicochemical characterization of the ribonucleic acid-antigen complex persisting in the liver of immunized rabbits. *Arch. Biochem. Biophys.* **105**, 179.

Salpeter M. M. and Bachmann, L. (1964). Autoradiography with the electron microscope. A procedure for improving resolution, sensitivity and contrast. *J. Cell Biol.* **22**, 469.

Saunders G. C. and King, D. W. (1966). Antibody synthesis initiated in vitro by paired explants of spleen and thymus. *Science* **151**, 1390.

Schechter, I., Bauminger, S., and Sela, M. (1964a). Induction of immunological tolerance towards a peptide determinant with a non-immunogenic polypeptide. *Biochim. Biophys. Acta* **93**, 686.

Schechter, I., Bauminger, S., Sela, M., Nachtigal, D., and Feldman, M. (1964b). Immune response to polypeptidyl proteins in rabbits tolerant to the protein carriers. *Immunochemistry* **1**, 249.

Schlossman, S. F. (1967). The immune response. Some unifying concepts. *New Engl. J. Med.* **277**, 1355.

Schlossman, S. F., Yaron, A., Ben-Efraim, S., and Sober, H. A. (1965). Immunogenicity of a series of αN-DNP-L-lysines. *Biochemistry* **4**, 1638.

Schlossman, S. F., Ben-Efraim, S., Yaron, A., and Sober, H. A. (1966). Immunochemical studies on antigenic determinants required to elicit delayed and immediate hypersensitivity reactions. *J. Exp. Med.* **123**, 1083.

Schlossman, S. F., Herman, J., and Yaron, A. (1969). Antigen recognition in vitro studies on the specificity of the cellular immune response. *J. Exp. Med.* **130**, 1031.

Schwartz, R. S. (1966). Specificity of immunosuppression by antimetabolites. *Fed. Proc.* **25**, 165.

Schwartz, R. S. and Damashek, W. (1963). The role of antigen dosage in drug-induced immunological tolerance. *J. Immunol.* **90**, 703.

Scothorne, R. J. and McGregor, I. A. (1955). Cellular changes in lymph nodes and spleen following skin homografting in rabbit. *J. Anat.* **89**, 283.

Scott, D. W. and Waksman, B. H. (1968). Tolerance in vitro. Suppression of immune responsiveness to bovine γ-globulin after injection of antigen into intact lymphoid organs. *J. Immunol.* **100**, 912.

Scott, D. W. and Waksman, B. H. (1969). Mechanism of immunologic tolerance. 1, Induction of tolerance to bovine γ-globulin by injection of antigen into intact organs in vitro. *J. Immunol.* **102**, 347.

Segal, S., Globerson, A., Feldman, M., Haimovich, J., and Givol, D. (1969). Specific blocking *in vitro* of antibody synthesis by affinity labelling reagents. *Nature (London)* **223**, 1374.

Sela, M. (1966). Immunological studies with synthetic polypeptides. *Advan. Immunol.* **5**, 29.

Sela, M., Fuchs, S., and Arnon, R. (1962). Studies on the chemical basis of the antigenicity of proteins. V. Synthesis, characterization and immunogenicity of some multichain and linear polypeptides containing tyrosine. *Biochem. J.* **85**, 223.

Sell, S. (1967). Studies on rabbit lymphocytes *in vitro*. V. The induction of blast transformation with sheep antisera to rabbit IgG subunits. *J. Exp. Med.* **125**, 289.

Sell, S. (1968). Studies on rabbit lymphocytes *in vitro*. VIII. The relationship between heterozygosity and homozygosity of lymphocyte donor and per cent blast transformation, induced by antiallotype sera. *J. Exp. Med.* **127**, 1139.

Sell, S. and Gell, P. G. H. (1965a). Studies on rabbit lymphocytes *in vitro*. I. Stimulation of blast transformation with an antiallotype serum. *J. Exp. Med.* **122**, 423.

Sell, S. and Gell, P. G. H. (1965b). Studies on rabbit lymphocytes *in vitro*. IV. Blast transformation of the lymphocytes from newborn rabbits induced by antiallotype serum to a paternal IgG allotype not present in serum of the lymphocyte donors. *J. Exp. Med.* **122**, 923.

Sell, S., Rowe, D. S., and Gell, P. G. H. (1965). Studies on rabbit lymphocytes *in vitro*. III. Protein, RNA and DNA synthesis by lymphocyte cultures after stimulation with phytohemagglutinin, with staphylococcal filtrate, with antiallotype serum, and with heterologous antiserum to rabbit whole serum. *J. Exp. Med.* **122**, 823.

Shellam, G. R. (1969a). Mechanism of induction of immunological tolerance. V. Priming and tolerance with small doses of polymerized flagellin. *Immunology* **16**, 45.

Shellam, G. R. (1969b). Mechanism of induction of immunological tolerance. VI. Tolerance induction following thoracic duct drainage or treatment with antilymphocyte serum. *Immunology* **17**, 267.

Shellam, G. R. and Nossal, G. J. V. (1968). Mechanism of induction of immunological tolerance. IV. The effects of ultra-low doses of flagellin. *Immunology* **14**, 273.

Shortman, K. (1966). The separation of different cell classes from lymphoid organs. I. The use of glass bead columns to separate small lymphocytes, remove damaged cells and fractionate cell suspensions. *Aust. J. Exp. Biol. Med. Sci.* **44**, 271.

Shortman, K. (1968). The separation of different cell classes from lymphoid organs. II. The purification and analysis of lymphocyte populations by equilibrium density gradient centrifugation. *Aust. J. Exp. Biol. Med. Sci.* **46**, 375.

Shortman, K. (1969a). The separation of lymphocyte populations on glass bead columns. *in* "Modern Separation Methods of Macromolecules and Particles—Progress in Separation and Purification" (T. Gerritsen, ed.), p. 91. Wiley (Interscience), New York.

Shortman, K. (1969b). Equilibrium density gradient separation and analysis of lymphocyte populations. *in* "Modern Separation Methods of Macromolecules and Particles—Progress in Separation and Purification (T. Gerritsen, ed.), Vol. 2. Wiley (Interscience), New York.

Shortman, K. D., Diener, E., Russell, P., and Amstrong, W. D. (1970). The role of non-lymphoid accessory cells in the immune response to different antigens. *J. Exp. Med.* **131**, 461.

Silverstein, A. M. and Prendergast, R. A. (1970). Lymphogenesis, immunogenesis and the generation of immunotopic diversity. *in* "Development Aspects of Antibody Formation and Structure" (J. Sterzl and M. Riha, eds.), Vol. I, p. 69. Publ. House Czech. Acad. Sci., Prague.

Silverstein, A. M. and Kramer, K. L. (1965). Studies on the autogenesis of the immune response. *in* "Molecular and Cellular Basis of Antibody Formation" (J. Sterzl, ed.). Academic Press, New York.

Simonsen, M. (1962). Graft versus host reactions. Their natural history and applicability as tools of research. *Progr. Allergy* **6**, 349.

Simonsen, M. (1969). *in* "Immunological Tolerance—A Reassessment of Mechanisms of the Immune Response" (M. Landy and W. Braun, eds.), p. 74. Academic Press, New York.

Siskind, G. W. and Benacerraf, B. (1969). Cell selection by antigen in the immune response. *Advan. Immunol.* **10**, 1.

Siskind, G. W., Paul, W. E., and Benacerraf, B. (1966). Studies on the effect of the carrier molecule on antihapten antibody synthesis. I. Effect of carrier on the nature of the antibody synthesized. *J. Exp. Med.* **123**, 673.

Sjovall, H. (1936). "Experimentelle untersuchungen über das Blut and die blutbildenen organe—besonders das lymphatische Geweke—das Kaminchens bei wiederholten Aderlässen." Hakan Ohlssons Boktryckeri, Lund.

Smith, C. (1964). The microscopic anatomy of the thymus. *in* "The Thymus in Immunobiology. Structure, Function and Role in Disease" (R. A. Good and A. E. Gabrielsen, eds.), p. 71. Harper (Hoeber), New York.

Smith, J. W., Barnett, J. A., May, R. P., and Sandford, J. P. (1967). Comparison of the opsonic activity of γ-G- and γ-M- anti-Proteus globulins. *J. Immunol.* **98**, 336.

Smith, R. T. (1961). Immunological tolerance of non-living antigens. *Advan. Immunol.* **1**, 67.

Smith, R. T. and Bridges, R. A. (1958). Immunological unresponsiveness in rabbits produced by neonatal injection of defined antigens. *J. Exp. Med.* **108**, 227.

Smyth, D. S. and Utsumi, S. (1967). Structure at the hinge region in rabbit immunoglobulin G. *Nature (London)* **216**, 332.

Snook, T. (1964). Studies on the perifollicular region of the rat's spleen. *Anat. Rec.* **148**, 149.

Söderström, N. (1967). Post-capillary venules as basic structural units in the development of lymphoglandular tissue. *Scand. J. Haematol.* **4**, 411.

Söderström, N. (1968). The free cytoplasmic fragments of lymphoglandular tissue (lymphoglandular bodies). A preliminary presentation. *Scand. J. Haematol.* **5**, 138 (1968).

Solomon, J. B. (1966). The appearance and nature of opsonins for goat erythrocytes during the development of the chicken. *Immunology* **11**, 79.

Sorkin, E. (1964). On the cellular fixation of cytophilic antibody. *Int. Arch. Allergy* **25**, 129.

Spector, W. G., Walters, M. N., and Willoughby, D. A. (1965). The origin of the mononuclear cells in inflammatory exudates induced by fibrinogen. *J. Pathol. Bacteriol.* **90**, 181.

Speirs, R. S. and Speirs, E. E. (1963). Cellular localization of radioactive antigen in immunized and nonimmunized mice. *J. Immunol.* **90**, 561.

Spiegelberg, H. L. and Weigle, W. O. (1965). The catabolism of homologous and heterologous 7 S gamma globulin fragments. *J. Exp. Med.* **121**, 323.

Spiegelberg, H. L., Miescher, P. A., and Benacerraf, B. (1963). Studies on the role of complement in the immune clearance of *Escherichia coli* and rat erythrocytes by the reticuloendothelial system in mice. *J. Immunol.* **90**, 751.

Staples, P. J., Gery, I., and Waksman, B. H. (1966). Role of the thymus in tolerance. III. Tolerance to bovine gamma globulin after direct injection of antigen into the shielded thymus of irradiated rats. *J. Exp. Med.* **124**, 127.

Sterzl, J., Mandel, L., Miler, I., and Riha, I. (1965). Development of immune reactions in the absence or presence of an antigenic stimulus. in "Molecular and Cellular Basis of Antibody Formation" (J. Sterzl, ed.), p. 351. Publ. House Czech. Acad. Sci., Prague.

Stevens, K. M. and McKenna J. M. (1958). Studies in antibody synthesis initiated *in vitro. J. Exp. Med.* **107**, 537.

Stewart, J. M., Young, J. D., Benjamini, E., Shimizu, M., and Leung, C. Y. (1966). Immunochemical studies on tobacco mosaic virus protein. IV. The automated solid-phase synthesis of a decapeptide of tobacco mosaic virus protein and its reaction with antibodies to the whole protein. *Biochemistry* **5**, 3396.

Strober, S. and Law, L. W. (1969). Further studies on the role of circulating lymphocytes in the initiation of primary antibody responses to different antigens. *Proc. Nat. Acad. Sci. U.S.* **62**, 1023.

Sulitzeanu, D., Rasooly, G., Benezra, D., and Gery, I. (1969). Autoradiographic follow-up of antigen during the induction of a secondary response *in vitro. Israel J. Med. Sci.* **5**, 443.

Sutherland, D. E. R., Archer, O. K., and Good, R. A. (1964). Role of the appendix in development of immunologic capacity. *Proc. Soc. Exp. Biol. Med.* **115**, 673.

Suzuki, T. and Deutsch, H. F. (1966). Dissociation, reaggregation and subunit structure studies of some human γM-globulins. *J. Biol. Chem.* **242**, 2725.

Svedberg, T. and Pedersen, K. O. (1940). "The Ultracentrifuge," Oxford Univ. Press (Clarendon) London & New York.

Sweet, L. C., Abrams, G. D., and Johnson, A. G. (1965). The fate of radioactive bovine γ-globulin during the primary antibody response in the mouse. *J. Immunol.* **94**, 105.

Szenberg, A. and Warner, N. L. (1963). Breakdown of polyvalent tolerance in the chicken by thymic grafts. *Nature* **198**, 1012.

Takahashi, M., Yagi, Y., Moore, G. E., and Pressman, D. (1969a). Pattern of immunoglobulin production in individual cells of human hematopoietic origin in established culture. *J. Immunol.* **102**, 1274.

Takahashi, M., Takagi, N., Yagi, Y., Moore, G. E., and Pressman, D. (1969b). Immunoglobulin production in cloned sublines of a human lymphocytoid cell line. *J. Immunol.* **102**, 1388.

Tao, T. W. and Uhr, J. W. (1966a). Capacity of pepsin-digested antibody to inhibit antibody formation. *Nature* (*London*) **212**, 208.

Tao, T. W. and Uhr, J. W. (1966b). Primary type antibody response *in vitro. Science* **151**, 1096.

Taylor, R. B. (1969). Cellular cooperation in the antibody response of mice to two serum albumins: specific function of thymus cells. *Transplant. Rev.* **1**, 114.

Till, J. E., McCulloch, E. A., and Siminovitch, L. (1964). A stochastic model of stem cell proliferation based on the growth of spleen colony-forming cells. *Proc. Nat. Acad. Sci. U.S.* **51**, 29.

Tizard, I. R. (1969). Macrophage cytophilic antibody in mice. Differentiation between antigen adherence due to these antibodies and opsonic adherence. *Int. Arch. Allergy Appl. Immunol.* **36**, 332.

Tong, W., Taurog, A., and Chaikoff, I. L. (1954). The metabolism of ^{131}I-labeled diiodotyrosine. *J. Biol. Chem.* **207**, 59.

Trainin, N. and Linker-Israeli, M. (1967). Restoration of immunologic reactivity of thymectomized mice by calf thymus extracts. *Cancer Res.* **27**, 309.

Traub, E. (1938). Factors influencing the persistence of choriomeningitis virus in the blood of mice after clinical recovery. *J. Exp. Med.* **68**, 229.

Uhr, J. W. (1965). Passive sensitization of lymphocytes and macrophages by antigen-antibody complexes. *Proc. Nat. Acad. Sci. U.S.* **54**, 1599.

Uhr, J. W. and Baumann, J. B. (1961a). Antibody formation. I. The suppression of antibody formation by passively administered antibody. *J. Exp. Med.* **113**, 935.

Uhr, J. W. and Baumann, J. B. (1961b). Antibody formation. II. The specific anamnestic antibody response. *J. Exp. Med.* **113**, 959.

Uhr, J. W. and Möller, G. (1968). Regulatory effect of antibody on the immune response. *Advan. Immunol.* **8**, 81.

Uhr, J. W. and Weissmann, G. (1965). Intracellular distribution and degradation of bacteriophage in mammalian tissues. *J. Immunol.* **94**, 544.

Uhr, J. W. and Weissmann, G. (1968). The sequestration of antigens in lysosomes. *J. Reticuloendothel. Soc.* **5**, 243.

Unanue, E. R. (1968). Properties and some uses of anti-macrophage antibodies. *Nature (London)* **218**, 36.

Unanue, E. R. and Askonas, B. A. (1968a). The immune response of mice to antigen in macrophages. *Immunology* **15**, 287.

Unanue, E. R. and Askonas, B. A. (1968b). Persistence of immunogenicity of antigen after uptake by macrophages. *J. Exp. Med.* **127**, 915.

Unanue, E. R. and Cerottini, J. C. (1971, in press). Fate and immunogenicity of macrophage associated hemocyanins. *in* "Developmental Aspects of Antibody Formation and Structure" (J. Sterzl and M. Riha, eds.), Vol. 2. Publ. House Czech. Acad. Sci., Prague.

Unanue, E. R. and Dixon, F. J. (1967). Experimental glomerulonephritis. Immunological events and pathogenetic mechanisms. *Advan. Immunol.* **6**, 1.

Unanue, E. R., Cerottini, J. C., and Bedford, M. (1969a). The persistence of antigen on the surface of macrophages. *Nature (London)* **222**, 1193.

Unanue, E. R., Askonas, B. A., and Allison, A. C. (1969b). A role of macrophages in the stimulation of immune responses by adjuvants. *J. Immunol.* **103**, 71.

Ungar-Waron, H., Hurwitz, E., Jaton, J. C., and Sela, M. (1967). Antibodies elicited with conjugates of nucleosides with synthetic polypeptides. *Biochim. Biophys. Acta* **138**, 513.

Valentine, R. C. and Green, N. M. (1967). Electron microscopy of an antibody-hapten complex. *J. Mol. Biol.* **27**, 615.

van Furth, R. Schuit, H. R. E., and Hijmans, W. (1966a). The formation of immunoglobulins by human tissues *in vitro*. III. Spleen, lymph nodes, bone marrow and thymus. *Immunology* **11**, 19.

van Furth, R., Schuit, H. R. E., and Hijmans, W. (1966b). The formation of immunoglobulins by human tissues *in vitro*. IV. Circulating lymphocytes in normal and pathological conditions. *Immunology* 11, 29.

Volkman, A. and Gowans, J. L. (1965a). The production of macrophages in the rat. *Brit. J. Exp. Pathol.* 46, 50.

Volkman, A. and Gowans, J. L. (1965b). The origin of macrophages from bone marrow in the rat. *Brit. J. Exp. Pathol.* 46, 62.

Walsh, T. E. and Smith, C. A. (1951). The influence of polymorphonuclear leukocytes and macrophages on antibody production. *J. Immunol.* 66, 303.

Warner, N. L. and Szenberg, A. (1964). The immunological function of the bursa of Fabricius in the chicken. *Ann. Rev. Microbiol.* 18, 253.

Warner, N. L., Szenberg, A., and Burnet, F. M. (1962). The immunological role of different lymphoid organs in the chicken. I. Dissociation of immunological responsiveness. *Aust. J. Exp. Biol. Med. Sci.* 40, 373.

Warner, N. L., Byrt, P., and Ada, G. L. (1970). Antigens and lymphocytes *in vitro*. Blocking of the antigen receptor site with anti-immuno-globulin sera. *Nature (London)* 226, 942.

Webster, R. G. (1968a). The immune response to influenza virus. II. Effect of the route and schedule of vaccination on the quantity and avidity of antibodies. *Immunology* 14, 29.

Webster, R. G. (1968b). The immune response to influenza virus. III. Changes in the avidity and specificity of early IgM and IgG antibodies. *Immunology* 14, 39.

Weigle, W. O. (1958). Elimination of antigen-antibody complexes from sera of rabbits. *J. Immunol.* 81, 204.

Weigle, W. O. (1961). The immune response of rabbits tolerant to bovine serum albumin to the injection of other heterologous serum albumins. *J. Exp. Med.* 114, 111.

Weigle, W. O. (1965). The immune response of rabbits tolerant to one protein conjugate following the injection of related protein conjugates. *J. Immunol.* 94, 177.

Weiler, I. J. and Weiler, E. (1965). Association of immunologic determination with the lymphocyte fraction of the peritoneal fluid cell population. *J. Immunol.* 95, 288.

Weiss, L. (1964). The white pulp of the spleen. The relationships of arterial vessels, reticulum and free cells in the periarterial lymphatic sheath. *Bull. Johns Hopkins Hosp.* 115, 99.

Weissman, I. L. (1967). Thymus cell migration. *J. Exp. Med.* 126, 291.

Wellensiek, H. J. and Coons, A. H. (1964). Studies on antibody production. IX. The cellular localisation of antigen molecules (ferritin) in the secondary response. *J. Exp. Med.* 119, 685.

White, R. G. (1963). Functional recognition of immunologically competent cells by means of the fluorescent antibody technique. *Ciba Found. Study Group No. 16.* p. 6.

White, R. G., Jenkins, G. C., and Wilkinson, P. C. (1963). The production of skin sensitizing antibody in the guinea pig. *Int. Arch. Allergy* 22, 156.

White, R. G., French, V. I., and Stark, J. M. (1967). Germinal center formation and antigen localisation in Malpighian bodies of the chicken spleen. *in* "Germinal Centers in Immune Responses" (H. Cottier, N. Odartchenko, R. Schindler, and C. C. Congdon, eds.), p. 131. Springer-Verlag, New York.

Wiener, E. and Levanon, D. (1968). Macrophage cultures: an extracellular esterase. *Science* **159**, 217.

Wigzell, H. and Andersson, B. (1969). Cell separation on antigen coated columns. Elimination of high rate antibody-forming cells and immunological memory cells. *J. Exp. Med.* **129**, 23.

Williams, G. M. (1966a). Antigen localization in lymphopenic states. I. Localization pattern following chronic thoracic duct drainage. *Immunology* **11**, 467.

Williams, G. M. (1966b). Antigen localization in lymphopenic states. II. Further studies on whole body X-irradiation. *Immunology* **11**, 475.

Williams, G. M. (1966c). Ontogeny of the immune response. II. The development of antibody-forming capacity and immunological memory. *J. Exp. Med.* **124**, 57.

Williams, J. M. and Ada, G. L. (1967). Antigen in tissues. III. The separation of antigen-containing components from lymphoid tissues. *Immunology* **13**, 249.

Williams, G. M. and Nossal, G. J. V. (1966). Ontogeny of the immune response. I. The development of the follicular antigen-trapping mechanism. *J. Exp. Med.* **124**, 47.

Williamson, A. R. and Askonas, B. A. (1967). Biosynthesis of immunoglobulins. The separate classes of polyribosomes synthesizing heavy and light chains. *J. Mol. Biol.* **23**, 201.

Wistar, R. and Shellam, G. R. (1969). Immunoglobulin levels during thoracic duct drainage in the rat. *Int. Arch. Allergy* **36**, 323.

Wofsy, L., Metzger, H., and Singer, S. J. (1962). Affinity labeling—a general method for labeling the active sites of antibody and enzyme molecules. *Biochemistry* **1**, 1031.

Wolstenholme, G. E. W. and Porter, R. Eds. (1966). *Ciba Found. Symp. Thymus—Exp. Clin. Studies.* Churchill, London.

World Health Organization Bulletin. (1967). The suppression of Rh immunization by previously administered human immunoglobulin (IgG) anti-D (anti-Rh).

Wormall, A. (1930). The immunological specificity of chemically altered proteins. Halogenated and nitrated proteins. *J. Exp. Med.* **51**, 295.

Yoffey, J. M. and Courtice, F. C. (1956). "Lymphatics, Lymph and Lymphoid Tissue," 2nd ed. Edward Arnold, London.

Yoffey, J. M. and Courtice, F. C. (1970). "Lymphatics, Lymph and Lymphoid Tissue," 3rd ed. Edward Arnold, London.

Young, J. D., Benjamini, E., Shimizu, M., and Leung, C. Y. (1966). Immunochemical studies on the tobacco mosaic virus protein. III. The degradation of an immunologically active tryptic peptide of tobacco mosaic virus protein and the reactivity of the degradation product with antibodies to whole protein. *Biochemistry* **5**, 1481.

Young, J. D., Benjamini, E., Stewart, J. M., and Leung, C. Y. (1967). Immunochemical studies on tobacco mosaic virus. V. The solid-phase synthesis of peptides of an antigenically active decapeptide of tobacco mosaic virus protein and the reaction of these peptides with antibodies to the whole protein. *Biochemistry* **6**, 1455.

Zaalberg, O. B. (1964). A simple method for detecting single antibody-forming cells. *Nature (London)* **202**, 1231.

POSTSCRIPT

Advances in immunological research continue to occur, if anything at an increased rate. The time which elapsed between submission of the manuscript of this monograph and correction of the proofs, though relatively short, has seen a spate of new discoveries. Some of these have been published, others presented at Meetings and others still in the "pipeline." It seemed worthwhile to mention a few so that readers will be made aware of recent trends and what to expect. Our choice is inevitably biased. As full documentation cannot, at the time of writing, be given for many, this postscript will be in the form of informal statements. We hope various authors will forgive this liberty.

Immunoglobulin molecules are yielding more of their secrets. Amino acid sequences of antibodies have been described which appear to be the combining sites for some antigenic determinants. As expected, those described so far are in the variable region of the light and/or heavy chains. The recent availability of homogeneous antibodies to known antigenic determinants will greatly speed these investigations and open up the way for detailed conformational studies. At the other end of the molecule, there is a renewal of interest in macrophage cytophilic antibody and a re-investigation of the existence of cytophilic antibody for lymphocytes.

At the time of writing this monograph, a variety of reasons caused us to restrict our attention to one major aspect of the immune response—antibody formation and tolerance. In the future such a restrictive approach will not be valid as there is increasing evidence for an intimate relationship between humoral antibody formation and cell-mediated responses. An exciting development is the effect of antigen modification so that an antigen which was previously a powerful immunogen can be converted to a tolerogen with however the ability to sensitise the recipient animal to give an *enhanced* cell mediated response to the original unmodified antigen. If it is proved possible to modify antigens in general so as to alter the subsequent immune response to them—so called immunological engineering, the potential importance to practical immunology in areas such as tumour biology, vaccination against bacterial and viral diseases, and tissue transplantation seems high.

The evidence that two types of lymphocytes—one thymus derived (T cell) and one bone marrow derived (B cell)—are involved in the antibody response to many antigens continues to grow. The topic is now a dominant theme in "academic" immunology and the implication of the findings are beginning to extend into more applied investigations. In some laboratory animals and for some antigens, the fact that cell co-operation occurs is now beyond reasonable doubt. Investigation into the role each cell type plays in antibody production, in tolerance and in cell mediated immunity will be greatly enhanced by the availability of two specific antisera—the isoantisera (anti-θ) reactive against the T cell of CBA mice and a heteroantiserum which appears to specifically react against bone marrow derived cells. After exposure to these antisera, cells of the appropriate antigenic specificity are lysed by complement. The use of these antisera has provided some of the strongest recent evidence for cell co-operation in the antibody response and has confirmed the importance of T-cells in the recovery of mice from a viral infection. Furthermore, it appears that the cellular lesion in high and low zone tolerance to some antigens differ. It is reported that the state of low zone tolerance to a given antigen in mice but not high zone tolerance to the same antigen can be abrogated if the mice receive spleen cells from X-irradiated, syngeneic mice previously injected with thymus cells and the antigen; *ie.*, the tolerant mice receive "thymus educated cells." The earlier finding (Chapter 9) that spleen lymphocytes from normal mice can be specifically inactivated by coating with antigen labelled to high specific activity with iodine-125 has been confirmed and extended to spleen cells from primed animals. Furthermore, using a hapten-carrier protocol with primed cells or a "thymus dependent" antigen with unprimed cells it has been shown that both T and B cells can be inactivated in this way. This represents an additional way to manipulate cell populations.

There are several reports of antibody production by spleen cells in tissue culture to hapten-carrier conjugates, thus opening the way to detailed investigation of the mode of action of T and B cells. Such investigations will be greatly aided if cell populations, enriched to a specific antigenic determinant or immunogen, can be readily obtained. An improved method for cell depletion with some encouraging cell enrichment, using antigen-coated polyacrylamide beads has been described. The phenomenon in vivo of low zone tolerance to flagellar antigens has now been reproduced in tissue culture and shown to be antibody mediated.

Finally, there are many recent reports which relate to the traffic of cells through the body. Some of these study cell migration to particular areas of lymphoid tissues, making use of cannulation of afferent lymph vessels. Others report on the origin of cells in lymphoid tissues. For example, it is reported that lymphocytes present in the primary follicles of the lymph node cortex are of bone marrow rather than recent thymic origin. Some studies have described the transport of aggregated globulin (and hence possibly antigen) to the germinal centre areas of mouse spleen. These approaches will help to elucidate the roles which antigen present in lymphoid follicles may play.

AUTHOR INDEX

Numbers in italics refer to the pages on which the complete references are listed.

SUBJECT INDEX

thymidine, 100, 154
thymus lymphocytes, 88
Hapten, 6, 9, 39, 98–100, 174, 180
    "carrier" and, 98, 164
    dinitrophenol (DNP), 254
    inhibition studies, 192–193
    lactic dehydrogenase subunits, 215
    poly-γ-D-glutamic acid, 164, 244
Hemocyanin, 16, 45, 52, 112, 118, 132,
    158, 213
Hemolytic focus assay, see Techniques
Hemolytic plaque test, see Techniques
Homoreactant, 152

I

IgA, 24–25
IgG, 24–28, 32, 48–49, 151–152, 157,
    162–163, 175–176
    fragments, 26–27, 32
    opsonization and, 32
    in primary immune response, 103–104
    receptors, 31
    suppression of antibody formation and,
        35
IgM, 24, 28–32, 151, 157, 162–163, 175,
    178, 247
    antibody, 200, 237
    in primary immune response, 103–104
    response, 185
    suppression of antibody formation and,
        35
Immune absorbants, lymphoid cell sus-
    pensions, 191–192
Immune response
    afferent, central and efferent, 2–5
    amplification mechanisms of, 246–247
    antibodies and, in vivo, 24, 33–37
    inductive mechanisms of, 128–130
    presence of antigen during, 171
    primary
        IgM and IgG, 103
        secondary and, antigen retention in,
            126
    polymorphonuclear leucocytes and,
        143
    postulated mechanisms of, 242–245
    thymus and bursa of Fabricius and,
        66–68

in vitro, 234
in vivo differences, 95
    x-irradiation and, 127–128
Immuno cytoadherence, 171–173, 176
Immunofluorescent technique, see Tech-
    niques
Immunogens, 5–7
    artificial and synthetic, 7–9
    detection of, 18–21
    immunogenicity of, 17
    naturally occurring, 9–16
    tolerogen or, 243–245
Immunoglobulins, see also IgA, IgG, IgM
    amino acids in, 27, 253
    chains
        light and heavy, 25–29
        light and ribosomes for synthesis of,
            91
    classes of, 24
    cyanogen bromide cleavage of, 26
    follicular localization of antigen and,
        126–127, 130, 151–152
    on lymphocyte surface, 178–179
    lymphocyte surface receptors and,
        170–171
    structure, 24
    subunits
        CNBr and peptic fragments, 26–27
        Fab, 149–152
        Fc, 27, 31, 109, 151–152, 248
        Fd, 26–27
        synthesis in vitro, 179
Immunoregulation, 259
Irradiation, 47, 62, 68, 105, 155–156
    antigen retention and, 127–128
    hemolytic focus assay of ARC and,
        93
    injection of thymus cells and, 88
    macrophages and, 159
    spleen cell function and, 233
    thymus-bone marrow interactions and
        "carrier effect" and, 98
    tolerance in adults and, 197
    transfer of cells to, 182, 192, 223
    x-irradiated hosts, for detection of de-
        layed antibody response, 223
    x-irradiated syngeneic recipients,
        223–226
    x-irradiation and peritoneal cells, 148